D1360268

SHADOW
MEDICINE

—

JOHN S. HALLER JR.

SHADOW MEDICINE

—

The Placebo in

Conventional and

Alternative

Therapies

COLUMBIA UNIVERSITY PRESS
NEW YORK

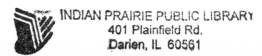

Columbia University Press
Publishers Since 1893
New York   Chichester, West Sussex
cup.columbia.edu
Copyright © 2014 Columbia University Press

Library of Congress Cataloging-in-Publication Data
Haller, John S., Jr., 1940–   author.
Shadow medicine : the placebo in conventional and alternative therapies /
John S. Haller Jr.
Includes bibliographical references and index.
ISBN 978-0-231-16904-2 (cloth : alk. paper) — ISBN 978-0-231-53770-4 (ebook)
I. Title. II. Title: Placebo in conventional and alternative therapies.
[DNLM: 1. Placebos. 2. Complementary Therapies. 3. Evidence-Based Medicine.
4. Placebo Effect. WB 330]
R733
615.5—dc23
2013048051

Columbia University Press books are printed on permanent
and durable acid-free paper.
This book is printed on paper with recycled content.
Printed in the United States of America
c 10 9 8 7 6 5 4 3 2 1

Cover design: Mary Ann Smith

References to websites (URLs) were accurate at the time of writing.
Neither the author nor Columbia University Press is responsible for URLs that
may have expired or changed since the manuscript was prepared.

For Clio,
my feline companion
and ever-present muse

There is no alternative medicine. There is only scientifically proven, evidence-based medicine supported by solid data or unproven medicine, for which scientific evidence is lacking.

—Phil B. Fontanarosa and George D. Lundberg,
"Alternative Medicine Meets Science" (1998)

The only solid piece of scientific truth about which I feel totally confident is that we are profoundly ignorant about nature. . . . It is this sudden confrontation with the depth and scope of ignorance that represents the most significant contribution of twentieth-century science to the human intellect.

—Lewis Thomas, *The Medusa and the Snail* (1979)

CONTENTS

ACKNOWLEDGMENTS

Special thanks go to Michael Flannery, professor and associate director for historical collections at the Lister Hill Library at the University of Alabama at Birmingham; Dennis B. Worthen, former Lloyd Scholar at the Lloyd Library and Museum in Cincinnati; Kyle Perkins, associate dean for academic affairs at Florida International University; and Marc Katchen and Debra Katchen, who gave generously of their time for support and guidance. My gratitude extends as well to Columbia University Press editor Patrick Fitzgerald, assistant editor Bridget Flannery-McCoy, copyeditor Annie Barva, and the press's anonymous reviewers, all of whom saw merit in my approach not to lay waste one side or the other in the ongoing feud between proponents of evidence-based medicine and those supporting unconventional therapies. Others to whom I am indebted include former colleagues David Werlich, John Dotson, Howard Allen, Mark Foster, Don Rice, and David Wilson; the librarians and staff of the Lloyd Library and Museum in Cincinnati, the Morris Library of Southern Illinois University at Carbondale, the Southern Illinois University School of Medicine in Springfield, the National Library of Medicine, Boston Medical Library, Harvard College Library, the Francis A. Countway Library of Medicine at Harvard Medical School, the John Crerar Library of Chicago, the New York Academy of Medicine Library, New York Public Library, Northwestern University, the Stanford University Library, the University of Illinois Library at Champaign-Urbana, the University of Wisconsin Library, the University of Kansas Library, the

University of Michigan Library, the Yale University Cushing/Whitney Medical Library, Google Books, and JSTOR.

As always, I am grateful to my wife, Robin, who offered inspiration, encouragement, criticism, and substantial assistance, including the reading of numerous drafts and the indexing of the book. Those errors of fact or interpretation that remain are mine alone.

ABBREVIATIONS

AIDS	acquired immunodeficiency syndrome
CAM	complementary and alternative medicine
EBM	evidence-based medicine
FDA	US Food and Drug Administration
HIV	human immunodeficiency virus
IOM	Institute of Medicine
NCCAM	National Center for Complementary and Alternative Medicine
NIH	National Institutes of Health
OAM	Office of Alternative Medicine
RCT	randomized clinical trial

INTRODUCTION

onsider for a moment these varying scenes: a graduate of Barbara Ann Brennan's School of Healing draws upon the forces in the universe to balance the multilayered fields of aura emanating from a patient; a homeopath, after a lengthy consultation, treats the symptoms of alopecia with sulfur serially diluted and succussed to 30°C to release its dynamized energies; a nurse creates an energy exchange using therapeutic touch to restore a patient's self-healing abilities; and, finally, a chiropractor applies spinal manipulative therapy to treat a child with attention deficit hyperactive disorder. Each of these modalities is representative of unconventional healing practices common across the United States. Whereas reductionist biomedicine draws its authority from the randomized clinical trial (RCT) and laws embedded in the natural sciences, these and other unconventional therapies rely on a philosophy of organism known as "vitalism," which explains life not by the laws of physics and chemistry, but by a principle, force, or spiritlike power that comes from beyond the material world to animate organic matter.[1]

In large measure, the differences separating biomedicine from these and other unconventional therapies concern the question of whether the body has a fundamentally different nature than the soul or whether the body, along with its brain/mind, should be considered as nothing more than extended matter. The French philosopher, scientist, and mathematician René Descartes (1596–1650) gave expression to this dichotomy and the nature in which the nonmaterial soul inhabited or found expression in a mechanical body with his aphorism "cogito ergo sum": "I think, therefore I am." This dualism gave birth to two polar traditions in Western medicine: one that constructed scientific models of thera-peutics using purely reductionist or biochemical processes; another that explained healing in terms of the soul's effect on the body—namely, a soul–body intervention. The former represented the course taken by reductionist science, and the latter was home to religion and became home to unconventional medicine. In the tradition of Descartes, ortho-dox medicine maintained a separation between body and soul, scorn-fully dismissing any and all metaphysical subtleties by viewing the body as a construct of material forces. In contrast, unconventional medicine embraced a variety of half-formed aspirations designed to escape the rationalist-empiricist heritage derived from Francis Bacon and invigo-rated by Isaac Newton and John Locke.[2]

Serving as a counterforce to conventional medicine's reliance on aca-demically trained physicians whose therapies are based principally on the materia medica (pharmacopoeia), unconventional medicine chooses a healing encounter that defines health in a psychological and spiritual manner attuned to notions of patient individualization and self-healing. Scarcely hidden in this encounter is a significant change in the healer's role. Rather than someone with access to rational scientific knowledge, training, and competence in special skill sets, the unconventional healer is someone who relies on intuitive insight and at the same time encourages a more egalitarian relationship with his or her patients—replacing reduc-tionist thinking with notions of spirituality, meditation, insight, attitude, and behavioral modification. In this new setting, the patient's experience becomes intensely personal and compares strikingly to certain types of spiritual awakening outside the material world of reductionist science.[3]

Overtly metaphysical in their view of the causal forces, unconven-tional healers conceive of a spiritual encounter that includes the indi-vidual's inner capacity to find harmony with nature. This has become the countervailing voice of unconventional medicine in its stand against the medical establishment with its empirically tested system of medicine. For unconventional medicine, nonmaterial (paranormal) agents work in unison with the body to achieve an inner harmony. In sharp con-trast to orthodox medicine, it encourages practitioners to exercise their metaphysical imaginations, identifying with a thinly veiled vitalism that not only reduces the universe to a single set of governing principles but articulates a philosophy that aligns the patient's recuperative powers with providential laws and purposes.

During the late eighteenth and early nineteenth centuries, the secular proponents of unconventional medicine relied principally on the assumptive world of animal magnetism, an etheric medium ritualized by the German physician Franz Anton Mesmer (1734–1815) in which all living and nonliving objects were thought to exist. For those more attuned to the spiritual and angelic aspects of Christianity, the mystical worldview of the Swedish scientist and theologian Emanuel Swedenborg (1688–1772) served as a metaphor for the primacy of spirit over matter. In both spheres, health and wellness depended on the individual's inner harmony and a resonance between the physical and metaphysical orders of reality. There was, in essence, a fundamental correspondence between the human mind and the universal mind, however defined.[4]

Having shared in Europe's inheritance, Americans felt at home as the body–mind dichotomy played out in the succeeding centuries. Through the nation's formative years, unconventional healers treated disease and illness with a variety of therapies designed to expunge from the mind those forces that supposedly engendered the body's infirmities. Numerous Old World practices (i.e., king's evil, the royal touch, mesmerism, phrenology, homeopathy, etc.) mutated into therapies (i.e., Perkinism, phrenopathy, physiomedicalism, osteopathy, chiropractic, etc.) tailored to the American scene. Some died out, but others, more adaptive to the changing environment, continued into later periods.[5]

Among the therapies to emerge out of this phenomenon was New Thought, which stood for a grab bag of techniques (i.e., suggestion, hypnosis, right thinking, visualization, relaxation, silence, affirmation, self-help, positive thinking, etc.) intended to bring mental and physical equilibrium to the individual. Utilizing a variety of mind-cure techniques, noted celebrities such as pioneer author of mental science Warren Felt Evans (1817–1889), founder of Christian Science Mary Baker Eddy (1821–1910), spiritual author and teacher Emma Curtis Hopkins (1849–1925), author and occultist William Walker Atkinson (1862–1932), author and philosopher Horatio W. Dresser (1866–1954), philosopher and mystic Ralph Waldo Trine (1866–1958), and minister, author, and positive thinker Norman Vincent Peale (1898–1993) offered a potpourri of therapies designed to overcome life's infirmities—whether physical, spiritual, or material. Combining elements of liberal Christianity, transcendentalism, Emersonianism, spiritualism, mesmerism, and Swedenborgianism, the proponents of New Thought created a philosophy that was middle class in character and focused on healing in the broadest sense of the word and that illuminated the more pragmatic side of the American character. Its revelators spoke of a harmony unfolding between the individual and the universe, be it God or some indeterminate force or energy. The outcome of their collective efforts was a hybrid philosophy simultaneously religious, synoptic, idealistic, optimistic, transformative, and eclectic. Making the best of their interwoven beliefs, they displayed an openness to the benefits of the material world while at the same time allowing for an inner mental and spiritual causation for disease.[6]

The physician and psychologist William James (1842–1910) referred to this phenomenon as the religion of "healthy-mindedness," a term that broke into the postmodernist world as a form of holistic therapy, implying an orientation toward the whole individual and multiple levels of health and well-being—an individualized diagnosis and treatment that encompassed the patient's physical, mental, and spiritual characteristics. James viewed disease as much the outcome of physical forces as the result of the mind and emotions. His interest in healthy-mindedness, which he described as "the only decidedly original contribution of the American people to the philosophy of life," stemmed from the fact that, pragmatically speaking, these nonreductionist healing therapies sometimes "worked."[7]

Today, the umbrella of New Thought is global in its reach, connecting celebrity healers such as Catherine Ponder, Barbara Brennan, Michael Beckwith, Eckhart Tolle, Rhonda Byrne, Mary Manin Morrissey, and Caroline Myss to millions of believers through books, videos, and the Internet and recycling age-old healing techniques intended to complement and sometimes even replace conventional medicine. Anne Harrington writes of "the medicalization of positive thinking," suggesting that many contemporary modalities (i.e., jogging, biofeedback, acupuncture, and even laughter) are actually techniques pulled from the past to fill the armamentarium of contemporary therapies. Books such as Herbert Benson's *The Relaxation Response* (1975) and *The Mind/Body Effect* (1979); Larry

Dossey's *The Extraordinary Healing Power of Ordinary Things* (2006) and *The Power of Premonitions* (2009); and Bernie Siegel's best-selling *Love, Medicine, and Miracles* (1986) are arguably modern-day throwbacks to a host of therapies that emerged out of the nineteenth century.[8]

Notwithstanding the dualism that pervades Western thought and culture, conventional medicine has not been immune to the limitations of reductionist science. On the one hand, factors such as character, education, social status, and environment have long weighed in the intuitive and clinical nature of the physician–patient encounter. On the other hand, it is fair to say that the effects of emotion, habit, trust, doubt, faith, hopefulness, apprehension, imagination, suggestion, and other direct and indirect forms of conscious human behavior have been often poorly appreciated, much less understood. An additional complicating factor has been the lack of precision in the definition of human behavior and its relationship to sociology, cultural anthropology, and psychology. For much too long, these elements have remained within the province of the theologian, philosopher, politician, and unconventional healer.

The history of medicine from ancient times through the first third of the twentieth century suggests recognition among physicians that their patients often became well in spite of their treatment. According to the psychiatrist Arthur K. Shapiro (1923–1995), of the 4,875 different remedies and 16,842 prescriptions used by healers over the course of recorded history, only a handful were actually effective. His hypothesis contends that, for all practical purposes, the minerals, herbs, and animal excretions used to purge, blister, sweat, and puke patients were nothing more than surrogates for the placebo effect. With the exception of cinchona or Jesuit's bark (containing quinine) for intermittent fever, foxglove (digitalis) for dropsy, mercury for syphilis, iodine for goiter, ipecac for dysentery, colchicum for gout, Edward Jenner's vaccination for smallpox, James Lind's demonstration of lemons for scurvy, and a few other interventions, no truly effective pharmacotherapeutic drugs appeared until the sulfonamides in the 1930s.[9]

Although the placebo found a role in the physician's handbag (albeit as a nuisance or dark secret), none anticipated the prominence it would garner in the mid–twentieth century when the Harvard anesthesiologist Henry K. Beecher (1904–1976) announced in his classic article "The

Powerful Placebo," published in the *Journal of the American Medical Association* in 1955, that in clinical trials the effects of the placebo often exceeded the effects of a pharmaceutical drug when dealing with symptoms of pain, headache, and nausea. His thesis hinted at the medicalization of phenomena that had thrived over the generations under terms such as *verbal affirmation, visualization, suggestion, relaxation, positive thinking,* and so on. In other words, the placebo threatened the very foundation blocks supporting the edifice known as conventional medicine. His findings also challenged the therapeutic efficacy and limits of the double-blinded, placebo-controlled RCT, recognized as the "gold standard" within conventional medicine's evidence-based pyramid.[10]

In addressing the standoff between the dueling protagonists of conventional and unconventional medicine, the placebo has served as both mediator and judge, challenging both in a variety of unforeseen and unanticipated ways. It also has raised numerous questions that demand a response. Must complementary and alternative therapies provide plausible proof of their efficacy before they are given legitimacy equal to that of biomedicine? How much evidence is required and in what form? Should the RCT be the only avenue for therapies to gain scientific acceptance, or are there other options that can and should be available? Must individualized therapies conform exactly with the more standardized clinical trial to justify their theories? How much deviance can or should normative science tolerate? If complementary and alternative modalities remove individualization and move toward standardization, what is left of their original principles? Is it reasonable to argue that the positive effects of complementary and alternative treatments are the result of a collection of separate processes, one or more of which is connected to the placebo response? Are the neural correlates the same as the placebo effect? Is the placebo effect the bridge spanning psychological and neurobiological processes? Does the placebo effect reduce the perceived effectiveness of conventional medicines? Is the placebo simply another name for the myriad unconventional "pathies" that have emerged over the years?[11]

To answer these questions and others throughout the text, I have chosen to address the subject in six chapters.

Chapter 1, "Evidence-Based Medicine," recounts the emergence of orthodox medicine and the importance it placed on various evaluative methods that compose the evidence-based pyramid. It begins with the development of the simple statistical comparative study whose history is centuries old and moves on to the blind or masked (placebo) assessment that emerged in the late eighteenth century, followed by the introduction of Pierre Charles Alexandre Louis's numerical analysis initially to dismantle the rationalistic beliefs embedded in the practice of bleeding and the heroic uses of calomel and tartar emetic. From there, the discussion turns to examples of placebo assessments carried out in the late nineteenth and early twentieth centuries and the introduction of the double-blind trial, followed by randomization. The chapter explains how the double-blinded, placebo-controlled RCT became the "gold standard" for evidence-based medicine (EBM) and was further enhanced by the so-called Cochrane Collaboration, which incorporated meta-analysis (i.e., using analyses of the research literature to build combined data resulting from independent trials) to strengthen the plausibility of the RCT's predictions. The chapter ends with an examination of the ethical challenges that helped to define as well as to limit the application of the RCT.

Chapter 2, "Postmodernist Medicine," examines the rise of postmodernism in the second half of the twentieth century and the myriad epistemological challenges it forced upon the core values of scientific positivism. Postmodernism viewed objectivity as an illusion, a set of images or metanarratives that fragmented both reason and meaning. Applied to medicine, it questioned the "truth" of the physician's reductionist account of illness, including those conclusions drawn from EBM. From there, the chapter tracks the resulting revolt against patient objectification and its replacement with complementary and alternative medicine's (CAM) more intuitive and individualized approach to medicine. This new representation of illness, employing social, psychological, and cultural components, facilitated the resurgence of CAM. Using the history of psychosomatic medicine as an example, the chapter explains how the discipline changed from being predominantly academic in nature to being laitized by a broad band of paraprofessionals, celebrity healers, and self-help gurus. The chapter traces the growth and popularity of CAM in the United States and Europe through the analysis of national surveys, including questionnaires sent to all 125 conventional medical schools in the United States. It also looks at efforts to categorize the different types of CAM therapies and the migration of select therapies into the medical school curriculum as well as into managed care.

Chapter 3, "'The Powerful Placebo,'" examines the consequences of the mind–body dichotomy on European science and of conventional medicine's choice to separate the functioning body from the conscious and unconscious self, a decision that both triggered unparalleled advancements in reductionist science and technology and opened opportunities for the philosophy-based system of CAM. After tracing the placebo's early status as a control procedure in clinical trials, the chapter takes note of Beecher's 1955 article "The Powerful Placebo," which viewed the placebo as a form of "therapy" and therefore challenged its very definition as an inert entity. From there, the discussion turns to efforts at redefining the parameters of placebo phenomena, including the suggestion that some forms of placebo are initiated by endogenous opioids (endorphins). The chapter looks at two specific factors essential for placebo action—namely, the suitability of the disease and the physician–patient relationship. Then, the narrative addresses the potential connection between the placebo and personality traits, the doctor as a form of "drug," the factor of trust, and the power of suggestion. The chapter examines the veracity of Beecher's conclusion that approximately 35 percent of a placebo control group show signs of improvements and whether the placebo is too often confused with other nonspecific elements (i.e., the disease's natural history, regression toward the mean, the Hawthorne effect, etc.), suggesting that the placebo effect is much more variable that previously thought. Finally, the chapter looks into some of the newer interpretations of the placebo effect, Sissela Bok's ethical challenge to the use of the placebo in clinical practice, and the importance of culture in the subjective perceptions that enrich the clinical outcome.

Chapter 4, "Politics of Healing," recounts the political pressures leading to the creation of the Office for the Study of Unconventional Medical Practices and its successors, the Office of Alternative Medicine (OAM) and the National Center for Complementary and Alternative Medicine (NCCAM) within the National Institutes of Health (NIH) in the United States. It traces the political issues that challenged each of these centers' directors, their dealings with CAM's proponents, and the resistance they faced from EBM researchers. The chapter examines the work of several commissions appointed to provide guidelines and methodologies for CAM validation, recounts the numerous challenges to the RCT by CAM proponents, and the efforts undertaken to reach consensus on how to "level the playing field" on which all therapies—conventional and unconventional—can be judged.

Chapter 5, "Complementary and Alternative Medicine's Challenge: A Case Study," offers an in-depth analysis of homeopathic theory and practice, including its laws of *similia* and dynamization; the RCT's implications for classical homeopathy; and the various hypotheses used to explain the modus operandi of homeopathy's dynamized medicines—explanations that begin with mesmerism and extend to Swedenborgianism, atomic energy, water memory, and the more recent quantum theory. The chapter recounts the differences that separate homeopathy from biomedicine and the mounting evidence arising from clinical trials that challenge homeopathy's claim to plausibility. In many ways, homeopathy is the poster child of CAM in that it faces the dilemma of justifying itself as a faith-based system, a form of psychotherapy or chaplaincy, a paranormal system that will eventually be explained to the satisfaction of reductionist science, or simply the equivalent of the placebo effect. The chapter concludes by suggesting that the tension between homeopathy and conventional medicine is essentially that of two epistemologically different systems: one whose view of disease causation begins at the metaphysical level, the other whose view begins at the cellular level.

Chapter 6, "Reassessment," explores CAM's continued popularity despite its poor performance in clinical trials; the close relationship between religiosity and physical health; the minimal expectation for CAM to justify its existence through replication; and the overriding evidence that most CAM modalities appear to work only marginally better than the placebo. It concludes with a set of observations on the relationship of CAM therapies to reductionist science, suggests areas of future study, and ends with a postscript on the exacting demands placed on the skeptic in the postmodern world.

Numerous scholars have examined alternative systems and the epistemological divisions that divide conventional and unconventional medicine. One key work is James C. Whorton's *Nature Cures: The History of Alternative Medicine in America* (2002),[12] which offers an outstanding overview of alternative systems, illuminating the philosophy of natural healing that has dominated their respective belief systems, including some, such as osteopathy, that relinquished their vitalistic theories and migrated into mainstream medicine. Another is Norman Gevitz, who edited *Other Healers* (1988), a set of ten essays on subjects ranging from how orthodox medicine defined, interpreted, and reacted to unconventional healers to how contemporary scholarship has reshaped thinking about unorthodox therapies.[13]

Building off these two works as well as numerous individual studies of unconventional therapies, the therapeutic revolution, and the beginnings of EBM, one has a better understanding of the origins, features, and accomplishments of research on evidence-based health care and clinical epidemiology over time. William Rothstein's *American Physicians of the Nineteenth Century* (1972) provides an insightful sociological perspective on the rebellion against so-called medical orthodoxy even though it actually formed a sect not too unlike its competition, an indication of medicine's impotence prior to the diagnostic and therapeutic revolution that occurred in the last quarter of the twentieth century. Paul Starr's stellar book *The Social Transformation of American Medicine* (1982) traces the emergence of medicine as a profession and its exponential growth in the twentieth century, stressing the elements of authority, economic power, and political influence. Without defacing medicine's scientific advances, Starr recounts how this physician-shaped profession was, in turn, subject to the changing needs of the marketplace and government policy. John Harley Warner's *The Therapeutic Perspective* (1986) links actual medical practice with medical science and professional identity, showing how changes in established therapies affected not only medicine's self-image, but its professional behavior, including its ethical obligations. In *No Other Gods: On Science and American Social Thought* (1997), editor Charles E. Rosenberg provides formidable examples of how American science, social thought, and values helped forge institutions in the late nineteenth and early twentieth centuries, emphasizing in particular the relationship between science (i.e., the ideal of research) and the nation's social thinking.[14]

These works lead one quite deliberately to Jeanne Daly's *Evidence-Based Medicine and the Search for a Science of Clinical Care* (2005),[15] in which she traces the transition from the practice of medicine based on authority, intuition, and clinical practice to the adoption of EBM and its companion, the Cochrane Collaboration. Particularly striking in Daly's history is her frequent and provocative questions concerning the dangers of overreliance on EBM at the expense of patient-centered care. Another important contributor to the subject is J. Rosser Matthews, whose *Quantification and the Quest for Medical Certainty* (1995)[16] recounts the notable undertakings of the Paris Academy of Medicine in the 1830s, the demands of experimental physiologists in their search for a truly scientific medicine based on physiological phenomena, and the contrasting visions of British epidemiologist and statistician Major Greenwood (1880–1949) and bacteriologist and immunologist Sir Almroth E. Wright (1861–1947) on whether scientific medicine could or should be centered in the laboratory. Matthews explains the ascendancy of the clinical trial in the 1960s, prompted in large part by the need for the regulation of highly active drugs, and shows quite persuasively that the issues involving the role of quantification and statistical inference persist into the present time, raising significant questions concerning objectivity and the meaning of medical science. With the RCT elevated to the gold standard for clinical science, Harry Marks's *Progress of Experiment* (1997)[17] points to its inherent problems amid efforts to rationalize medicine using laboratory and statistical measures. Marks insists that the RCT remains a social process and part of the postmodernist critique of science's presumed unassailability. Each of these books explores biomedicine's search for identity, the contested areas of private practice and clinical trials in the evolving therapeutic perspective, the limits of clinical epidemiological findings, and the challenge of looking beyond reductionist science to a sense of medical pluralism with its diversity of healing beliefs and practices.

Besides those who have questioned the RCT as biomedicine's stamp of identity, there are critics such as Marcia Angell and Arnold S. Relman, who from 1977 to 2000 filled the top editorial positions at the *New England Journal of Medicine* and repeatedly took the medical-industrial complex (i.e., Big Pharma) to task for manipulating clinical researchers and the RCT for its own entrepreneurial ends. Their editorials and publications were replicated by Jerome Kassirer, whose book *On the Take: How Medicine's Complicity with Big Business Can Endanger Your Health* (2005) sounded the alarm of pernicious financial conflicts of interest between Big Pharma and the independence of the medical researcher. Using dramatic headings such as "Can We Trust Our Researchers," "Your Doctor's Tainted Information," and "Money-Warped Behavior," he explained the publication of articles favorable to a given drug in non-peer-reviewed journals, industry-funded studies and speaker bureaus, and other murky relationships between academic medical centers and the medical industry. Similarly, Richard Smith, editor of the *British Medical Journal* for twenty-five years, noted the corrupting influence of Big Pharma in his explosive article "Medical Journals Are an Extension of the Marketing Arm of Pharmaceutical Companies" (2005). Identifying questionable ways in which the pharmaceutical companies obtain the results they want, he suggested that journals should critique trials, not publish them.[18]

Others focused their studies on the placebo, beginning with John Harley Warner, whose 1977–1978 article " 'The Nature-Trusting Heresy': American Physicians and the Concept of the Healing Power of Nature in the 1850's and 1860's" traces the dichotomy between biomedicine's association with traditional medical therapies whose locus is the materia medica and the more complicated but indeterminate capacity of individuals to heal themselves. Arthur K. Shapiro and Elaine Shapiro's *The Powerful Placebo* (1997) stirred an international conversation on the etymology of the term *placebo* (i.e., whether the definition includes both active and inert substances) and whether it encompasses both physiological and psychological interventions. Knowing the nonspecific nature of the placebo, they asked whether a physician should consciously make it part of his or her armamentarium. The Shapiros gained the honor of challenging the fundamental premises of scientific medicine by suggesting that the placebo—a factor that arguably defies rational therapeutics—can assume an integral role in scientific medicine. The authors also brought to the fore the ethical issues raised by the placebo's use in both research and general practice, a subject that endures to the present due largely to recent revisions in the Declaration of Helsinki (written originally in 1989) and the troubling questions raised by Sissela Bok, a philosopher and senior fellow at the Harvard Center for Population and Development Studies, in her book *Lying: Moral Choice in Public and Private Life* (1978).[19]

Anne Harrington's book *The Cure Within* (2008) and edited volume *The Placebo Effect: An Interdisciplinary Exploration* (1997)[20] complement the Shapiros' work with a multidisciplinary approach that emphasizes the clinical role (i.e., the physician–patient encounter's including the factors of trust, suggestion, and empathy) of the placebo beyond simply serving as a research tool for purposes of drug comparison. Those scholars who have contributed to the discussion (Robert A. Hahn, Howard Brody, Donald D. Price, Robert Ader, David B. Morris, Irving Kirsch, Howard L. Fields, Howard Spiro, and the Shapiros) have sought to narrow the gap between the patient's subjective experience and the disease's objective process. They not only look to what has been gained from such therapies but take their discussions to newer thresholds with questions that are ethically charged and more importantly challenge the epistemological edifice with questions that offer rich opportunities for future scholars.

Other books have also contributed to the role of placebos in medicine. Howard Spiro's *The Power of Hope* (1998) provides compelling reasons for the use of the placebo beyond its surrogate role in the randomized clinical trial. W. Grant Thompson's *The Placebo Effect and Health* (2005) explains that although placebos carry no intrinsic benefits, they nonetheless play into the physician–patient encounter in a manner that compels a new look at the healing virtues of evidence-based medicines. A gastroenterologist, Thompson compliments the pharmaceutical trial and the role played by the placebo in adding to the physician's materia medica. Richard Kradin, former director of the Mind/Body Institute at the Beth-Israel Deaconess Medical Center and author of *The Placebo Response and the Power of Unconscious Healing* (2008), sees the placebo as an added component in all therapeutics. In *The Healing Arts* (1986), Ted Kaptchuk and Michael Croucher expound on the diversity of healing systems in the world today and of biomedicine's many strengths and weaknesses. Nevertheless, they point to a serious deficiency in biomedicine in its failure to address the whole patient. What is unclear from the book is what standards alternative therapies should be judged by—a question that begs an answer. Kaptchuk's *The Web That Has No Weaver* (2000) contrasts Chinese and Western medicine, providing lucid explanations of Eastern cosmology and its relationship to the harmony affecting the body in health. One might conclude from the book that the author is suggesting that biomedical reductionism would do well to turn back to the principles found in its own philosophical traditions.[21]

Much of this scholarship was the result of Beecher's article "The Powerful Placebo," which forced a paradigmatic change in the how the placebo should be viewed and interpreted. Together, these authors account for contemporary society's interest in the placebo effect; its place in history, including twentieth-century clinical trials; the significance of the double-blind, placebo-controlled RCT; the putative pathways of the placebo response in sickness and healing; the doctor as a therapeutic agent; disagreements concerning placebo response, including ethical controversies; and the challenge of understanding and harnessing the placebo for future use.

Numerous other books are helpful in meaningful ways, including Robert Burton's *The Anatomy of Melancholy* (1621), John Lukacs's *At the End of an Age* (2002), Irving Kirsch's *The Emperor's New Drugs* (2010), Michel Foucault's *The Birth of the Clinic* (1973), Thomas Kuhn's *The Structure of Scientific Revolutions* (1962), and Susan Lederer's *Subjected to Science: Human Experimentation in America Before the Second World War* (1995), which focuses on the moral assumptions that American doctors shared regarding experimentation on humans and animals before World War II (i.e., Nuremburg) and that accompanied the emergence of laboratory science. R. Barker Bausell, a former research director of an NIH-funded CAM research center, editor of *Evaluation and the Health Professions*, and author of *Snake Oil Science: The Truth About Complementary and Alternative Medicine* (2007), clearly stands his ground against the claims of unconventional therapies. From each of these authors, one can learn the value of skepticism when it comes to the subject of scientific objectivity and the equally important need to appreciate the views evinced by opposing paradigms.[22]

Despite claims to the contrary, the body–mind or body–spirit dualism remains the defining element in biomedicine's physician–patient relationship, a bifurcated model that is seldom present in non-Western cultures, where human life is perceived in a less restrictive fashion. But, as Ted Kaptchuk has recently observed, it is time for conventional and unconventional medicine to find common ground. This means finding "how one reconciles solid objectivity arrived at independent of belief and culture with the absolute uncontestable importance and meaningfulness of subjectivity."[23] All this helps to explain why the proponents of CAM have urged a reexamination of their many claims, including their insistence that the RCT ought not to be the only standard for evaluating their therapies.[24] "The reductionist approach of the randomized controlled trial," Iain Smith explained in the *British Medical Journal* in 1995, "may fail to allow for the holistic effect that is central to the philosophy of most complementary therapies." The RCT should compare "whole treatments" rather than individualized components, he reasoned. Doing so "would allow inclusion of the things that matter to patients rather than just those that matter to the investigators."[25]

For too many years, the weight of reductionist logic has posed an insurmountable barrier to consciousness research, challenging any suggestion of a teleology of the body. Yet CAM continues to rely on a teleological tradition, something that reductionist science finds hard to take seriously—whether that tradition's source is some external or human-centric force. That said, the phenomenon of the subjective experience in healing remains a vast unknown. Although reductionism has diminished the mind to something akin to "scientific" matter (i.e., behaviorism and functionalism), it does not represent a final unassailable view. Its attempt to ground everything in matter fails to capture the whole person. The challenge for medical science is to address the mind–body problem in a manner radically different from what has dominated past conversations—that is, to build a bridge between objectivity and subjectivity that will stand the test of replication. Achieving this will no doubt require a revolution in thinking.

This book represents the culmination of several decades of research on unconventional therapies. Despite what I find to be CAM's many serious and substantive shortcomings, I have tried earnestly to be fair in dealing with its supporters' claims and aspirations. In my opinion, CAM has much to teach those who stand firmly in the biomedical camp. Resolution of the issues between EBM and CAM will not be easy, yet common ground exists between them in that they both bring legitimate issues to the discussion. One way to begin this dialog is to realize that postmodernist medicine is a *process* whose goals may be evident, but whose methods remain elusive.

SHADOW
MEDICINE

—

1

EVIDENCE-BASED MEDICINE

Before you are useful, be sure you are harmless.

–Hippocrates

Much of what passes today as orthodox medicine struggled to define itself in the early nineteenth century by separating its beliefs and practices from those of the competition. The task was neither easy nor inevitable. Until the therapeutic revolution in the second half of the century and the triumph of clinical medicine, the prevailing characterization of healing had been its diversity because wide differences existed in clientele, philosophy, treatment, training, professional status, regulation, and licensing. Even though the medical majority used political muscle to oppose its competitors by blocking them from equal access to the law, Abraham Flexner astutely identified the majority as just another medical sect in this period.[1] To be sure, conventional doctors were in the clear majority, but what separated them from their competitors was sometimes difficult to determine given the breadth of their own therapeutic theories and practices, many of which showed distinctive regional preferences. Armed with a mere handful of effective medicines, most doctors focused their efforts on palliative treatment, a phenomenon that reflected the idiosyncratic nature of the healing arts.[2]

With improvements in the basic medical sciences and the migration of experimental findings into bedside practice, proto-orthodoxy eventually learned how to track the course of disease, test information, and invite attention to newer treatments and strategies.[3] Not until the last quarter of the nineteenth century did medical care and medical education emerge as a scientific enterprise, helped along by advances in germ theory, antiseptic techniques, hygiene, anesthesia, and surgery. The publication of William Osler's *The Principles and Practice of Medicine* (1892) symbolized the validation and clarity of conventional medicine, marking the triumph of proto-orthodoxy's break from dogma and its transition to a more rigorous scientific approach to medicine.[4]

By the turn of the twentieth century, orthodox medicine's hold on both the public and the halls of government had succeeded in eliminating or corralling a number of fringe therapies and, by strategically revising its code of ethics in 1903, coaxed some of the more respected sectarians (mostly eclectics[5] and homeopaths who were licensed as doctors of medicine) to abandon their distinctive systems and unite under the banner of regular or conventional medicine. By the time the American Medical Association's Council of Medical Education announced in 1935 that it would no longer rank sectarian schools, regular medicine had obtained a virtual dominance over all other forms of practice. A year later, the New York Homeopathic Medical College and Hahnemann Medical College of Philadelphia relinquished their homeopathic status, and in 1939 the last eclectic school closed after graduating its final class.[6] "As the sole arbiter of science," explains sociologist Terri Winnick, "regular medicine was able to blithely dismiss competing philosophies and treatments as unscientific. More importantly, they [*sic*] were also able to align themselves with the state and seek its protection over their work."[7] Buttressed by its allegiance to scientific knowledge, defended by the courts, and legitimized by a supportive educational system, conventional medicine enjoyed an overpowering presence in American culture. Its identification with science gave it a level of self-justification, identity, and protection unequaled by any of its competitors.[8]

By the mid–twentieth century, the new biologically grounded healthcare system had transformed the physician, in matters of health and disease, into an academically trained and diagnostically skilled clinician whose qualities were inspirational, dominant, and authoritative.[9] In a quite literal sense, explains historian Charles Rosenberg, an "insulating sacredness" was applied to the hospital and, by inference, to the physician who labored there. Clearly, qualitative differences existed within the profession between specialists and general practitioners, between hospital and non-hospital clinicians, and between urban and rural doctors. Nevertheless, the public appeared to ignore such distinctions. To the degree that religious symbolisms were not explicitly evident in the public's image of this emerging reductionist culture, there was nonetheless a vision of a new and idealized authority figure who carried within his or her persona a transformative influence on patients' bodily infirmities. As an authority figure, the physician not only projected a certain level of scientific legitimacy but purported to have legal authority, political privilege, and cultural acceptance—entitlements that also came with obligations that included training, uniform standards, accreditation, licensing, and regulation.[10]

NORMATIVE SCIENCE

Rationalism in medicine is identified with the search for the basic mechanisms of disease, whereas empiricism is best represented as an emphasis on the outcomes for individuals or groups of patients. The tension between these two approaches has been explosive over the centuries. Through most of antiquity, the dominant influence was rationalism, best expressed in the doctrine of the humors (blood, phlegm, yellow bile, and black bile) first taught by the Pythagorians, who explained health and disease in terms of humoral balance or imbalance. Rationally based treatments used agents whose modus operandi was justified prior to their clinical application. The empiricists protested these formalized abstractions, stressing instead specific symptoms, remedies, and outcomes. With breakthroughs in clinical pathology and germ theory in the second half of the nineteenth century, a truly scientific medicine evolved using the power of observation, fact finding, the development of a working hypothesis, experimentation, and an outcome. Both rationalism and empiricism proved essential ingredients in modern medicine—the beginnings of a combined rationalist-empiricist tradition.[11]

Early in medical orthodoxy's rise to power, what would become known as "evidence-based medicine" challenged philosophy-based practice as

the highway to success. Trust in the intuition and informed personal judgment of an experienced clinician, whose diagnosis and treatment encompassed such variables as sex, race, temperament, and even the environment, fell before the weight of a newer clinical judgment obtained from
"independent" science as embodied in experimentation, quantitative precision, and evidence. Unlike unconventional healers, most of whom had
acquired their knowledge through the *practice* of healing and who offered
only metaphysical explanations for their modus operandi, biomedicine
identified reductionist baselines against which to measure its therapies.
Whereas unconventional medicine adhered to vitalistic theories to construct a philosophy of organism, biomedicine looked to physiological,
pathological, and eventually biochemical and molecular processes derived
from physical matter and to treatment based on the calculus of probabilities. That is not to say that biomedicine rejected spirituality altogether; it
simply chose not to incorporate metaphysical elements into either disease
etiology or treatment. Instead, its therapeutics was derived from laws and
methods that were drawn from the natural sciences and that explained
the body in biological terms that could be generalized from one person to
another rather than as untested spiritual or intuitive conjectures idiosyncratic to each individual. Unlike unconventional medicine's more doctrinaire character, biomedicine was steeped in a positivistic uncertainty that
forced both observation and reasoning to the very center of the discovery
process. At its best, biomedicine encouraged a healthy sense of skepticism
and urged various forms of sampling, to be followed by repeated experimentation to reaffirm a hypothesis. Biomedical science flourished in
this new environment, making its discoveries all the more significant by
throwing into question competing epistemological approaches as neglect-
ful, if not outright fraudulent.[12]

Biomedicine's professional identity was thus based on the unambigu-
ous application of normative science whose laws interpreted the body as
a materialistic system that could be reduced and analyzed according to
its component parts. Likewise, it treated disease as a biochemical phenomenon that could be classified into discrete categories of causation
using standardized, objectified, and technologically validated biochemical treatments and mechanisms. It was guided not only by the fact that
its active pharmaceutical substances "worked" (even when the patient

was unaware of its administration or doubted its effectiveness), but by the assumption that their effects could be demonstrated, measured, and replicated. Admittedly, biomedical knowledge was—and is—seldom value free, being interspersed with numerous socioeconomic components, but, historically, the rigor of its research optimally changed opinions, beliefs, and practices.[13]

The evolving use of clinical trials to evaluate therapeutic and prophylactic agents formed an important part of biomedicine's professional identity, particularly in the role of a spoiler in its war against the claims of unconventional competitors.[14] Conducted with help from individual investigators, governments, hospitals, and public-health agencies, these trials involved the use of comparative statistics and studies; masked assessment to ensure that the subjects (single-blind) or both subjects and investigators (double-blind) were unable to identify the experimental from the control group; and randomization, meaning that subjects were allocated to a group in a random manner to avoid conscious and unconscious bias.[15]

The simple statistical comparative approach looks at existing evidence or generated new evidence designed to inform on the effectiveness, benefits, or harmful effects of different treatment options. Referenced as far back as the ancient Babylonians and found as well in the Old Testament, it continued to surface over the centuries, including mortality statistics documenting the effectiveness of smallpox inoculation, lemons in the treatment of scurvy, Jesuit's bark in treating intermittent fevers, different therapeutic treatments for cholera and yellow fever, and the effects of antisepsis in amputations.[16] An analysis carried out in the 1840s by the Hungarian physician and pioneer of antisepsis Ignaz Semmelweis (1818–1865) at the Lying-in Hospital in Vienna tested his theory of the cause of puerperal fever among women who had just given birth at the hospital by comparing the practices of two groups who attended the women: one of physicians and their medical students who, in addition to their obstetrics duties, were in frequent contact with cadavers on account of their pathological studies; the other of midwives who were not.[17]

Statistical comparative approaches include the following types:

- *Clinical series.* A clinical series is simply a record of clinical experience, a comparatively inexpensive analysis drawn from a single (anecdotal) case report (i.e., the discovery of diethytstilbestrol administered during pregnancy[18]) or from a number of case studies. Its benefit comes from reporting the effects of a new application or technique and assessing it against its use with other patients in a clinic or medical facility. These case studies are often based on a computerized set of medical records from a hospital records room (i.e., Medicare claims for performing a surgical procedure) and used to achieve some level of error reduction. The comparison is usually made without the benefit of large numbers of patients, randomization, definition of objective, or generalizable information. The issue is more a question of internal validity rather than external validity. A clinical series is seldom an indicator of effectiveness because the variables between and among the cases studied may differ in numerous ways—that is, diagnosis criteria, eligibility, outcome, and so on. Despite these inadequacies, the clinical series is inexpensive and easy to prepare, and it provides information that may prove helpful in the application of a new technique or set of complications.[19]

• *Retrospective (case–control) study.* This type of study is somewhat unique in that the event being investigated occurred before the initiation of the investigation. An example is the National Halothane Study addressing the safety of the anesthetic agent halothane as compared with other agents used in the 1960s. The study eventually included 850,000 surgical procedures in thirty-four hospitals.[20] Another example might be a study of registries that record a particular epidemic whose repetition is separated by long periods of time and where treatments (including the hypothesized cause and therapeutics are very different) are spaced years and even decades apart. Although the retrospective study is cost effective, its value is often illusory due to the challenge of providing convincing evidence of causal relationships. Such studies rely on data that are subject to errors in their collection, errors in patient recall, the lack of a design study, selection bias, and the absence of a control group.[21]

• *Historical control study.* This alternative assumes the predictive value of past data based on the fact that all patients were assigned a standard treatment, with results that were known and subsequently reported in a manner easily understood. Such studies are usually part of an evolving research program and require repeated trials by other investigators who treat the same types of patients, but with newer treatments. In other words, historical control studies are used to compare past patients with patients who have been given a newer treatment—a protocol that avoids potential ethical issues. The fundamental problem is that the historical controls are confounded by context. Among the variables that define this form of study are the indeterminate size and length of trials; adaptations to new diagnostic and prognostic techniques; and nature of patient selection. Notwithstanding complaints from those who criticize patient bias in the selection of those to receive the newer treatment (i.e., the comparable nature of the treated subject and the variables that might affect the outcome), historical control-group studies have proven popular in the research of cancer and other diseases with high mortality where patients refuse to accept randomization and their likely assignment to a control group. In addition, the studies are shorter in length compared to the RCT and considerably less expensive.[22]

• *Contemporaneous control study.* This form of study is a preferred alternative to the historical study because it creates a separate control group that receives the standard treatment alongside a group that receives the most contemporaneous form of treatment. It thereby avoids unlikely differences or surprising results that may have emerged over time.

• *Observational study.* In this form of nonrandom study, such as comparing the risk of lung cancer between smokers and nonsmokers, both treatment and control groups are considered part of the study. In such cases, researchers have no control over the composition of the control group or, for that matter, over whatever treatments the group may be taking. The objective is to provide insight into cause–effect relationships without constructing an expensive and cumbersome RCT. Burdened with numerous ambiguities, most observational studies (i.e., the approximately four hundred trials on cigarette smoking that stretched out more than a decade) are slow to come to a final conclusion. In its suggestion of a cause–effect relationship, the observational study has the least degree of control because there is no way for the researcher to know the subjects' full background and whether other factors might be involved or not. Nevertheless, because patients enrolled in randomized trials are often different from those treated in clinical practice (i.e., women , elderly, ethnic groups), observational data are sometimes viewed as more relevant.[23]

• *Prospective (cohort) study.* Sometimes referred to as a "quasi-experimental study," this type of study represents a subset of the observational study and is a close cousin to the RCT. It is an epidemiological analysis intended to evaluate the relationship of an otherwise healthy cohort formed in a nonrandom manner to study a specific condition or set of conditions and characteristics shared by some members of the group and studied according to a hypothesized cause or treatment. In many instances, the study group is drawn from within a cohort of the general population that has been exposed to a specific condition (i.e., cigarette smoking), a situation that requires researchers to attempt some separation of the total group into meaningful subgroups to analyze exposure, age, sex, race, and other characteristics in the outcomes. Such studies may involve a few or many variables in an attempt to demonstrate a causal relationship. Problems with this type of study involve the logistics of tracking those involved in the study; the frequency of drop-outs from the study; and the fact that individuals may change treatments during the period of the study.[24]

The addition of blind or masked assessment to the statistical comparison, including the use of a sham device or placebo, has been around at least since the eighteenth century, when human subjects were first known to be tested under conditions of intentional ignorance to ensure the objectivity of a particular intervention. Intended initially to detect medical fraud, the masked assessment was employed in a notable series of examinations to test the validity of the energy force known as *animal magnetism* that the Swabian physician Franz Anton Mesmer claimed to envelop the universe with a scope and intensity that affected all living and nonliving matter. Mesmer's medical training caused him to view this fluid as the ultimate power or reality behind the universe and a potential source for healing illnesses. He and his devotees held that medical science, moral improvement, and even social progress could be engineered through the prudent control of this force.[25]

Given the spread of Mesmer's discovery across Europe and the extraordinary cures that allegedly ensued, the French government established two separate commissions in 1789 to examine his claims. The first consisted of members of the Faculty of Medicine and the Royal Academy of Sciences; the second was formed of members of the Royal Society of Medicine.

In testing the effects of animal magnetism and the "crises" that affected Mesmer's patients, the commissioners underwent treatment themselves but reported feeling no sensation or influence. They then performed blind trials to determine the degree to which some contamination of the mind had influenced the effects attributed to magnetism. In one experiment, a patient was brought before five trees presumed to have been magnetized. As the patient approached the first four trees, he fell into a "crisis" even though the only tree reputedly mesmerized had been the fifth. Other experiments involved having a patient drink water from cups, some of which were allegedly magnetized, and others not, and deceiving the patient into believing he was receiving mesmeric treatment when he was not. The commissioners, including the scientist, inventor, and statesman Benjamin Franklin (1706–1790), concluded that the presumed cures from animal magnetism could be better explained as the product of imagination.[26] For R. Barker Bausell, writing more than two hundred years later, Mesmer's treatments also represented "demonstrations of how susceptible both patients *and* practitioners are to allowing their expectations (and the suggestions of others) to cloud their judgment."[27] The commission's findings signaled Mesmer's fall from grace, but they did not bring an end to the coterie of his disciples, who proceeded to move beyond the theory of animal magnetism to develop what became known as "hypnotism," the power of suggestion, and the beginnings of modern psychotherapy.[28]

The self-doubts and uncertainties harbored among physicians in the late eighteenth and early nineteenth centuries served as catalyst to the introduction of the numerical analysis (*la méthod numérique*) and the construction of a new consensus around what constituted orthodox medicine. Motivated by the Napoleonic legacy of data collection to provide a more reassuring basis for scientific and philosophical thinking, medical men such as Philippe Pinel (1745–1826), August François Chomel (1788–1858), Gabriel Andral (1777–1876), Jean Baptiste Bouillaud (1796–1881), and Pierre Charles Alexandre Louis (1787–1872) chose to bring the calculus of probabilities, statistical analysis, and basic numerical methods into the study of disease by observing facts and then collating and analyzing them. Louis's emphasis upon observation, classification, and numerical analysis weighed heavily among the members of the Paris Clinical School, including many American students, and helped to dismantle the rationalistic beliefs propounded by Scottish physicians William Cullen (1710–1790) and John Brown (1810–1882), American physician Benjamin Rush (1746–1813), French physician François J. V. Broussais (1772–1838), and other authority figures. In the battles that ensued, the practice of bleeding as well as many of the mainstays of the materia medica, including the widespread use of calomel and tartar emetic, declined in usage as appreciation for numerical analysis and systematic methods of investigation led to a more "expectant" regimen of healing.[29]

Louis's numerical analysis ironically also became the method of choice among the century's unconventional healers, who believed they could demonstrate the superiority of their own medicines over allopathic (nonhomeopathic) treatment. This group included the Thomsonians and eclectics, whose journals made frequent comparisons of mortality rates of patients treated with articles from their herbal-based materia medica and patients treated with those heroic treatment favorites (i.e., bleeding, tartar emetic, calomel) preferred by medical orthodoxy. It also included homeopaths, whose high-energy remedies were obtained through *trituration* (the potentization of an insoluble raw material that is ground in a mortar and pestle with sugar of milk and attenuated serially to create a medicated pellet) and *succussion* (the potentization of a serial dilution by shaking in order to create a spiritlike healing essence). Devised in Germany, homeopathy spread through Europe and then America, becoming a popular alternative at a time when medicine's proto-orthodoxy faced serious questioning from its own professional elite. During outbreaks of cholera and yellow fever, homeopathy's minute doses of camphor, cuprum, and veratrum, along with careful adherence to hygienic rules, compared favorably to regular medicine, whose harsh regimens complicated treatment, disturbed the natural processes of cure, and retarded recovery. Homeopathic infirmaries and hospitals were careful collectors of statistical records, and in the mid-1860s the American Institute of Homeopathy established its own bureau of statistics to support the validation of its claims. Not surprisingly, the number of patrons of homeopathy grew during these epidemics, including numerous regular physicians who had despaired of their own therapeutic measures. Homeopaths, to their credit, encouraged simple rules—a good diet, fresh air, cleanliness, and no mixing of medicines—to accompany their highly attenuated medicines.[30]

On the basis of these claims, a series of experiments was undertaken in the 1830s to examine the validity of homeopathic practice. These experiments included the work of homeopathic physician Jacques A. Guerard (1796–1874) at the Hôtel Dieu de Lyon in 1832, who prescribed homeopathic medicines for various febrile diseases over a period of seventeen days, but with no perceptible improvement in the patients' conditions; Gabriel Andral at the Hôpital de la Pitié in Paris, who tested homeopathic medicines on 140 patients diagnosed with various diseases; Victor Baillie (n.d.), Leon Simon (1798–1867), and Paul Francis Curie (1799–1853), who treated patients at the Hôtel Dieu with homeopathic medicines over a five-month period; and commissions formed in 1835 by both the king of Naples and the Prussian government to test homeopathic treatment. In all these early experiments, the results were mixed, with both homeopathy and medical orthodoxy claiming victory.[31]

Several of the more interesting clinical trials of homeopathy were performed by French internist Armand Trousseau (1801–1867), who adopted a combination of blind assessment and the use of a placebo bread pill to test the efficacy of medicines that patients believed were homeopathic. In his 1834 article "Expériences homéopathiques tentées a l'Hôtel-Dieu de Paris" and in subsequent publications, he reported testing rhus tox, nux vomica, ignatia, belladonna, arsenicum, and ipecac with mixed results.[32] One unanticipated outcome of these experiments was for academic homeopaths to minimize the centrality of their doctrine of *similia* (i.e., the use of medicines that when given to a healthy person create a symptom complex of physical and emotional characteristics similar to that of the suffering patient) while stressing instead the lower dilutions common among regular physicians.[33] This helps explain why, as early as the 1840s, Sir John Forbes (1787–1861), physician to Queen Victoria's household, criticized the high dilutions of homeopathic medicine as an "outrage to human reason," explaining its successes simply as the result of self-limiting diseases.[34]

By the end of the nineteenth century, blind assessment had even entered the armamentarium of the Society for Psychical Research in Britain and that of its cousin the American Society for Psychical Research to test the claims of spiritualism, whose "sensitives" reputedly read minds (telepathy), saw and interpreted auras surrounding living and nonliving objects, spoke with ghostly apparitions, caused inexplicable movements of lifeless objects, interpreted the "rappings" of otherworldy spirits, and read books while blindfolded.[35]

The vision of objectivity that had loomed large in the thinking of Louis and his disciples helped transform medicine into a science, validated by therapeutic results. Only later did the "science" of medicine move from the bedside to the laboratory of a hospital or research institute. To the extent that doctors adopted physiology as a scientific discipline independent of clinical practice, medicine was seen as advancing beyond conjecture by becoming a scientific certainty (absolute objectivity) and not simply a probability. It was this challenge that appealed to Claude Bernard (1813–1878) and his vision of medical objectivity as well as to Carl Wunderlich (1815–1877), who sought to establish fixed laws of temperature; Gustav Radicke (1810–1883) with his endorsement of medical instrumentation; and others who eschewed "averages" for "laws" arrived at with pathological precision. Helped further along by statisticians such as George Udny Yule (1871–1951) at Cambridge University, Raymond Pearl (1879–1940) at Johns Hopkins, Karl Pearson (1857–1936) at University College London, and Major Greenwood (1880–1949) at London Hospital Medical School, statistical methods became an integral part of medical instruction, migrating eventually into all aspects of medicine—both clinical and laboratory. Many, of course, would object to the exclusive reliance on either the clinical or the laboratory approach, convinced that both rested on the uncertainty of medical inference.[36]

Examples of late-nineteenth- and early-twentieth-century employment of nontherapy assessments include Austin Flint's (1812–1886) work at Bellevue Hospital testing various drug efficacies for rheumatism using diluted tincture of quassia as his "placeboic" remedy of choice;[37] Charles Édouard Brown-Séquard's (1817–1894) comparison of water injections to rabbit and guinea pigs' testicular extracts in the 1890s;[38] the work of Emil Behring (1854–1917) and his colleagues at the Robert Koch Institute in Berlin in the 1890s evaluating diphtheria antitoxin serum extracted from the blood of horses and tested against a "reference material" of an earlier serum; Johannes Fibiger (1867–1928) of Copenhagen, who in 1896–1897 tested the efficacy of diphtheria antitoxin on 484 patients at Blegdamshospitalet using alternate-day allocation;[39] E. L. Thorndike (1874–1949) and

R. S. Woodworth's (1869–1962) study of mental functions in 1901;[40] and W. H. Winch's 1908 study of memory improvement in schoolchildren.[41] Later, in 1916, David I. Macht (1882–1961) at Johns Hopkins compared the analgesic efficacy of morphine to that of a saline solution;[42] and in 1918 Adolf Bingel (1879–1953) employed a controlled comparison of antitoxin serum and normal horse serum. This comparison was followed by trials testing opium alkaloids and several tests of xanthines thought to be effective for angina pectoris.[43]

The methods for conducting these clinical trials, especially in the selection of patients, varied among researchers and institutions, leaving significant differences in the results. Those who realized this impediment, such as Fibiger, suggested alternation, where patients' treatment depended on the day of their admittance, receiving either standard treatment or standard treatment plus serum. The trial was considered quasi-randomized, not blinded. During the 1930s, the UK Medical Research Council headed by Major Greenwood recommended this method for clinical trials. Accordingly, alternation was used to evaluate serum treatment for pneumonia in 1934 and treatment of the common cold in 1944. Ever so slowly, alternation became the accepted standard through the 1940s.[44]

The fact that researchers generally knew which treatment potential patients would receive or what existing patients were receiving lent an element of bias to the investigation. Out of this impediment emerged the principle of randomization, first formulated by Ronald A. Fisher (1890–1962) in *Statistical Methods for Research Workers* (1925) and *The Design of Experiments* (1935) for agricultural experimentation and later put into practice by Austin Bradford Hill (1897–1991), whose articles for the *Lancet* and book *Principles of Medical Statistics* (1937) became the bible for those working in medical problem solving.[45] In them, Hill led readers through the different aspects of statistical analysis, variability, standard deviation, and common fallacies. Intended to rule out conscious and unconscious bias on the part of the patient or investigator that entered into the results, randomization eventually became the standard for satisfying licensing authorities, consumers, pharmacy manufacturers, ethicists, and attorneys.[46] Indeed, the ascendency of the double-blind, placebo-controlled RCT provided conventional medicine with its most effective weapon.

In the RCT, subjects are assigned randomly either to a group receiving a specific treatment or to a control group whose members are given no treatment, a placebo, or another standard treatment. The object is to minimize bias by equalizing the conditions of those receiving the specific treatment with those in the control group. With a level of constancy maintained in the trial or study, the results are intended to show statistically the difference in efficacy between the specific treatment and non-treatment, placebo, or other treatment in the control group.[47] Its requirements include a precise statement of the problem that the study intends to answer; the identification of groups of similar patients to be observed under similar circumstances and differing only in the specific treatment; the random sorting of patients for their group assignment; and, finally, disguising and blinding (single or double) the procedures used in the treatment. In double-blinding, patients, providers, and evaluators are unaware of the nature of the treatment; in randomization, there is assurance that the groups undergoing treatment are handled identically; and in the use of the placebo, scientists can assess whether the treatment has specific effects attributable to the tested intervention that are distinct from the effects associated with the placebo.[48]

Not until 1946 did Hill judge that the time was right to advocate for randomization as a means of eliminating bias. The first trial to use randomization tested the efficacy of immunization (using a pertussis vaccine) for whooping cough, a trial that was eventually published in 1951.[49] A few months after the trial commenced, Philip D'Arcy Hart and Marc Daniels began a trial of streptomycin (first isolated in 1943 at Rutgers University) for the treatment of pulmonary tuberculosis. The results were reported in 1948, three years before the whooping cough trial was published.[50] According to Iain Chalmers, director of the Cochrane Centre at Oxford between 1992 and 2002, "The only reason that allocation schedules based on random numbers are to be preferred to those based on strict alternation is because they are easier to conceal, not because they are any better at abolishing selection bias." This was the reason, Chalmers explained, that "a schedule based on random numbers was used for the streptomycin trial, and why the study is a methodological landmark."[51]

Another example of randomization occurred in trials undertaken in the 1950s to test bilateral internal mammary artery ligation surgery as a treatment for angina pectoris (lack of blood to the heart). In two double-blind trials, with fourteen subjects given a sham operation and twenty-one receiving actual ligation, it was shown that the ligation had no greater effect on angina pectoris than the placebo.[52] In his provocative article "Surgery as Placebo," published in 1961, Henry K. Beecher used the bilateral ligation example to advocate for the RCT, insisting upon the process of "blinding" to remove the potential effects of bias. As Scott Podolsky explains, Beecher's paper served as "an apotheosis of concerns which dominated Beecher's thinking and writing throughout the 1950s: the quantification of subjective responses, the need for the elimination of bias from therapeutic investigations, and an appreciation for the placebo effect."[53] However, until randomization became the centerpiece of trials used for the approval of new drugs, its acceptance proved slow, due mainly to the fact that it required large numbers of patients to demonstrate a quantitatively measured conclusive outcome.

The predominance of the RCT led to the establishment of a new hierarchy for determining quality evidence and forced a massive change in the way evidence-based research was incorporated into clinical medicine. The new evidence pyramid had case reports at the bottom, with observational studies and other forms of evidence only slightly higher. "If you find that the study was not randomized," advise the authors of *Evidence-Based Medicine: How to Practice and Teach EBM*, "we suggest that you stop reading it and go on to the next article."[54]

Proponents insist that the value of the RCT and its fundamental role in basic science has changed the very face of medicine. In effect, the properly controlled RCT remains the principal tool for testing the safety and efficacy of a drug compound or treatment. Its utility versus other modalities is to eliminate confounding and bias. The question asked by the researcher is very basic: "Is the state of the patient different, having been treated, than he would have been otherwise?"[55] Trials are intended to serve as a form of guidance when doubts exist about the best treatment to reduce the effects of a disease or illness. Effective trials take months and sometimes even years to complete. For that reason, sufficient cause is needed for the medical community to entertain such a trial in place of a nonrandomized observational study. Are there moral and professional obligations why a clinical trial should be undertaken or repeated? Are there important medical and/or public-health issues that justify the clinical trial? The answers to these questions are what have driven the RCT to its ascendant role in EBM.[56]

A good example of the RCT's effectiveness occurred during clinical trials run by Merck Research Laboratories in New Jersey in the late 1990s of the drug known as MK-869, an eagerly anticipated addition to psychopharmacology's fight against depression. To the industry's surprise, Merck revealed that patients receiving an inert placebo during its clinical trials did almost as well as those using the new drug. Although the outcome was surely a disappointment for Merck, it served as an enticement for psychiatrists and clinical psychologists to reflect on the power of the placebo effect. For them, this result was not as much an embarrassment as it was for Merck, but a matter of increasing importance and insight into the pedigree of the placebo itself and its potential role in healing. In fact, it encouraged some to argue that many of the popular antidepressant drugs on the market were nothing more than expensive placebos. In this context, the placebo effect has been a hazard for drug developers insofar as it challenges the scientific basis of the multibillion-dollar antidepressant market. Afflictions with a significant psychological component (i.e., pain, anxiety, depression, etc.) are especially affected by the placebo, creating a challenge when proving the efficacy of an active substance. "Frequently, the differences between the two groups are so small as to be statistically insignificant," observed Martin Enserink in *Science* magazine.[57]

BIG PHARMA

With EBM's intent to assess the relative safety and efficacy of pharmaceutical products and methods, the RCT emerged as a significant factor in conventional medicine's consolidation and power. Its methodology stood in stark contrast to the less documented claims of unconventional practitioners with their anecdotes and their historical, case, and observational studies. For conventional medicine and its pharmaceutical industry, the RCT became a profitable way to introduce new drugs into the market by demonstrating statistical improvements over existing remedies or the placebo or both. Guided by the statistical probabilities of evidence-based data, physicians found it less necessary to comprehend the complexity of the clinical judgment, a factor that continues to weigh against the RCT because there is the assumption that patients in the different groups are generally "the same."[58]

In April 1961, Senator Estes Kefauver (D–TN) introduced a bill into the Eighty-Seventh Congress in an effort to amend the antitrust laws regarding the prescription drugs industry and thereby to prevent monopolistic abuses in drug marketing. The bill, the result of hearings held by the Senate Judiciary Committee's Subcommittee on Antitrust and Monopoly, derived from numerous complaints regarding patent laws, the manipulation of drug research, the industry's hostility to generic drug names, the abuse of trademarks, and the shifting of drug research from public to private channels. By the time the amended bill passed through both houses and became law on October 10, 1962, what became known as the Kefauver–Harris Amendment was a shadow of its former self. Nonetheless, helped along by the public outcry following the thalidomide tragedy in late 1961, the act did bring reform, albeit weak, to the behemoth known as Big Pharma.[59]

What began as a research-and-development mechanism to legitimize the effectiveness of new and existing drugs against a control group devolved in the post–Cold War era into Big Pharma's reaching out to capture a global market share through buyouts, takeovers, and double-digit profits. In doing so, Big Pharma proceeded to commercialize scientific research through the creation of privatized contract research organizations, rule changes that shortened the average time for drug approval, and lobbying of governments to continually bend the laws to meet the biopharmaceutical industry's demands. To make matters worse, the contract research organizations took over the bulk of clinical drug trials, making them proprietary and inaccessible to disclosure, skewing published research with results favorable to drugs owned by the research sponsor, creating embarrassing conflicts of interest between drug companies and the authors of scientific review papers, and supporting "ghost" or "honorary" authorship of papers that distorted clinical summaries to highlight a particular drug's or company's results. All of this suggests that in the RCT's climb to prominence within the EBM pyramid, it underwent an unanticipated commercialization, placing medical schools, clinicians, and academic researchers in the virtual pocket of the pharmaceutical industry.[60] This ethically troublesome relationship helps explain why research into the placebo itself has been conspicuously ignored in deference to research into expensive new drugs. In fact, some drug companies (i.e., Lilly and Pfizer) have even attempted to exclude placebos altogether from their drug trials.[61]

In spite of Big Pharma's shadow role in the prominence of the RCT in medicine, most researchers continue to hold to the belief that the RCT is the only true standard for EBM because they consider it "clear, clean, and crisp."[62] As John Tukey explained in 1977, "The *only* source of reliable evidence about the usefulness of almost any sort of theory . . . is that obtained from well-planned and carefully conducted randomized . . . clinical trials."[63] Sheila Gore reinforced this point in 1981, writing that "randomized trials remain *the* reliable method for making specific comparisons between treatments."[64]

COCHRANE COLLABORATION

One additional explanation for the broad acceptance of EBM and the RCT can be traced to a ninety-two-page book titled *Effectiveness and Efficiency: Random Reflections on Health Services* (1972), written by epidemiologist Archie Cochrane (1909–1988). As a doctor in a German prisoner-of-war camp during World War II, Cochrane had kept meticulous records of the sick and wounded, accounting for medicines and procedures that did or did not work in the treatment of his patients. Based on his wartime experiences and his subsequent work as director of the Medical Research Council Epidemiology Unit in Wales, Cochrane called for a better quality of reasoning than what currently passed as evidence-supported practices. Having schooled himself in medical statistics and epidemiology, he became fascinated with the relationship between tuberculosis and disabling lung disease (progressive massive fibrosis) among coal miners in the Welsh mining valley and deeply troubled by the types of treatments prescribed by general practitioners. He was also concerned with the lack of logic used in the treatment of maternity care and hypertension. Noting that doctors were using numerous interventions of unknown safety and efficacy, he argued for a better means of evaluation using the most unbiased methods. Cochrane was not alone in his criticism; individuals such as Tom McKeown and Ivan Illich, among others, pointed to evidence that medical care was oftentimes doing more harm than good.[65]

Suspicious as to how certain practices either came about or persisted despite newer information, Cochrane sought to introduce epidemiology and biostatistics into the medical school curriculum as well as to build an evidence-based library organized around a synthesis of worldwide literature on clinical research.[66] The application of quantitative methods to clinical practice marked a paradigm shift by ruling out a host of preconceptions that had for so long marked clinical practice and against which Cochrane had railed. His work culminated in the Cochrane Collaboration and the use of meta-analyses to establish a secure knowledge basis for making more informed clinical decisions.[67] The meta-analysis is a statistical method intended to review related research studies—both large and small—for the purpose of identifying consistent and reliable effects. For example, by merging a group of nonrandomized but similar studies, the meta-analysis extracts marks or indicators of similarity that provide for a broader acceptance of conclusions derived from individual studies. Notwithstanding the intent, there is no value in using the meta-analysis to correct bad science; bad data continue to make for bad outcomes.[68]

The meta-analysis represents a form of reductionism used by "lumper" scientists who choose to rely on an estimate drawn from all available studies taken together.[69] By contrast, "splitter" scientists choose to match the characteristics of patients to various subgroups within trials. Splitters prefer narrow approaches that show efficacy in a single disease, whereas lumpers prefer the broader analysis.[70] Splitters argue persuasively on the basis of greater accuracy, but the methodological obstacles to splitting give the clear advantage to the lumpers. "A broad meta-analysis increases power, reduces the risk of erroneous conclusions, and facilitates exploratory analyses which can generate hypotheses for future research," argues Peter Gøtzsche, director of the Nordic Cochrane Center in Copenhagen. Because of the high probability that many clinical trials are sullied by indeterminate elements, including social and cultural components that are beyond the reviewer's control, Gøtzsche reasons that patients and clinicians are "better served" by drawing generalizations from the broad meta-analysis than by splitting trials into smaller and smaller units, such as strategies to reduce the uncertainties in the tension that confronts the clinician who is faced with making a clinical judgment in the face of uncertainty.[71] Nevertheless, meta-analyses are often criticized for including too broad an array of treatments and diseases.[72] Statistically, explains Michael Foley at James Cook University Hospital in Middlesborough, some trials will show benefit "even when the real effect of the treatment is zero, and these are the trials that are most likely to be published."[73]

Cochrane's ideas set off shockwaves across the medical world, and in 1993 the first Cochrane Center opened in Oxford, cofounded by a group of seventy-seven doctors from eleven countries and based on the premise that "limited resources should be used to provide forms of health care that have been shown to be effective by properly controlled research."[74] The center's director, Iain Chalmers, inaugurated this collaborative effort with the initial examination of the research findings of forty-eight journals to foster the exchange of ideas. Beginning with clinical issues, the center has since incorporated in its purview such themes as health services research, health policy, analysis, and educational medicine.[75] By 2003, the collaboration had expanded to fifty review groups, eleven methods groups, ten fields and networks, and fifteen centers around the world.[76]

According to Chalmers, the science of research synthesis involves several steps to avoid bias and the effects of chance:

- Stating the objectives of the research.
- Defining eligibility criteria for studies to be included.
- Identifying (all) potentially eligible studies.
- Applying eligibility criteria.
- Assembling the most complete data set feasible.
- Analyzing this data set, using statistical synthesis and sensitivity analyses, if appropriate and possible.
- Preparing a structured report of the research.[77]

Today, the Cochrane Collaboration, supported by more than 650 international organizations, involves multiple centers and more than twenty thousand volunteers from a hundred or more countries who review the results of different medical interventions. At each of its centers, Collaborative Review Groups conduct systematic reviews of both published and unpublished research reports with the intent to share what "works" in the health sector based on high-quality evidence. Rather than conducting original research, the volunteer scientists and physicians review the safety and efficacy of a drug or other treatment drawn from hundreds of individual studies—both small and large—and scrutinize each for methodological weaknesses or biases. Although RCTs are considered the most reliable, nonrandomized observational studies are sometimes used when randomized experiments are lacking.[78] As a statistical method for making accurate predictions based on the combined data results of several independent studies (i.e., clinical trials, observational studies, and individual patient records), such reviews have also proven useful in determining if a specific research hypothesis is effective when the results from the reports appear ambiguous or lacking in standardized methodologies.[79]

The United States has been an active contributor to the Cochrane Collaboration, with representatives attending its first colloquium in 1993, the establishment of the Baltimore Cochrane Center that same year, and the opening of centers in San Francisco, San Antonio, and New England. Support from the National Library of Medicine and its MEDLINE database records has also contributed to the development of the Cochrane Central Register of Controlled Trials. Several Cochrane entities are presently registered in the United States—three Cochrane Review Groups (Prostatic Disease, HIV/AIDS, and Neonatal); one Methods Group (Screening and Diagnostic); one Field Group (Complementary and Alternative); one Branch Group (San Francisco); and one Cochrane Review Group Satellite (Eyes and Vision). According to David Tovey, editor of the Cochrane Library, and Robert Dellavalle at the University of Colorado in Denver, the United States has the largest number of the library's users, amounting to 1.8 million visits in 2009, constituting a third of its activity. In addition, the nation's top-ten medical schools and forty of the top fifty are licensed to the Cochrane Library. The nation's researchers also produce the highest proportion of publications in the issues of the *Cochrane Database of Systematic Reviews*.[80]

The need for making the canon of evidence-based research literature accessible to health-care practitioners resulted in the creation of the National Institute for Clinical Excellence and the Agency for Healthcare

Research and Quality. Besides the *British Medical Journal*, the *Journal of the American Medical Association*, *Annals of Internal Medicine*, and the *New England Journal of Medicine*, which remain the mainstays of EBM, several newer publications supporting review and EBM were begun, including *Oxford Database of Perinatal Trials* (1988), *ACP Journal Club* (1991), *Clinical Practice Guidelines* (1992), *Evidence-Based Medicine* (1995), *EMB Online* (1995), *Evidence Based Obstetrics and Gynaecology* (1997), *Evidence-Based Complementary and Alternative Medicine* (2004), *Bandolier Journal* (2008), *Journal of Evidence-Based Medicine* (2008), and *EM Practice Guidelines Update* (2009).

COCHRANE COMPLEMENTARY MEDICINE

In 1996, an evidence-based complementary-medicine field known as the Cochrane Complementary Medicine Field was funded by the NIH's OAM to produce, maintain, and disseminate systematic reviews on topics in health care. Focusing on complementary-medicine topics, the outcomes of the Cochrane Collaboration were included in the database of reviews listed in the Cochrane Controlled Trials Registry. By 1998, the Cochrane Complementary Medicine Trials Registry held more than 3,500 RCTs, only 33 percent of which had been identified in a MEDLINE search or by the OAM. Some, in fact, had never been published in any journal because they were part of a conference or dissertation. The extent to which this so-called gray literature has been accepted as "evidence" has caused conventional researchers to raise concerns with regard to not only how much real evidence supports complementary medicine, but how to evaluate it. For the proponents of CAM, however, there is the presumption that any qualitative or methodological problems would be offset by the number and consistency of the results.[81]

Given these combative issues, the University of Maryland Center for Integrative Medicine was established to examine and identify the results of systematic trials of alternative therapies and to disseminate them to health-care providers and the public. In addition, symposia were organized in various countries to discuss meta-analytic processes, design issues in CAM research, and disseminate reviews of CAM therapies.

Early efforts centered on botanicals, vitamins, and traditional Chinese medicine, including efficacy analyses of twenty-six trials and more than three thousand patients treated with acupuncture (P6 stimulation) for adult postoperative and chemotherapy-induced nausea and vomiting. The pooled data indicated the superiority of P6 stimulation over sham treatment. Given the success of the acupuncture trials in holding to qualitative evidence, the center received a $2.1 million research grant from NCCAM in 2007 to extend the work of the Cochrane Complementary Medicine Field.[82]

Even with the expansion of the Cochrane Registry into complementary medicine, alternative practitioners continue to argue that RCTs fail to evaluate the efficacy of their therapies, which they insist are "so complex or esoteric" as to require a wholly different methodology. Many CAM manufacturers, for example, complain that they cannot afford to conduct RCTs and that other means, including evidence-based practice, should be used to demonstrative drug effectiveness. By integrating individual clinical expertise with external clinical evidence from systematic research, critics of the RCT feel they have a likely alternative to clinical trials where certain populations are prevented from participating and where effectiveness is gauged within normal practice conditions. This alternative creates a hierarchy of evidence that involves a variety of non-randomized subjects.[83]

Despite CAM's continued criticism of it, the Cochrane Collaboration includes several notable achievements: escape from the uncertainty of traditional clinical authority; the value of collectively produced evidence; greater transparency among clinicians, consumers, and policymakers; increased academic research; facilitated access to research literature; changes in health-care practice; and additional evidence for clinical decision making.[84] By the same token, several detractions remain unresolved: clinicians and patients' continued resistance to change; the daunting task of summarizing evidence (i.e., knowledge translation); quality-of-life issues; the challenge of moving from evidence-based research to clinical practice; lack of consistency in practice guidelines; inequalities in the availability of services; issues of cost containment; sufficiency of evidence for policymaking; continued bias among consumers; shift of power away from clinicians to researchers; unnecessary government intervention and regulation; and vulgarized understanding of EBM in treatment decisions. There also remains the challenge of converting EBM into clinically relevant answers.[85] Thanks to the work of Alvan Feinstein in defining the principles of quantitative clinical reasoning and David Sackett for his teaching of critical appraisal, EBM and the Cochrane Collaboration have become core concepts in undergraduate, postgraduate, and continuing medical education.[86]

Evidence-based medicine, a concept guided by the belief that clinical practice should be based on scientific evidence and buttressed by a meta-analysis of RCTs providing high-probability estimates, became the model for reductionist medicine in the twentieth century and continues to be so in the twenty-first. Its outcomes provide for a uniform set of guidelines by which studies are conceived and how outcomes and recommendations are obtained. Together, these guidelines provide the practitioner with the most credible information to take into the clinical encounter.

ETHICS AND EQUIPOISE

The early success of the clinical trial came without ethical committees or research councils to lay down procedural guidelines. Medical ethics, such as it was, relied upon the Hippocratic Oath, which, for all practical purposes, left the definition of "ethical behavior" in the eyes of the beholder. Trials were not only too small to be truly effective in detecting the efficacious nature of new drugs, but many were administered in an overtly dangerous and even life-threatening manner.[87]

Historically, the process of obtaining patient consent to participate in clinical trials has been fraught with issues, not the least of which is the morality of giving an inert substance to someone who is expecting (or hoping for) an effective treatment for a disease or illness.[88] Doctors remain uncomfortable with this aspect of such trials because it implies some degree of deception toward the patient.[89] The "blind" aspect of the RCT involving an active experimental drug is difficult to ensure under the best of intentions and is frequently deemed unethical when the health of the subjects is either endangered or if the experimental drug is of questionable scientific value when compared against existing treatments—a matter not only of clinical importance, but of public policy as well.[90]

If the purpose of a clinical trial is to generate unbiased groups of suitable patients for comparison against interrelated drug actions or procedures, and if some treatments are hazardous, then under what circumstances can a physician give or withhold treatment while preserving the ethical standards that are demanded by the profession? Can a new treatment be ethically withheld from a patient in a doctor's care? Is a proposed treatment safe or at least unlikely to do harm? Is consent necessary for a patient's inclusion in a controlled trial? What factors should determine whether a patient can be brought into a controlled trial? Are there any reasons why a patient brought into a controlled trial should not be allocated randomly to different treatments? Given the procedures that control a double-blind test, is it ethical for a doctor not to know the specific treatment administered to a patient? When is the evidence from an RCT judged to be statistically significant? With what level of evidence can it be said that there is no real difference in the therapeutic effects of two treatments in an RCT? At what point can we conclude that the statistical results of an RCT outweigh any unknown factors that might play a causal role in the experimental and control groups?[91]

On August 19, 1947, the so-called Doctors' Trial at Nuremberg had concluded with an opinion by presiding Judge Walter Beals that addressed not only the accusations of war crimes against Nazi doctors accused of using their knowledge of medicine to perform gruesome experiments on prisoners, but also the defense's claim that there was no law to differentiate between legal and illegal experimentation. The trial ended with the adoption of a set of ten points that became known as the Nuremberg Code. Along with the Declaration of Helsinki, promulgated in 1964, it became the basis for the *Code of Federal Regulations Title 45*, which has governed research on and off in the United States and other nations.[92]

The first of the Nuremberg Code's ten principles, stating that "the voluntary consent of the human subject is absolutely essential," alarmed medical researchers in the immediate years after the war as needing further clarification.[93] As a result of this alarm, physicians proceeded to draft their own statement, which some hoped would permit them to conduct certain types of research without obtaining consent.[94] This document, known as the Declaration of Helsinki, was prepared by the World Medical Association's Committee on Medical Ethics, which began its work in 1953. Unlike the Nuremberg Code, it was intended as a guideline designed by physicians for physicians. Formulated in 1964, it has undergone seven revisions, the most recent occurring in 2013.[95] It too, however, excludes research done without obtaining consent. Both the Nuremberg Code and the Declaration of Helsinki state that any voluntary subjects of human experimentation must be informed of the duration, methods, risks, and purpose of the experiment. Anything less is deceit and therefore morally unacceptable. "Physicians who combine medical research with medical care should involve their patients in research only to the extent that this is justified by its potential preventive, diagnostic or therapeutic value," the declaration states, "and if the physician has good reason to believe that participation in the research study will not adversely affect the health of the patients who serve as research subjects." As for the placebo, the declaration accepts its use only in those instances "where no proven intervention exists" or where for compelling scientific reasons it is necessary "to determine the efficacy or safety of an intervention." In either case, however, patients receiving a placebo must "not be subject to additional risks of serious or irreversible harm as a result of not receiving the best proven intervention."[96]

Don Marquis addressed these ethical issues in a 1983 essay, "Leaving Therapy to Chance," suggesting that although the RCT can be interpreted as a form of therapy and therefore compatible with the physician–patient relationship, there should nevertheless be a single ethic for both the clinical trial and the therapeutic physician–patient relationship.[97] Several years later Benjamin Freedman presented the principle of *clinical equipoise*. With this term, Freedman argued that the use of the placebo in the RCT was ethical provided the professional community had not as yet reached a consensus on a standardized treatment. Clinical equipoise was "grounded in the normative nature of clinical practice, the view that a patient is ethically entitled to expect treatment from his or her physician—an entitlement that cannot be sacrificed to scientific curiosity."[98] Only when there is a clear lack of consensus among experts regarding the comparative merits of existing treatments can an RCT be justified. Any RCT that exposes a patient to an inferior intervention is unethical.[99]

Even after Marquis and others took this position, public-health researchers suggested that the benefits of some research, particularly if the intent is to help the greater good, outweighs the risks it presents to individuals.[100] But for critics such as Wendy Mariner, professor of health law at Boston University, "the problem with using intent as the touchstone of the definition of research is [that] it does not address the difficulty many researchers have in being honest about their own intentions." For this reason, she insisted that public researchers "should be held to at least as high an ethical standard as medical researchers." Pointing to any number of well-intentioned projects that used human beings without their knowledge or consent, she urged the public-health community "to voluntarily adopt higher ethical standards for all its activities."[101]

To be ethically justifiable, every clinical trial should satisfy at least three thresholds: first, the research question should have value; second, the research should be designed so that an outcome is likely to be obtained; and third, the participants' rights must be protected.[102] Because vulnerability is closely tied to trust and confidence in the healer, the matter of informed consent obligates physicians to make a very explicit disclosure of the risks, dangers, and choices attendant to any proposed therapy. As Wake Forest scholar Mark Hall explains, "The intensity and emotional content of trust in physicians can lead patients to be extraordinarily forgiving, but also to experience extreme feelings of betrayal once the limits of trust are breached."[103]

Through its several revisions, the Helsinki Declaration moved inexorably to underscore the role of research ethics involving human subjects. In its fourth revision (1996), the document noted that "in [medical] research on [human subjects] considerations related to the well-being of the human subject should take precedence over the interests of science and society." In its 2000 version, it stated that "no national ethical, legal or regulatory requirement should be allowed to reduce or eliminate any of the protections for human subjects set for in this Declaration." This language stemmed from clinical trials funded by the NIH's Centers for Disease Control in which patients with human immunodeficiency virus (HIV) in the United States were given unrestricted access to drugs, but patients from developing countries were excluded from the trials in spite of the fact that one of these drugs, zidovudine, had been identified as an effective antiretroviral treatment.[104]

The latest language of the Helsinki Declaration allows a researcher to offer enrollment to patients *only* when there is uncertainty in the community of expert practitioners about the efficacy of the preferred treatment. For an RCT to be considered ethical, the declaration states that a condition of *equipoise* must prevail, meaning that sufficient doubt exists within the clinical community as a whole to the value of an existing treatment, so there is no reason to prefer any particular arm of a proposed trial.[105] Furthermore, the authors of the declaration chose not to distinguish between therapeutic and nontherapeutic research. When physicians combine their research with clinical care, the physician remains bound to "fully inform the patient which aspects of the care are related to research."[106]

Exemplary of the challenge brought about by the equipoise condition was the multicenter RCT that compared the drug Sunitinib against a placebo in patients diagnosed with the almost always fatal metastatic and inoperable gastrointestinal stromal tumor. Researchers at the University of Michigan Cancer Center declined to participate in the trial, arguing that there was no way a placebo could be helpful to people in such a dire situation and therefore that the trial was morally unjustified. The core issue for researchers was the lack of connection between the purposes of clinical research and the obligations of physicians to their patients. Given Article 28 of the Declaration of Helsinki (2000), it is clear that "the physician may combine medical research with medical care, only to the extent that the research is justified by its potential prophylactic, diagnostic or therapeutic value."[107]

■ ■ ■

The RCT has understandably been acknowledged as the most valid method for interpreting the efficacy of a given treatment because its technique of patient randomization—its most defining characteristic—presumably reduces bias by giving both the group receiving an active drug and the control group equality within a protocol that differs only in the type of treatment. The outcome of that special feature is thought to illuminate a statistical difference that measures the comparative efficacy of each treatment. Depending on the size of the experiment and the range of restrictions used to identify the choice of participants in the study, the results can vary in the definitive nature of the outcome. The values derived from the RCT have been numerous, not the least of which is demonstrating if the experimental treatment is less, equal, or superior to a nonspecific placebo. Provided that the study is well designed, the results, including both positive and adverse effects stemming from a new drug or treatment, can be significant.[108]

Nevertheless, the canonization of the RCT is perhaps presumptive on the part of its uncritical admirers because its raison d'être (i.e., better evidence) is only one of many values used in an evaluation. Seen in the full context of the philosophy of medicine and health care, the RCT's ultimate accomplishments remain uncertain, not because of its goal of effectiveness and efficiency, but because so much of what happens in the clinical trial fails to capture the many biological, social, and cultural processes that intrude into the physician–patient encounter. Healing is a complex process that is weakened or strengthened by a multitude of independent and related variables, including differences across countries and cultures, any one of which can affect the intended outcome.[109]

Not surprisingly, some of the harshest criticism of the RCT has come from those who were its founders and who recognized that the aggregate of information comprising the evidence rarely covers all the decision moments in the physician–patient encounter. Alvan Feinstein at McMaster University, for example, accused the RCT's supporters of being obsessed with it, a condition he called "randophilia." "Instead of taking on the challenges of developing a clinical taxonomy, they have just promulgated randomized trials," he complained. "And when you couldn't do randomized trials on the big scale, you did N-of-one randomized trials. And when randomized trials couldn't give you the answer, you then did meta-analysis. I mean it just shocks me."[110] For Feinstein, Sackett, and others among EBM's founding fathers, however, the RCT informs individual clinical expertise; it does not replace it.[111]

"Evidenced-based medicine has produced important new information about clinical interventions," explains Jeanne Daly in *Evidence-Based Medicine and the Search for a Science of Clinical Care.* "The question is whether these approaches provide sufficiently versatile methods for resolving the range of problems found in clinical care. Have other, broader approaches been sidelined? If so, why, and what are the implications?" In the use of the term *evidence*, she concludes, "the hierarchy of evidence can be invoked but without the disclaimer that it applies only to the task of assessing the effectiveness of interventions. The risk now is that the notion of evidence from evidence-based medicine may disseminate far beyond its roots, to the extent that it loses scientific credibility." She argues persuasively that there has been an "overestimation of the capacity of trials alone to resolve the fundamental problems of clinical medicine." There is now, she insists, a need to shift to broader goals and to recognize that the RCT is only one of many methods to address medicine's multifactorial issues.[112]

There is little question that the double-blind, placebo-controlled RCT has greatly improved drug research and medical care, but also that it has done little to contextualize the positive results in a clinical trial by combining its "active" therapies with the nonspecific components of healing. Long revered as the gold standard of EBM, it is now criticized for excluding any number of variables that might potentially distort its methodology. It was this sense of ambiguity that caused the objective and verifiable world of EBM to be challenged by postmodernism beginning in the 1960s. Relying on a form of literary analysis intended to question the linear history of modern art and culture, with multiple narratives that constructed a perspective on what is taken to be reality, postmodernism came to view EBM as simply one narrative among many. Its knowledge base was relative, socially constructed by normative science's power structure, and, by implication, no more reliable than the personal anecdote.

2

POSTMODERNIST MEDICINE

We are ignorant about how we work, about where we fit in, and most of all about the enormous, imponderable system of life in which we are embedded as working parts.

–Lewis Thomas, *The Medusa and the Snail* (1979)

Medicine's golden age of modernity came to an end in the late 1960s and early 1970s when its authority was challenged by an amalgam of diverse cultural trends, heady intellectual discourse, consumerism, a service and information economy, a culturally based approach to knowledge, and a shift in autonomy from doctors to patients. As in literature, art, history, philosophy, architecture, and even fiction, the assumed certainty of an objective reality came under fire with new interpretations intent on substituting unrepresentable intuitions in place of ultimate principles. In this new age of postmodernism, nothing was beyond questioning; no principle was self-sustaining. The so-called modern mind, once viewed as the culmination of reductionist thinking—the child of the Enlightenment—found itself abandoned by a combination of skepticism and relativism that questioned past authorities, including the sciences. The autonomous individual, once the source of meaning and truth, dissolved into a collage of subject and object, self and other, anarchistic in its diversity and meaningfulness. Assumptions long held involving the potential of human reason, the inevitability of human progress, and even scientific positivism fell victim to quarrelsome theories that viewed objectivity as an illusion and science as little more than an ideological argument subverted by the conflicting elements of age, class, ethnicity, and gender. For the postmodernist, there was no rational basis for the existence of an objective reality. What existed as reality was relative to the observer and molded by culture and social influences.[1]

Efforts to ascribe a conceptual coherence to postmodernism appear to violate its very premise that terms such as *boundaries, core human values,* and *scientific positivism* lack an objective reality. Instead, postmodernism's argument—both epistemological and ideological—is grounded on subjectivity, viewing objectivity as an illusion, the outcome of what Friedrich Nietzsche (1844–1900) once described as "a sum of human relations, which have been enhanced, transposed, and embellished poetically and rhetorically, and which after long use seem firm, canonical, and obligatory to a people."[2] From the writings of Nietzsche to those of Jacques Derrida (1930–2004), Michel Foucault (1926–1984), Jean Baudrillard (1929–2007), Clifford Geertz (1926–2006), and contemporary scholars such as John Lukacs (b. 1924), the attainment of a truly objective scientific method has been judged impossible, fragmented by social contexts and multiple levels of reasoning and meaning. Knowledge is a set of images or metanarratives that over time partnered with social, cultural, and political power to pass as authoritative, stable, and timeless concepts. All knowledge is historically and culturally based—that is, a discourse mediated by time-bound narratives existing within a culture. The postmodernist sees truth as a consensus of ideas agreed upon within a society at a particular period of time.[3]

Applied to medicine, postmodernism infers that the "truth" of an illness is no longer in the physician's objectivist and biomedical account, but in the patient's narrative, which is not only distinctive, but often confusing, if not self-contradictory.[4] The implication for EBM is that because society's current value system can and will alter with our changing understanding of nature, EBM should not be viewed as the only (or even preferred) basis for judgment. That said, biomedicine and its RCT felt the full brunt of the uncertainties that accompanied postmodernism and its multiple versions of fractured truths. The objective, verifiable, and replicative nature of EBM, supported by the RCT and expanded with the meta-analysis, was dismissed as a construct of myths that had wrongly been touted as unchangeable and universally applicable.[5] As Paul Hodgkin explained in the *British Medical Journal*, "To the postmodern eye truth is not 'out there' waiting to be revealed but is something which is constructed by people, always provisional and contingent on context and power."[6] David P. Frost of University College London reinforced this view as well: "All meaning is constructed by a hermeneutic process and . . . all theories are metaphors which evolve as sociohistorical movements, selected by their rhetoric[al] strength rather than [by] any concept of proof."[7]

While biomedicine touted an objectivist account of disease, its high-tech changes had come with the loss of the human touch, evidenced by what many understood to be shorter physician–patient encounters and the greater use of intermediary health professionals interacting with patients through lab tests, magnetic resonance imaging, computerized tomography scans, and other innovative technologies. The truism that physician–patient encounters were growing shorter in the postmodernist era—a belief reinforced by Ian Morrison and Richard Smith in 2000, who observed that patients were not experiencing sufficient quality time with their doctors—was refuted, however, by David Mechanic, Donna D. McAlpine, and Marsha Rosenthal, who showed that quality time with patients had actually increased in both the United States and the United Kingdom due to a continuity of care that included email communications with patients following their time with the physician.[8]

Notwithstanding these two contending positions, advances in treating infectious disease using vaccines, antibiotics, surgical management of trauma, and chemical manipulation of body functions came at the cost of increased health-care fees, expensive technology, questionable drug side effects, and depersonalization. Thus, although biomedicine showed impressive gains, especially in acute disease, it was noticeably deficient in areas of chronic or complex etiologies. Given the evidence of greater patient autonomy and interest in a more integrated approach, postmodernist medicine offered a new representation of illness involving social, psychological, and cultural components; innovative new discourses on pain, suffering, and empathy; and perceived limitations of the dominant biomedical model. Despite the continuing authority of reductionist science, patient interest in nontraditional therapies grew exponentially. The so-called art of medicine—namely, those aspects of the clinical encounter marginalized by the overlay of laboratory science and technology—found a supportive environment among CAM practitioners, who arguably have little to offer patients other than empathy and interventions that carry only minor validity beyond a range of anecdotal support.[9]

The challenge for conventional medicine, explained Michael A. Kottow of Olga Children's Hospital in Stuttgart in the early 1990s, was patient objectification that focused on statistical generalities rather than on the sick individual. Being inductive and based on probabilities, science seldom offered room for individualized medicine. Biomedicine was scientific in both its diagnostic and therapeutic approach, whereas alternative medicine gave little regard to standardized diagnostics, replacing diagnostic evaluation with a subjective process focused on symptoms. Biomedicine centered its energies on "disease-eradicating therapy," whereas alternative therapies looked instead at attacking symptoms and addressing patient well-being. As Kottow explained, "Alternative medicine does not cure but rather peripherally changes patients' attitudes towards the natural event of their disease."[10]

In the fabric of postmodernism's conception of the universe, the lines of distinction between real science and pseudo- or deviant science remain blurred. At what point, the postmodernist asks, can deviant or pseudoscience be given an "alternative" or "complementary" status to normative science? What is to say that deviant or pseudoscience won't at some time become normative science? Then again, is there sufficient reason to examine more closely the claims of deviant science? Is there enough disagreement with the orthodox viewpoint to question the consensus against which deviant science is judged? Does the fact that conventional medicine is showing greater favoritism to complementary and integrative approaches provide evidence of either disagreement or rival factions within orthodoxy? Is this evidence of what Thomas Kuhn called a "crisis" in normative science?[11]

In the wake of what appeared to be a crisis in the reductionist world of science, a host of CAM therapies emerged, many of which were fashioned from debunked systems hoping for a second chance. Taking advantage of the changing health-care environment, advances in pharmacology (in particular psychotropic medications), increased signs of outpatient treatment of depressive disorders, and the rise of third-party payers, those who espoused these therapies set out to capture what they considered to be their fair share of the marketplace.

PSYCHOSOMATIC MEDICINE

Evidence of this new construct was the direction taken by psychosomatic medicine in the postmodernist age. The term *psychosomatic*, which derives from the Greek words *psyche*, meaning "to breathe," and *soma*, meaning "body," represents the interface between the behavioral side and biomedical side of medicine. The power of suggestion in the doctor–patient relationship had once been integral to the ancient Greeks' humoral theories in their regard for maintaining a proper balance of the body's fluids (i.e., "passions"). The Greeks accepted the notion of the influence of emotions on physical health and illness, and this belief grew progressively over the centuries. It was also apparent to the English scholar Robert Burton (1577–1640), who in his best-known classic *The Anatomy of Melancholy* (1621) observed that "the mind most effectually works upon the body, producing by his passions and perturbations miraculous alterations, as melancholy, despair, cruel diseases, and sometimes death itself."[12]

Nevertheless, this interface lost much of its gravitas in the post-Enlightenment era when Cartesian dualism gave the mind (spirit) an entirely separate existence from the body. Despite the later work of French neurologist Jean-Martin Charcot (1825–1893), who used hypnosis to demonstrate the role of psychological factors in modifying the course of physical symptoms, the mind–body dichotomy remained prevalent in mainstream medicine and was given added empowerment with the advent of cellular pathology in the late nineteenth century. The advances made in bacteriology, biochemistry, and disease specificity had a disproportionate influence on medical practice, thereby prolonging the yet unresolved mind–body dichotomy.[13] Austin Flint's *Principles and Practice of Medicine* (1881) left room for doctors to find a connection between the emotions and the disease, but, symbolic of medicine's reductionist emphasis, William Osler's *Principles and Practice of Medicine* (1892) gave unrelenting attention to biomedical science, with little left over for the functional disorders of the nervous system.[14]

This emphasis on the physiological factors in human behavior emerged as a movement in the late nineteenth century when German physician, psychologist, and physiologist Wilhelm Wundt (1832–1920) chose to abandon introspection as the principal means of understanding mental processes and turned instead to the study of physically observable behaviors. Wundt's *Principles of Physiological Psychology* (1874), which explored the feelings, emotions, and volitions of consciousness, marked a significant departure from the more mystical, religious, philosophical, and mechanistic approaches that had dominated in previous centuries. In that earlier era, both chronic and functional disorders were treated with specific therapies, and elements of "obscure pain" and addictions were most often classified as "moral deficits" of the soul and "shamefully disregarded." In essence, physicians were "locked in by the limitations of the prevalent physiochemical views" of their discipline, and rare was the individual who attempted to transcend those limitations. Wundt's American disciples included psychologist James McKeen Cattell (1860–1944), who contributed to the development of intelligence theory and testing; G. Stanley Hall (1844–1924), known for his prodigious scholarship in adolescence behavior; Hugo Münsterberg (1863–1916), famous for his contributions in applied psychology; psychologist and educational reformer Charles Hubbard Judd (1873–1946); Lightner Witmer (1867–1956), known for his work in clinical psychology; and Edward Bradford Titchener (1867–1927), who contributed to the development of intelligence theory.[15]

Those changes that emerged to emphasize the unconscious aspects of doctor–patient interaction went unexplored until the psychological studies of Sigmund Freud (1856–1939), Carl Jung (1875–1961), and Pierre Janet (1859–1947) in Europe and those of William James (1842–1910), James Mark Baldwin (1861–1934), Charles Hamilton Hughes (1839–1916), and Ernst Meyer (1904–2005) in America. Each in his own way reported that the range of humankind's knowledge of the mind was like a small island whose visible portion was just the top of a great coral mountain chain hidden by the ocean. Their collective exploration gave new meaning to the subconscious and, in turn, to the full range of the mind in its relation to disease and healing. Yet even into the 1930s few medical students were exposed to more than a smattering of these ideas, which lacked a disciplinary basis in the medical student's curriculum. This meant that the subconscious, when discussed, was usually treated as an aside and couched in skeptical or even derisive terms.[16]

Men such as Austrian psychotherapist Alfred Adler (1870–1937), best known as the founder of individual psychology; Paul M. Schilder (1886–1940), author of popular *The Image and Appearance of the Human Body: Studies in the Constructive Energies of the Psyche* (1935); Roy R. Grinker (1900–1993), one of Freud's last patients and founder of the Institute for Psychosomatic and Psychiatric Research and Training at Michael Reese Hospital; and Yale anthropologist–linguist Edward Sapir (1884–1939) eventually provided substantial new underpinnings along with interdisciplinary connections to the field of clinical psychiatry. Then, too, the work of physiologist Walter Bradford Cannon (1871–1945), professor and chair of the Department of Physiology at Harvard Medical School; neurologist Stanley Cobb (1887–1968), director of the Department of Psychiatry at the Massachusetts General Hospital in Boston; and pioneering endocrinologist Hans Selye (1907–1982) at the Université de Montréal laid the groundwork for the acceptance of behavioral components such as emotions, appetites, and stress as contributing factors in disease. Cannon's *The Wisdom of the Body* (1932), Cobb's *Borderlands of Psychiatry* (1943) and *Foundations of Neuropsychiatry* (1952), and Selye's *The Stress of Life* (1956) questioned long-held distinctions between mental and physical symptoms, between psychic and somatic causes, and between psychology and physiology.[17]

The outbreak of World War II gave new impetus to psychosomatic medicine due to the traumas experienced by wartime casualties. Roy R. Grinker and John P. Spiegel's *War Neuroses in North Africa* (1943) and *Men Under Stress* (1945) provided important new information on war trauma and treatment using an integrated biopsychosocial approach to human behavior. By the end of the war, a paradigm shift was under way to recognize psychological and socioenvironmental determinants in understanding human illness.[18]

The late 1940s and early 1950s witnessed a general engagement of the behavioral sciences in medicine. In 1949, for example, the Russell Sage Foundation as well as the Josiah Macy Foundation instituted symposia to help formulate an interdisciplinary exchange among behaviorists and the hard sciences. Other encouragement came from the Center for Advanced Study in the Behavioral Sciences at Palo Alto, California, and from the Ford

Foundation, which supported studies on anxiety, depression, and other mental dispositions that became catalysts for dramatic growth in psychosomatic medicine. One byproduct of this interdisciplinary discussion was the question of whether these therapies had superior outcomes to that of the placebo, a query that led inevitably to furthering the evolution of placebo theory and the role of the physician's personality or behavior in the clinical encounter. Tried first in mental hospitals, the placebo soon migrated into general hospitals with the creation of psychiatric units. This latter phenomenon was short-lived, however, as hospitals moved toward a more technical laboratory-based and compartmentalized pattern of services.[19]

Psychosomatic medicine entered into the 1950s on its way to becoming an integral part of every medical specialty when, as medical historian Theodore M. Brown explains, it suddenly fell from grace. The reason for this eclipse, he suggests, was internal medicine's shift into numerous sub-disciplines as well as into a more biochemical and reductionist mode—directions that disconnected internal medicine from psychoanalytic and behaviorist therapies.[20] According to E. D. Wittkower in his 1960 presidential address to the American Psychosomatic Society, "There is a growing cleavage noticeable in psychosomatic publications between those with more and more psychiatry and less and less physiology, and those with more and more physiology and less and less psychiatry."[21]

As academic psychotherapy migrated toward psychoendocrinology and neurochemistry, seeking to build a connection between immune and neuroendocrine systems and opening a new field called *psychoneuroimmunology*,[22] the balance of psychotherapy fell into the hands of social workers, family doctors, celebrity physicians, healers, marriage counselors, psychiatrists, psychologists, self-help groups, and spiritualists, who turned the discipline into advice and self-help commentaries offered through workshops, books, TV shows, blogs, websites, and video packs, advocating new visions of health and happiness—a discourse that opened a wedge between biomedicine's cure-centered focus and postmodernism's definition of healing as a newfound wisdom regarding the quality of life.[23] As a cascade of changes impacted conventional medicine's authority and legitimacy, psychotherapy with its competing brand names became a large part of the discussion in the 1960s, looking at illness from both a patient perspective and a cross-cultural and comparative view. This process included a review of the placebo effect, psychological experiments in persuasion or thought reform, a new perspective on religion and cultural contexts of persons and groups, and myriad psychiatric theories. Of principal interest were the beliefs, expectations, images, and perceptions that structured a person's view of reality; the role of the healer or persuader in sanctioning or restructuring assumptive beliefs; and the role of the patient in internalizing and reevaluating those experiences.[24]

In 1987, Americans spent $4.2 billion on 79.4 million outpatient psychotherapy visits.[25] In a *Consumer Reports* study by Martin E. P. Seligman in 1995, no specific modality did better than any other for any disorder. Psychotherapy was a self-correcting discipline; that is, if one technique showed signs of not working, its mental health specialists moved quickly to other techniques. Psychotherapy was and is a field concerned principally, if not primarily, with improvement in patients' general functioning, and it is therefore hard to imagine it providing more than symptom relief to patients. For that reason, there remains the issue of empirically validating something that may be due to a specific problem as distinct from the patient's "satisfaction" or "overall emotional state" and of distinguishing between psychotherapy alone and psychotherapy plus medication.[26]

A number of individuals emerged as representatives of this holistic health/New Age movement, including psychic healers, lay practitioners, professionally trained heterodox practitioners, and even a few academically trained biomedical physicians. Among postmodernism's celebrity healers were some of the first academically trained physicians to venture beyond reductionist medicine to learn from non-Western healing modalities. David M. Eisenberg of Harvard's Osher Research Center was a medical exchange student to the People's Republic of China in the 1980s, where he went to study acupuncture, massage, herbal medicine, meditation, Tai Chi, and food as medicine. Other contemporaries included author and physician Andrew T. Weil, who was drawn to the study of plants; Jon Kabat-Zinn of the University of Massachusetts Medical School, who studied the application of Buddhist meditation to medicine; Dean Ornish of the Preventive Medicine Research Institute in California, who examined the correlation between lifestyle and coronary artery disease; and Ted Kaptchuk, who studied traditional Chinese medicine. Outside the United States were others such as Brian Berman of Ireland and David Reilly of

Scotland, who studied homeopathy; and Edzard Ernst of Austria and Dieter Melchart of Germany, who undertook various studies of complementary therapies. Altogether, their advocacy had the result of drawing a ragged boundary between metaphysics and the natural sciences, a testimonial perhaps to their willingness to entertain both a reductionist approach as well as an intuitive approach to health and healing.[27]

Within this group, two biomedically trained individuals stand out: Andrew Weil and Deepak Chopra. Both are arguably the most visible spokespersons for holistic medicine, encouraging the fuller integration of alternative modalities. Trained in conventional medicine, they practice a more integrative form of healing that draws from a succession of alternative therapies as well as from the inner sanctum of biomedicine.[28]

Andrew Weil (b. 1942) earned his medical degree from Harvard Medical School in 1968 before interning at Mt. Zion Hospital in San Francisco and then working briefly at the National Institute of Mental Health. He began experimenting with yoga and meditation and wrote *The Natural Mind* (1972), which reflected his growing disillusionment with conventional medicine. As director of the Center for Integrative Medicine at the University of Arizona and editor of the *Journal of Alternative and Complementary Medicine*, he has become a dispenser of New Age self-healing practices. His ten principles of health and illness include: (1) perfect health is not attainable; (2) it is alright to be sick; (3) the body has innate healing abilities; (4) agents of disease are not causes of disease; (5) all illness is psychosomatic; (6) subtle manifestations of illness precede gross ones; (7) everybody is different; (8) everybody has a weak point; (9) blood is a principal carrier of healing energy; and (10) proper breathing is a key to good health. At the basis of all good health, he argues, is attention to lifestyle.[29]

Like Weil, Deepak Chopra (b. 1947) was biomedically trained, at the All India Institute of Medical Sciences in 1968 and in residencies at the Lahey Clinic in Massachusetts and the University of Virginia Hospital before earning board certification in internal medicine and endocrinology. He, too, became disenchanted with conventional medicine, turning to transcendental meditation and establishing the Maharishi Ayurveda Health Center for Stress Management in Massachusetts. In 1993, he moved to California to become director of the Sharp Institute for Human Potential and Mind/Body Medicine. In 1996, he opened the Chopra Center for Well Being in La Jolla, California, where he and David Simon led seminars on energy-based wholeness, Ayurveda, meditation, yoga, and other fulfillment exercises. As an advocate of a more metaphysical mind–body connection, Chopra insists that each body is an energy field and that aging is subject to each individual's mental state. A proponent of "quantum healing," he urges a form of positive or correct thinking as the motive force that governs each person's energy field.[30]

In the 1990s, Chopra took on the entrepreneurial mantra of the prosperity gospelers in *Unconditional Life—Discovering the Power to Fulfill Your Dreams* (1992) and *Creating Affluence—Wealth Consciousness in the Field of All Possibilities* (1993). His newfound interest represents a restatement of New Thought, whose writers, thinkers, and publicists adopt an idealistic view of the universe in which physical nature is a manifestation of the will of God and the world is as large and as immediate as consciousness can make it. This interest represents yet another effort to merge the spiritual insights of the East with the reductionist accomplishments of Western science.[31]

As noted earlier, most studies, including meta-analyses, have found little or no difference in effectiveness between the professional psychotherapist and the minions of paraprofessional therapists and counselors.[32] As late as 1997, the effectiveness of more than 90 percent of psychotherapy's more than four hundred modalities had not proven superior to the placebo.[33] This speaks to the deep concerns raised earlier by Erich Fromm in *The Crisis of Psychoanalysis* (1970) when he noted the possibility of psychotherapy's stagnation and potential death.[34] The question is thus raised whether, for example, there is a difference in effectiveness between the approaches taken in, say, Herbert Benson's *The Relaxation Response* (1975) and *Timeless Healing: The Power and Biology of Belief* (1996), on the one hand, and those taken in Rhonda Byrne's *The Secret* (2006) and *The Power* (2010), on the other.[35] Existing studies indicate little difference between professional and nonprofessional therapists or, for that matter, between psychotherapy administered by professionals and self-administered treatments resulting from self-help literature.[36] As Jerome Frank explains, "The placebo may be as effective as psychotherapy because the placebo condition contains the reasons, and possibly the sufficient, ingredient for much of beneficial effect of all forms of psychotherapy."[37] This suggests that much of what has trans-pired under the umbrella of psychotherapy is little more than a variation of the phenomenon identified earlier as New Thought, mind-cure, Christian Science, healthy-mindedness, and positive thinking.[38]

Today, psychosomatic medicine remains a gleam in the eye of its pro-ponents as they look to the biopsychosocial model set forth by the Ameri-can psychiatrist George Engel (1913–1999), who advocated the integration of the biological, psychological, and social factors in illness and healing. Former president of the American Psychosomatic Society and editor of its journal *Psychosomatic Medicine*, Engel never relinquished his vision of a medical education system that would promote the interrelationship of these factors in human health and disease. In an article titled "Realiz-ing Engel's Vision: Psychosomatic Medicine and the Education of Physi-cian-Healers," Dennis H. Novack, associate dean of medical education at Drexel University College of Medicine, enlisted Engel's vision to project the ideal medical school curriculum, whose components would include both an understanding of disease pathogenesis involving nonbiological determinants as well as physical examination and technical procedures.[39]

SPIRITUALITY

One particular marker of postmodernism was the positive relationship that emerged between spirituality and physical and mental well-being, a position that had already been well defined by William James in his 1902 book *The Varieties of Religious Experience*.[40] Spirituality may or may not connote a religious affiliation, tradition, or association; alternatively, it may merely suggest a more personal meaning, reflection, or wholeness irrespective of any external force or energy. In either case, however, there is the obvious possibility that it has the likely effect of a perception of healthy-mindedness. The mere expectation of relief for pain, for example, tends to relieve it. By contrast, administering a specific treatment with the attitude that it is either useless or might not work has the likely effect of a disappointing outcome. This more than suggests that a good communica-tive relationship between healer and patient fosters an effective outcome.[41] In the mid-1990s, cardiologist Herbert Benson, founder of Harvard's nonprofit Mind/Body Medical Institute at Beth Israel Deaconess Hospital in Boston, recommended improving health through "relaxation response"—a meditative process of word repetition that is remarkably similar to the late-nineteenth- and early-twentieth-century practices of New Thought mind-cure healers and self-help authors Charles F. Haanel (1866–1949), Frank Haddock (1853–1915), Emma Curtis Hopkins (1849–1925), Horatio W. Dresser (1866–1954), and Napoleon Hill (1883–1970). Today, Benson's relaxation therapies are commonplace in medical schools and hospitals.[42]

Those who advocate spirituality as a valid component of health care often criticize the biomedical model for viewing illness as a physical condition that can be logically analyzed and treated without incorporating the patient's psychological and social experiences (and by implication, spirituality) into the encounter.[43] Spiritual beliefs, they insist, remain important factors in some patients' perception, and clinical caregivers should take such things into account as they deal with disease or illness. Just as evident is the fact that professional ethics impose clear constraints on when and how this can or could be done. Religion has been historically connected with disease and illness from the earliest of times, but its intersection with medical science since the seventeenth century has been distant, each preferring to deal with the sick patient in an autonomous manner. Doctors and other health-care professionals, however, are increasingly including their patient's religious or spiritual beliefs in order to make available a wider range of support systems in the course of treatment. There has even been a "growing recognition that patients present themselves as integrated beings whose physical, emotional, and spiritual welfare are intertwined." However explained, spirituality's effect on healing is to create a sense of oneness in the patient—an intersection of mind and body that strengthens physical and mental wellness.[44]

Contemporary scholars are finding statistically meaningful evidence in a variety of clinical, community, cross-sectional, and longitudinal studies showing that spiritual involvement of various types or dimensions (i.e., prayer, meditation, religious services, study groups, etc.) can be beneficial to physical and mental health. Their studies have also attempted to factor in different health practices, social support, psychosocial resources, and belief structures. Mindful that communication is at the heart of the spiritual and religious component in health-promotion and prevention strategies, patient response might well be aligned to the communicative encounter itself irrespective of the particular subject matter. That said, research into health-related communication suggests a rethinking of the meaning, role, and importance of spirituality as distinct from provider–patient support or encouragement.[45]

OPEN DOOR

As a counterculture phenomenon in the United States, postmodernist medicine accommodates relationships with meditation, prayer, yoga, nutritional therapies, pop psychology, homeopathy, wellness, naturopathy, vegetarianism, and feminist theory. It represents health-care and healing modalities practiced outside and on the fringe of conventional medicine because of differences that may be cultural, economic, philosophical, scientific, medical, or educational in nature. In their accommodation to postmodernism, Americans learned about naturopathy, reeducated themselves about homeopathy, debated the relevance of orthodox medicine's superiority, demanded the coverage of chiropractic under Medicare, and rediscovered the potential of traditional, Native, and Eastern forms of healing. Most importantly, the unquestioned authority of scientific medicine diminished despite its ability to offer sophisticated technological solutions for acute and long-standing problems. Modern medicine, its authority embedded within an increasingly technological and mechanistic framework, was viewed as having faltered in its ability to address the personal side of health and illness. The consequence of these changing views was the forging of a new social contract that included the reemergence of alternative modalities whose theoretical and methodological approaches competed alongside the dominant system of conventional medicine. First chiropractors and then acupuncturists won access rights in the states as interest in their therapies captured the public eye. Both were early beneficiaries of the growing role of consumer power. Conventional medical doctors continued to enjoy status and income but found themselves sharing the marketplace with a broad assortment of licensed and unlicensed healers and facing an increasingly hostile attitude to their once-sovereign position.[46]

The uneasy relationship between CAM and conventional medicine has been due to the fact that although the origins of both disappear into the healing practices of ancient cultures, a distinction yet remains, with one having chosen to move forward on a materialistic path grounded in the natural sciences, and the other choosing a vitalistic path that connects cure to spiritual intuition and conjecture.[47] CAM's popularity is representative of the more mystical propensities of the postmodern world, as evidenced in books and digital media that address the paranormal and the proposition that such propensities may be filling a void left by the decline of more formalized religion. The connection between spirituality and physical health, a long-standing tradition among unconventional therapies, offers important insights into CAM's popularity.[48] As Brian M. Hughes at the National University of Ireland explains, given that patients tend to approach medicine on the basis of heuristic reasoning rather than logical rationalism, CAM is more often characterized "as a popular deconstruction of the hegemony of biomedical science, and a counter-cultural onslaught against modernist, technologically focused conceptions of progress." CAM substitutes mystical expressions of physical and mental health for the faith-based beliefs and practices of organized religion. "The attention given to CAM," Hughes suggests, "may be a displaced version of the attention previously devoted to orthodox religions." In a statistical comparisons of CAM and religious observance in Ireland (not including Dublin), he found that CAM usage was greater in those regions where religious observance had declined. This, he feels, explains why the interest in the paranormal has not diminished in Western societies despite that interest's more secular identity in the postmodern world.[49]

The elements that now underlie postmodernist thinking are a complex mixture of religion, mysticism, cosmic energy, disbelief in Western reductionism, and an increased fascination with Eastern philosophies. In medicine, this combination has involved a new approach to treating disease and illness that stands in sharp contrast to the biomedical model. Whether referring to the serial dilutions of homeopathy, the subluxations of chiropractic, Barbara Brennan's high-energy medicine, anthroposophy, therapeutic touch, or any number of other interventions, this discourse has encouraged a more metaphysical encounter with the world, one that questions the basic assumptions about the nature of reality. Rejecting the term *sectarian* as too pejorative, the vocabulary of postmodernism has welcomed the descriptions *unconventional, complementary, holistic,* and *alternative* into its lexicon—terms that are often politically or socially motivated, depending in large measure on the speaker and the audience. The term *alternative* suggests the exclusive use of nonorthodox therapies as substitutes for conventional ones, whereas *complementary* implies the use of nonorthodox therapies in conjunction with or supplementary to conventional medicine, suggesting in the process a more integrative approach to healing. Unfortunately, consumers have tended to use both terms simultaneously, a situation that suggests the more appropriate use of the term *complementary and alternative medicine.*[50]

Not all accept the label *CAM* as appropriate, however. David Eisenberg, Thomas Delbanco, and Ronald Kessler consider it pejorative and insist on substituting *integrative* as a more accurate term.[51] *Integrative medicine* is not intended as a synonym for *complementary medicine* but is indicative of treatments intended as adjuncts to conventional medical treatment that are not typically part of the medical school curriculum. Equally important is the fact that the term *integrative* focuses on health and healing rather than on disease and treatment. "It views patients as whole people with minds and spirits as well as bodies and includes these dimensions into diagnosis and treatment," explain Lesley Rees and Andrew Weil. "It also involves patients and doctors working to maintain health by paying attention to life-style factors such as diet, exercise, quality of rest and sleep, and the nature of relationships."[52]

Still others prefer the term *holistic medicine,* which implies giving the individual patient an instrumental role—both conscious and unconscious—in building and maintaining his or her medical landscape (physical, social, and mental well-being) through health promotion, treatment, healing, and disease prevention. In contrast to the positivistic framework of conventional medicine, holism looks beyond the formalized canon of reductionist science to the interrelationship of mind, body, and spirit as contributing factors in human wellness. It assumes, therefore, that each individual represents a complexity of interdependent functions that are affected by physical, mental, spiritual, and environmental factors, any one of which might negatively or positively influence the whole body as well as the individual part. In this postmodernist scheme of things, there is the assumption that individuals should trust their intuitions, experiences, feelings, and personal insight as a source of ultimate knowledge of the external world.[53]

Despite the lack of consensus on the proper terminology, the changes that accompanied this counterculture attitude led to the establishment of numerous lay and professional organizations operating on the periphery of academic medicine. Formed during the heyday of postmodernism, the National Center for Homeopathy (1974) and the American Holistic Medical Association (1978) served as catalysts to a consumer-driven movement to broaden the use of alternative therapies within the nation's health-care system. Other representative organizations include the International Veterinary Acupuncture Society (1974), the American Holistic Veterinary Medical Association (1978), the International Foundation for Homeopathy (1980), the American Holistic Nurses' Association (1981), the American Association of Naturopathic Physicians (1981), the American Veterinary Chiropractic Association (1987), and the Academy of Veterinary Homeopathy (1995).

Along with lay and professional associations came a plethora of journals. In the United States, some of the more popular include *Acupuncture and Electro Therapeutic Research* (1976), *Complementary Therapies in Medicine* (1986), *Journal of Alternative and Complementary Medicine* (1995), *Alternative Medical Review* (1996), *Journal of Body Work and Movement Therapies* (1996), *Evidence-Based Complementary and Alternative Medicine* (2004), and *Research Journal of Medicinal Plant* (2006). The higher-ranked journals from the United Kingdom include *Acupuncture in Medicine* (1983), *Complementary Therapies in Clinical Practice* (1995), *Journal of Ethnobiology and Ethnomedicine* (2005), *Chinese Medicine* (2006), *BMC Complementary and Alternative Medicine* (2009), and *Chiropractic and Manual Therapies* (2011). The popular journal *Evidence-Based Complementary and Alternative Medicine*, better known as *eCAM*, was founded by Edwin L. Cooper, who served as its editor in chief between 2004 and 2010. High in its impact-factor ratings released by Thomson Reuters in 2012 are publications on popular issues such as "acupuncture and herbal medicine for cancer patients," "integrative oncology," and "complementary and alternative therapies for liver diseases." On its agenda for future special issues are topics such as "spirituality and health," "scientific basis of mind–body interventions," and "evidence-based medicinal plants for modern chronic diseases."[54]

After much discord, the tensions exhibited over the respective merits of the nation's heterodox healing systems appear to have settled into détente. This uneasy coexistence is by no means the outcome of any mediation between the contending parties, but the consequence of increased patient empowerment, cost factors, medical consumerism, decision making in managed care, and changes in the nation's health-care delivery system. The debate is no longer one of legitimacy, but of the degree to which heterodox therapies should be either sanctioned or included within the fortress of biomedicine. Increased interest in the relationship between doctor and patient and the emerging science of psychoneuroimmunology has opened innovative pathways involving behavior, attitude, and the placebo effect, encouraging a new look at the individual's capacity for healing.[55]

CAM POPULARITY

The growth in CAM's popularity coincided with a decided increase in the cost of health care, which grew exponentially over the decades. Between 1965 and 1975, expenditures tripled in the United States, rising from $41 billion to nearly $130 billion; between 2000 and 2010, they rose from $1.2 trillion to more than $2.6 trillion.[56] During this period of rising costs and unintended consequences stemming from complicated new technology, the ineffectiveness in managing certain chronic conditions (i.e., lower back pain and fibromyalgia), the add-on costs of risk management, and the tragic story of birth defects due to thalidomide and other drug side effects, conventional medicine found itself competing with an emerging holistic health-care movement. Unconventional therapies, many of which had been around for centuries, claimed safer and less-expensive treatments.[57]

In studying citations in the five most influential US medical journals (*Journal of the American Medical Association, New England Journal of Medicine, American Journal of Medicine, Annals of Internal Medicine,* and *Archives of Internal Medicine*) over a thirty-five-year period from 1965 to 1999, Terri A. Winnick notes a "steady stream" of articles on unconventional medicine.[58] Many of the early citations concerned the issue of licensure and whether chiropractic should be included for payment in Medicare and Medicaid. Later, following the visit of President Richard Nixon to China in 1972, attention focused on Chinese medicine, opening a robust discussion of acupuncture and related modalities. Other popular topics covered Laetrile treatment for cancer and interest in herbal medicines. Not surprisingly, articles in the early years were arrogant, insulting, and "bitingly negative" toward unconventional medicine, especially regarding chiropractic, but they moderated over time to "measured discussion" and "objective disinterest." In this latter phase, occurring after the establishment of the OAM within the NIH in 1992, authors showed an enhanced awareness of unconventional medicine's appeal and a more realistic view of its place in a pluralistic, consumer-centered marketplace. There was even a decided increase in the use of terminology such as *holistic, holism, natural, gentle, nontoxic, whole patient, self-actualization*, and *nonpathologic goals*, all of which suggested a desire on the part of doctors and patients for a more inclusive, compassionate, and empathic approach to healing. Journal articles also focused increasingly on specific unconventional treatments and the results stemming from controlled trials. Choosing objectivity over ridicule, the journals mounted an effective educational campaign using the controlled clinical trial as its mechanism for establishing efficacy. "Evidence-based medicine" became the new watchword for validating unproven heterodox treatments. Here, the OAM and the NIH became useful vehicles to lead medical heterodoxy through the intricacies of scientific testing.[59]

CAM therapies encompass not only highly complex traditional health systems such as those found in Chinese, East Indian, and Native American cultures, but distinct entities such as dietary, spiritual, and botanical modalities; practices such as hypnosis and chiropractic taught in degree-granting institutions; and less-structured entities such as therapeutic touch, Reiki, anthroposophy, and crystal healing, to name just a few. Some modalities involve manipulations or applications to the body; others utilize discrete active or inactive organic and inorganic substances, the adjustment of paranormal forces that supposedly surround or enter the body, or mind–body activity originating from inside or outside the patient.[60]

Ethnographer Bonnie Blair O'Connor identifies seven categories of CAM in her 1995 book *Healing Traditions*: (1) alternative systems such as acupuncture, Ayurveda, and homeopathy; (2) bioelectromagnetic applications; (3) diet, nutrition, and lifestyle changes; (4) herbal medicine; (5) manual healing such as massage, osteopathy, and therapeutic touch; (6) mind–body control such as biofeedback and meditation; and (7) pharmacological and biological treatments.[61] The *Clinician's Complete Reference to Complementary and Alternative Medicine* (2000) adds two additional categories: community-based health-care practices and unclassified methods.[62] In all, virtually hundreds of healing modalities are in use today and employ a wide range of diagnostic and therapeutic methods. Of this number, many have cycled in and out of popularity. To the extent that these therapies have elements common with conventional medicine, they are more easily subject to examination and evaluation for their safety and efficacy. Others, in particular those more doctrinaire in their embrace of paranormal forces or energies, prove difficult to assess using normative science.[63] Most significantly, CAM has become a symbol of postmodernism with its skepticism of science and technology, its preference for spirituality and the natural environment, and its emphasis on choice and responsibility.[64]

Most states license some level of CAM. As of 2002, all states license chiropractic; a lesser number license acupuncture and massage therapy; eleven license naturopathy; and three (Connecticut, Arizona, and Nevada) license non-MD homeopathic practitioners. Ayurveda, however, is not licensed in any of the states even though it has existed as a healing system for more than a thousand years. Notwithstanding this situation, thousands of Ayurveda practitioners operate openly in the United States.[65]

Not only has there been a proliferation of new healing modalities and health delivery services in postmodernist medicine, there is also evidence of a rising proportion of women as healers contributing to the construct of medical values, identities, and practices.[66] In conventional medical schools, the percentage of women doctors increased from 5.8 percent in 1960 to roughly half in 2011.[67] Today 53 percent of family-practice residents, 63 percent of pediatric residents, and nearly 80 percent of obstetrics and gynecology residents are female.[68] The overall number of women in complementary and alternative medicine is even higher (72.2 percent of yoga practitioners;

77 percent of naturopaths; 85 percent of massage therapists; 58 percent of acupuncturists; and nearly 90 percent of homeopaths). Drawing wisdom from both the secular sciences and America's alternative spiritual traditions, women have become disproportionately central to maintaining the delicate balance between the healthy individual, the social environment, and the spiritual energies thought to course through the universe.[69]

The definition of CAM produced by the OAM in 1997 and later adopted by the White House Commission on Complementary and Alternative Medicine Policy in 2002 represents the product of competing social and political forces:

> Although heterogeneous, the major CAM systems have many common characteristics, including a focus on individualizing treatments, treating the whole person, promoting self-care and self-healing, and recognizing the spiritual nature of each individual. In addition, many CAM systems have characteristics commonly found in mainstream health care, such as a focus on good nutrition and preventive practices. Unlike mainstream medicine, CAM often lacks or has only limited experimental and clinical study; however, scientific investigation of CAM is beginning to address this knowledge gap. Thus, boundaries between CAM and mainstream medicine, as well as among different CAM systems, are often blurred and are constantly changing.[70]

Nevertheless, consensus remains problematic because *complementary and alternative medicine* is more an "umbrella" term for multiple modalities that operate beyond the borders of conventional medicine as well as several that are now being taught in regular medical schools. Given this reality, Edzard Ernst and his colleagues have suggested a new definition: "CAM is diagnosis, treatment and/or prevention which complements mainstream medicine by contributing to a common whole, by satisfying a demand not met by orthodoxy or by diversifying the conceptual frameworks of medicine."[71]

In essence, CAM conceptualizes the body, mind, and environment in an all-encompassing holistic relationship. In numerous surveys of CAM patients, statistics reveal that 80 percent or more of its users report leaving their treatments "emotionally stronger, less anxious, and more hopeful about the future." Much of their satisfaction is attributed to their ability to choose a therapist; the amount of time spent in the physician–practitioner encounter; the manner in which the illness is explained; the practitioner's focus on the patient's emotional state rather than on the underlying disease; the "low-tech" approach involving more physical contact; the individualized nature of the intervention (the holistic approach versus the disease approach of conventional medicine); and the setting (i.e., private and noninstitutional) in which they are treated. In the absence of organic disease, where both doctors and patients struggle to understand and "cure" ill-defined symptoms, CAM provides a valued set of palliative therapies.[72]

The first significant national survey of CAM usage by adults in the United States was carried out by David Eisenberg and his colleagues and published in the *New England Journal of Medicine* in 1993. Examining the usage of sixteen major CAM therapies, the researchers estimated that 34 percent of the adult population had used at least one complementary therapy in the previous year and that this segment of the population made an estimated 425 million visits to CAM practitioners. Surprisingly, the number of these visits roughly equaled visits to primary-care physicians. In spite of such robust figures, an estimated 90 percent of CAM patients were self-referred, which suggests a lack of knowledge or communication between patients and their primary-care physicians regarding the use of alternative treatment. No doubt, this phenomenon was reinforced by patients' reluctance to face their conventional physicians' hostility toward their choice of an unorthodox competitor.[73]

In a follow-up survey of trends, Eisenberg and his colleagues surveyed 1,539 adults in 1991 and 2,055 in 1997 to measure prevalence, cost, and disclosure of CAM therapies to conventional medicine. The findings were no less remarkable.

1. The use of some therapies increased from 33.8 percent in 1990 to 42.1 percent in 1997.
2. The probability of persons using alternative therapies increased from 36.3 percent in 1990 to 46.3 percent in 1997.
3. Alternative therapies were most frequently used for chronic conditions such as back problems, anxiety, depression, and headache.

4. Only about 38.5 percent of persons using alternative therapies chose to tell their primary-care physician.

5. The percentage of patients paying out of pocket for their alternative therapies decreased slightly from 64 percent in 1990 to 58.3 percent in 1997.

6. Visits to alternative-medicine practitioners increased from 427 million in 1990 to 629 million in 1997, a number that exceeded the total visits to conventional primary-care physicians.

7. Approximately 15 million persons took herbal remedies or high-dose vitamins along with their prescription medicines.

8. Expenditures for alternative therapies increased 45.2 percent between 1990 and 1997, when it was estimated at $21.2 billion.[74]

In an effort to correct sampling errors, the National Center for Health Statistics conducted a survey in 1999, providing respondents with a list of eleven potential therapies (acupuncture, relaxation techniques, massage therapy, imagery, spiritual healing or prayer, lifestyle diet, herbal medicine, homeopathy treatment, energy healing, biofeedback, and hypnosis), with the option of adding a therapy not on the list. With a response rate of 70 percent from a total of 30,801 adults, the survey revealed that 28.9 percent of US adults had used at least one CAM therapy during the previous year, a percentage that was higher for women (33.4 percent) than for men (24 percent) and higher among persons with health insurance than among those without it. When organized by groups, the most popular modalities were those considered body–mind interventions, such as prayer, relaxation, imagery, hypnosis, and biofeedback (16.4 percent). Other popular forms of CAM were herbal therapy (9.6 percent) and chiropractic (7.6 percent). The survey also showed that CAM was more popular in the Midwest and West than in the Northeast or South and more highly used among those who rated their health either poor or fair.[75]

In 2005, Hilary Tindle and her colleagues (including Eisenberg) returned to the original 1993 Eisenberg questionnaire to find comparability of information. In doing so, the researchers looked at eighteen CAM practices but excluded prayer. Their survey indicated that the most commonly used therapies were herbs (18.6 percent), followed by relaxation techniques (14.2 percent) and chiropractic (7.4 percent). The evidence suggested that the percentage of the population using at least one CAM modality in the previous year, 35.1 percent, indicated a stable environment for CAM between 1997 and 2002, except for yoga and herbal therapy usage, which showed disproportionate increases.[76] These and several other surveys reveal a number of characteristics that have appeared constant over the years.

- More than one-third of all Americans seek some form of CAM modality for their health and illness problems. Although some researchers attribute this statistic to the "tumultuous managed care environment," others are more inclined to attribute it to more esoteric body–mind constructs.[77]
- The majority of CAM users are women, Caucasians, and the more highly educated.[78]
- Those individuals most apt to utilize CAM are generally in poorer health, seriously ill, or suffering from pain, musculoskeletal problems, or anxiety-related issues. Less clear are the motivations that stem from dissatisfaction with conventional medicine because so many of those who use CAM do so in conjunction with conventional medical care.[79]
- Both the Mexican American and Hispanic populations are more prone to use CAM than other ethnicities. The same is true of the Native American population. All three groups are frequent users of spiritual-healing techniques, herbal remedies, and traditional healers.[80]
- CAM has brought health and religion into a partnership with concern for the environment, politics, autonomy, and natural products.[81]

AMERICAN MEDICAL SCHOOLS

According to an analysis published in 2005, the medical profession's response to the growth of CAM came in three distinct phases: in the first phase, from the late 1960s through the early 1970s, biomedical doctors condemned, ridiculed, and sought to contain the spread of CAM therapies by exaggerating their risks; during the second, from the mid-1970s through the early 1990s, conventional medicine looked inwardly at its own shortcomings due to increased evidence of patient dissatisfaction; and in the third, beginning in the mid-1990s, mainstream medicine chose a more integrative approach.[82] In reflecting on this phenomenon since the initial publication of the journal *Alternative Therapies in Health and Medicine* in 1995, Jeffrey Bland, chair of the Institute for Functional Medicine, remarked that numerous topics viewed as alternative years earlier had, after being examined through the lens of reductionist science, "moved into greater acceptance within the general healthcare system."[83]

Although surveys indicate that the majority of patients using CAM treatments do not inform their primary physician, there appears to be much less opposition among mainstream physicians to CAM therapies than in earlier decades. A 1992 survey of nearly six hundred family physicians queried by the Department of Family Medicine at the East Carolina School of Medicine in Greenville, North Carolina, indicated that 44 percent of the physicians reported being willing to work with CAM and that 23 percent believed that CAM could help where regular medicine had failed.[84] In Canada, a comparable survey of two hundred practitioners indicated that 54 percent had referred patients to CAM healers and 16 percent were actually practicing some type of CAM.[85] In other words, regular physicians were either referring patients to what they viewed as more or less respectable forms of CAM or adopting CAM in some manner in their own practices. Referral rates in 2000 ranged from 50 percent for chiropractic and 47 percent for acupuncture to 24 percent for massage, 10 percent for homeopathy, and 4 percent for herbal medicine.[86]

A 1996–1997 American Medical Association survey indicated that 46 of the 125 US medical schools included CAM topics in their curriculum. A subsequent survey in 1998 indicated that 75 were offering CAM electives or including CAM topics in existing courses. Exactly *how* CAM had been presented—namely, whether instructors encouraged CAM or accompanied their comments with a bias—was not determined.[87] In a 1998 survey of 1,297 faculty at six health science center schools, the highest use of alternative therapies reported was by allied health faculty (76 percent), followed by nursing (74 percent), dentistry (65 percent), pharmacy (56 percent), veterinary medicine (55 percent), and medicine (52 percent). Clearly, however, the question of educating medical students about CAM therapies without marginalizing them remains an issue, particularly if the goal is to include or integrate CAM into the full range of therapeutic modalities taught in the medical curricula. As yet, there is no clear set of objectives or competencies with respect to CAM therapies that medical students are required to learn for the US Medical Licensing Exam.[88]

Writing in 1998, Jay Udani, at the Health Services Research and Integrative Medicine program at Cedars-Sinai Medical Center in California, reported that equating alternative medicine to quackery was no longer accepted practice in US medical schools. He attributed this change to the increased use of the terms *complementary* and *integrative* and the fact that CAM modalities were most often performed as adjunct to conventional medicine. Udani noted that such therapies used in combination with conventional medicine had increased from 34 percent of the US population in 1990 to 69 percent in 1998 and that only 4 percent of the population chose to use such therapies exclusively.[89] The more popular of these nonconventional systems included chiropractic, acupuncture, vitamin and herbal treatments, homeopathy, biofeedback, massage, hypnotherapy, and yoga.[90] Even as the use of complementary medicine continued to grow in the 1990s, there remained a clear lack of standards or guidelines for how it could or should be integrated into conventional medicine. During the late 1990s, much of what was taught came in the form of continuing medical education.[91]

In response to a 2000–2001 questionnaire sent to all 125 conventional medical schools in the United States by the Liaison Committee on Medical Education, ninety-one schools reported including CAM in their required curriculum, sixty-four reported offering CAM as an elective, and thirty-two reported including CAM as part of an elective. It was still clear, however, that the content of these courses varied widely from one school to the next, with opinions ranging from neutrality to limited acceptance to outright scorn.[92] Included among those schools offering substantive teaching of CAM were Harvard Medical School, Albert Einstein College of Medicine, Columbia University, Duke University, Mount Sinai School of Medicine, Stanford University, University of Arizona, Georgetown University, Jefferson Medical College, University of Minnesota, and several of the University of California medical schools.[93]

Numerous suggestions for the inclusion of CAM in schools emerged from discussions among medical educators, including those listed here and published in the *Annals of Internal Medicine* in 2003.

1. Teach students to become knowledgeable about the therapies most used by patients. This includes chiropractic, spiritual healing, herbal remedies, dietary supplements, relaxation techniques, and massage.

2. Only one medicine should be taught in US medical schools. Recognizing a diversity of therapies, students should be taught that CAM therapies must be peer reviewed and evidence based before they can be given serious consideration within the curriculum.

3. Create opportunities for exchange programs between and among US medical schools and the schools of chiropractic, acupuncture, mind–body therapies, therapeutic massage, and naturopathy.

4. Encourage student and faculty interest groups to share information about CAM therapies and to participate in the evaluation of evidence.

5. In courses that include CAM therapies, students should be examined on their mastery of CAM content and about CAM options where appropriate.

6. Incorporate CAM in case histories used in the curriculum.

7. Offer a well-designed elective in CAM therapies, including relevant readings and a review of the scientific literature.

8. Give students the opportunity to observe local CAM practitioners and to experience CAM therapies themselves to provide depth to their understanding.

9. CAM education is needed at all level of medical education, including attendance at workshops, conferences, and informal sessions related to CAM issues.[94]

A major restructuring is now occurring in the way that CAM services are organized and delivered in an environment of managed care. In a 2001 survey, nearly 16 percent of the nation's community-based hospitals offered some level of CAM service. In addition, several major medical centers, including cancer centers, have integrated CAM therapies into their patient care: M. D. Anderson in Houston; Memorial Sloan-Kettering Cancer Center; Columbia–Presbyterian Medical Center in New York City; Duke University; and the Integrative Medicine Program managed by David Rakel at the University of Wisconsin.[95] At the Integrative Medicine Service unit at Memorial Sloan-Kettering in New York, practitioners utilize massage, music therapy, and acupuncture in their wards and offer outpatient referrals for relaxation, yoga, and Tai Chi classes.[96] What remains at issue is how the modern hospital, the bastion of biomedicine's specialty care, accommodates an umbrella health-care system with multiple providers offering competing modalities, some of which have radically different epistemologies and without clear scientific evidence of benefit. Should these modalities require the acceptance by conventional medicine and third-party providers before being made available? Should hospitals be required to address problems of health, illness, and healing in ways that challenge the reductionist view of the world? To date, hospitals appear not to encourage this type of discussion.

That said, much remains to be learned about what is being done in CAM practices, the conditions for which it is being done, by whom, and what education and training prepare practitioners to do it.[97] Both integrative and collaborative CAM programs are in their infancy. Their challenges over the next decades involve improved communication; training and certification; reimbursement; appropriate research models; comprehensive information for both the public and conventional practitioners; and appropriate education in all stages of conventional and CAM health-care training. Given the restrictions on licensing qualifications to all but a few CAM modalities, the training of alternative healers varies from bona fide medical degrees to self-identification of expertise among healers who operate on the fringes of the health-care industry.[98] Equally important with all of these factors is the daunting challenge for CAM to provide a "proof of efficacy"—beyond its exaggerated promotional literature—for its healing treatments given the fact that both the Kefauver–Harris Amendment of 1962, sometimes called the "Drug Efficacy Amendment," and the Dietary Supplement Health and Education Act of 1994 excluded herbal preparations, phytomedicinals, dietary, and food supplements from quality-control measures instituted by the US Food and Drug Administration (FDA). CAM manufacturers do not have to establish efficacy before they market their products. As a result, many CAM products are mislabeled, misidentified, and adulterated with different plants of unknown origin. Without enforced standardization, it is impossible to determine the active ingredients, much less their stability. The fact that so many patients combine their prescription drugs with herbals of unknown origin or efficacy creates serious risks-to-benefits ratios associated with patient outcome, a situation that raises the question of whether CAM treatments do more harm than good given the risks of misdiagnoses, contraindications, and the competence of nonmedically qualified practitioners.[99]

■ ■ ■

Beginning in the 1960s and 1970s, postmodernist healers emerged to challenge the muscular strength of conventional medicine's reductionist bias. Beset with a host of issues, including rising costs, inadequate insurance coverage, excessive use of antibiotics, exposés involving patient rights, and the decline of physician autonomy and authority, conventional medicine entered a period of self-doubt and introspection as it tried to reconcile its scientific achievements with a declining doctor–patient relationship. Postmodernism challenged conventional medicine's disease protocols, the RCT, and even the meta-analysis. The outcomes of the clinic and the laboratory also came into question as attitudes and expectations regarding the EBM underwent closer examination, transforming it into a "soft" science based on knowledge socially constructed to fit the needs of the culture. In this new setting, even the Cochrane Collaboration was made an object of derision, a storefront for housing "evidence" (i.e., different narratives) in the health sciences. To the extent that the collaboration "worked," it was said to function as a service to the culture's immediate needs. To the extent that postmodernism became the mindset of the age, it opened the door to an assault on the scientific method, offering entreé to CAM and open-mindedness to CAM's proposition that the RCT was little more than a cultural artifact.

By the early 1990s and the beginnings of managed care and efforts at cost containment, conventional medicine faced an even greater threat to its professional sovereignty and to the doctor–patient relationship as insurance providers chose to extend patient coverage to less costly alternatives. Along with these changes came the US Department of Education's decision to accredit numerous complementary and alternative healing programs, thus breaking conventional medicine's virtual monopoly on the practice of healing.[100] This change eventually led medical schools to include discussion of unconventional medical practices as part of their regular curriculum.[101] In more recent years, biomedical doctors have added elements of complementary and alternative treatments to their individual and corporate practices. Although not necessarily trend setting, these changes have suggested a willingness on the part of conventional medicine to accommodate epistemologically different healing systems.[102]

Even with the openness among many mainstream practitioners, conventional medicine has not found assimilation easy due to CAM's epistemological, ideological, and methodological differences. Postmodernism goes far to explain the popularity of unconventional therapies in that an increasing number of patients have come to reject the assumptive practices, quantitative methods, and overarching and objective certainties of reductionist medicine for their own intuitive and nonlinear truths. Nevertheless, CAM's modalities diverge so sharply from biomedical reductionism (i.e., in the nature of their evidence and the subjective manner of their production) that they defy explanation using the framework of scientific medicine. Methodological pluralism may open the gates to a new global medicine, but its usefulness in the creation of commonly shared evidence-based medical knowledge remains problematic.

Instead of fading away as an anachronism in the postmodernist world, CAM has experienced significant growth in both the United States and abroad. Nearly half of all Americans now use some form of CAM, including a considerable percentage of the well-educated middle class, who find themselves troubled by environmental issues, aware of the importance of individual choice, and anxious over the negative impacts of science and technology. In this regard, CAM's popularity has become as much a social movement as a reflection of individual choice. Nevertheless, issues remain regarding its safety, efficacy, and potential side effects. Consumers need to be better educated on their choices, and conventional physicians need to have a stronger relationship with their patients to better understand how patient choices may or may not benefit from a combination of CAM and more conventional therapies. Neither the unconventional healer nor the scientific community can view CAM therapies as simply a "fringe" interest among consumers. That said, CAM has yet to explain how its therapies work and for the reasons its proponents believe. As will be seen in chapter 3, the rapidly growing recognition of the placebo effect and the conditions under which it operates not only challenged normative science but also undermined CAM's reputation, if not its actual legitimacy.

3

"THE POWERFUL PLACEBO"

Faith is indeed one of the miracles of human nature which science is as ready to accept as it is to study its marvelous effects.

–William Osler, "The Faith That Heals" (1910)

As noted earlier, when Descartes conceived of the mind, whose essence is thought, as a nonphysical substance existing independently of the body, the mind–body dichotomy became one of the predominant features in European science and philosophy. It posed the question how an immaterial mind could cause any action in a material body and vice versa. Left without a satisfactory explanation for how two ontologically distinct entities could interact, Western science proceeded on a course that left a void between the body's physical or corporeal properties and the immaterial mind. Its choice of a more materialistic and depersonalized study of the human body underscored therapeutic theories and treatments that gave little attention to consciousness, motivation, and other nonspatial religious, philosophical, or mind–body interactions. As a result, the body was conceived of and treated as a reductionist organ system driven by mechanical causality—an "object-body" view of humankind that served as a dynamo for unparalleled advancements in science and technology but left the body bereft of its other half.[1]

In his 1916 presidential address before the zoological section of the British Association for the Advancement of Science, D'Arcy Thomson reinforced biomedicine's reductionist bias. "While we keep an open mind on this question of vitalism [and] the belief that something other than the physical forces animate the dust of which we are made, . . . it is the plain bounden duty of the biologist to pursue his course unprejudiced by vitalistic hypotheses, along the road of observation and experiment, according to the accepted discipline of the natural and physical sciences."[2] Even harsher judgment came from Abraham Flexner in 1910. "To plead in advance a principle couched in pseudo-scientific language, or of extra-scientific character is to violate scientific quality," he warned. "The tendency to build a system out of a few partially apprehended facts, deductive inference filling in the rest, has not indeed been limited to medicine, but it has nowhere else had more calamitous consequences."[3]

Conventional medicine's decision to separate the functioning body from the conscious and unconscious self generated an irreducible tension between the body's objectification and the patient's more subjective state, leaving religion and unconventional therapies free to promote themselves as paradigmatic alternatives to the reductionist model. Thus, despite the judgment of reductionist medicine, vitalism continues to dominate the unconventional medical mind, resisting the substitution of the *how* of natural science for the *why* of metaphysics. To this day, CAM remains an opinion-based system, but its apologists insist on calling it a philosophy-based system. Embedded in an esoteric and transcendent worldview, its therapies give patients a philosophical perspective that is exemplified by the harmony expressed in the forces of yin and yang, the life phases attributed to anthroposophy, the healing powers in nature ascribed by naturopathy, and the overpowering presence of universal energies thought to sustain a condition of healthy-mindedness. Not unlike faith healing, its therapies attribute failure to the patient's lack of belief. In this sense, explains ophthalmologist Michael Kottow, "alternative approaches bathe themselves in the self-fulfilling prophecy that he who believes in his own cure will actually get better."[4]

BEECHER'S DISCOVERY

Notwithstanding these subtle nuances between mind and matter, researchers concluded that the placebo effect, or positive patient expectancies, had become an unquestionable factor in Western medicine's success.[5] The editors of the *British Medical Journal* estimated that 10 percent of the 188 million prescriptions dispensed in Great Britain in 1949 were placebos. The same had been evident in British hospitals that maintained a stock of sugar pills and saline injections for patients who were unresponsive to pharmacologic regiments. This practice of using placebos was justified not only on economic grounds, but also because "they ha[d] in some cases a more powerful effect than known pharmaceutical agents."[6] As late as 2003, researchers found that 48 percent of Danish practitioners were giving placebo treatments ten or more times a year for therapies that they knew would have no effect on the patient's condition.[7]

As a product of postmodernist medicine, the placebo has undermined the positivist model of biomedicine by interjecting subjectivity, uncertainty, and ambiguity into the clinical encounter. In other words, the identification of a specific disease or illness does not exist apart from the manner in which the members of a society conceptualize it, react to its awareness, and the way they address it. Disease and illness exist in and through the lens of the culture and the particular values, limits, and contexts that have been assigned to it. As the culture of a people evolves over time, disease, like other elements in the society's lifespan, are encountered, perceived, and managed differently.[8]

So what do researchers know about the placebo effect? Is it real? How does it work? When does it work? On whom does it work? What are researchers' attitudes toward it? Is it ethical to use? What do these attitudes communicate to prospective subjects in clinical trials? To what extent is there deception in the process? Is the placebo effect the same or different from other therapeutic effects? If we think that a medical intervention causes a therapeutic effect (post hoc ergo propter hoc), is this not a false assumption? Can we be sure that what we attribute as the cause for a specific change is really the cause, or might there be multiple sources of the effect? Is it possible to have a placebo effect without some personal psychosomatic connection with the healer who administers it? Similarly, is it possible to have a placebo effect if the patient is in disbelief of the placebo's potential powers? And how does the placebo relate to unconventional therapies? Are the two different or simply the same?

Finally, it should be noted that if placebo treatments, as Henry Beecher's 1955 article suggests,[9] help upward of 35 percent of patients with their diseases and illnesses, is there reason to conclude that the placebo is powerless, or does it have a degree of real therapeutic effectiveness? In an analysis of 139 trials involving forty clinical conditions and a total of 8,525 patients, Asbjørn Hrøbjartsson and Peter Gøtzsche concluded that "the use of placebo outside the aegis of a controlled, properly designed clinical trial cannot be recommended." Compared with no treatment, the placebo did not have a significant effect on the outcome.[10]

The word *placebo* is found in the Latin translation of the Hebrew word *ethalekh*, meaning "I will go before," a phrase found in Genesis 33:12 ("And he said, Let us take our journey, and let us go, and I will go before thee"). It is also found in Psalm 116:9 ("I will walk before the Lord in the Land of the Living") and in the Vesper prayer, "Placebo domino in regione vivorum" ("I will please the Lord in the land of the living"). Each of these phrases, explains Patrick Wall in *Textbook of Pain*, was used centuries later to explain the practice of pre-Reformation priests and monks who sang prayers for the dead in return for a fee. When applied in its more modern usage, it suggests the use of a sham treatment before or until an active medical intervention was employed.[11]

In 1785, the word *placebo* appeared in George Motherby's *New Medical Dictionary*, where it was defined as a "commonplace method or medicine" used by practitioners who had nothing in their medical bag to address the disease or illness but who intended nonetheless to satisfy their patients' imaginations, beliefs, and expectations while nature took its course. This definition helps to explain why the word has been used principally to describe a dummy treatment and the positive effects that sometimes accompany its employment, which both ancient and modern physicians prescribed when nothing they did seemed to resolve the patient's complaint.[12]

According to anthropologist Daniel Moerman, healing occurs on three distinct levels. The first, *autonomous healing* (sometimes called *vis medicatrix naturae*, *self-limited disease*, or, as John Harley Warner put it, the *nature-trusting heresy*), implies that many acute diseases, illnesses, and injuries persist until the body, through processes that remain a puzzle to the reductionist mind, takes upon itself the suppression of the symptoms and recovers its normal state of equilibrium. The second, *active therapeu-*

tic, occurs when, for example, a physician employs an antibiotic to accelerate the healing process. And the third, the *placebo effect*, consists of a combination of the first two, in which the "act, though not the content of medicine, somehow triggers the body to autonomous healing."[13] It is this placebo effect or placebo response that Henry Beecher, Arthur Shapiro and Elaine Shapiro, Robert Ader, Arthur Kleinnman, Richard Kradin, W. Grant Thompson, Howard Brody, Ted Kaptchuk, Anne Harrington, and others have described as the ritual intersection of patient, doctor, and a substance or procedure known to be pharmacologically or physiologically inactive for the condition being evaluated. Much like a triptych of early Christian art whose panels broaden the landscape on which the subject or event is viewed, the placebo opens the narrow heuristic confines of healing to a wider clinical relationship—one in which not only the patient, but also his or her doctor, family, religion, values, and culture are simultaneously represented.[14]

As explained earlier, placebos were often administered as single-blind controls and later as double-blind controls in clinical trials. In both instances, the researchers' focus was on the active drug, not on the placebo. Reserved for status as a control in evaluating an agent or procedure in a clinical trial, it elicited little interest other than its inclusion in a derisive joke or epithet. Indeed, placebo literature is virtually nonexistent until the mid–twentieth century.[15] Thus, although much was being made of the placebo-based clinical trial, the actual *placebo effect* (i.e., the placebo as therapy) was ignored even when it was shown to result in remarkable benefits to the patient. As William Carpenter, director of the Psychiatric Research Center at the University of Maryland, remarked, the placebo effect was a "kind of a soft underbelly" that academics and the pharmaceutical industry were "more comfortable leaving out of sight."[16] This was particularly the case with pain, rheumatoid arthritis, hay fever, headache, cough, anxiety, depression, and other ills of an indefinite nature. Physicians and researchers essentially chose to relegate the placebo effect to an undefinable, unintended, and nonspecific category rather than to consider it a positive measurable response in its own right. Folded in with the body's self-healing capacity, spontaneous remission, natural history, and other indeterminate and unpredictable elements, the placebo effect was marginalized in the pharmacologically centered world of drug experimentation.

Also left unresolved was the interaction between patients and their environments, their individual histories and social circumstances, and their encounters with physicians that involved trust, hope, and myriad suggestions, feelings, and expectations that factored into the therapy in some manner.[17] "One would think that something as potent as the placebo effect would have been subject to at least as much study as most pharmaceuticals, but that is unfortunately not the case," commented Eric Cassell of the New York Hospital–Cornell Medical Center.[18]

All this changed following Beecher's 1955 article "The Powerful Placebo," in which he concluded from a study of fifteen different controlled trials involving more than a thousand patients that placebos provided significant effectiveness in approximately 35 percent of the cases where they were used. He suggested that placebos could work through physiological and biochemical mediators to the point of even exceeding the effects of an active pharmacological drug, a hypothesis that challenged the very definition of the placebo as an unreal or inert entity. Thus, the difference between the placebo as a control factor in a clinical study and that of a specific therapy revealed an uneasy tension within the medical community because it argued for a quite different role or purpose for the placebo and suggested a level of deliberate deception without proper consent.[19]

Until Beecher's work, few researchers had made a connection between the plethora of analgesic drugs on the market and the psychological and subjective aspects of pain. Beecher suggested that placebos worked effectively better on the anxiety component of pain and that no great differences existed across groups of different race, age, and education. Despite the fact that pain was a subjective experience subjectively evaluated, there was a constancy in the average response to morphine and to placebos that varied little across studies conducted by different researchers using large groups of patients, sophisticated and unsophisticated, and between clinical patients and volunteers in experimental studies. Implied in Beecher's research was the assumption that if patients could improve due to a belief they were receiving an active medicine, then any clinical trial that failed to use a placebo control group would find it difficult to demonstrate its effectiveness. Beecher's announcement brought the placebo out from its marginal place in therapeutic practice and onto center stage. When this occurred, the pharmacopoeia found that it had a more limited impact on disease and illness than previously thought.[20]

In 1956, Edward Wayne of Glasgow reinforced Beecher's hypothesis by carrying out a number of clinical trials employing inert "dummy" preparations that proved to exert "powerful therapeutic effects." In testing the treatment of asthma using a protein derivative, for example, he found no difference between it and a saline injection. Equally important, he found that "a considerable proportion of the subjects were improved by the inert therapy." For Wayne, this raised the question of whether it was appropriate for a physician to use a placebo deliberately, realizing that he was using "suggestion" as the only therapeutic agent. Wayne's argument, reiterated several decades later by Sissela Bok in her 1974 article "The Ethics of Giving Placebos," had the effect of ending the widespread use of placebos in patient care.[21]

Bok's article, plus her book *Lying: Moral Choice in Public and Private Life* (1978), set off a firestorm of discussion on the evils of dishonesty and why lying is bad. Although rejecting Kant's condemnation of *all* lies, she was equally adamant that utilitarianism provided little cover for lying as a way to explain the presumed benefits to the "greater good" resulting from its use. Explaining the damage done to the liar as well as the risk of underestimating the effects of lies and that such practices tend over time to become institutionalized, Bok provided ample demonstration that lies were seldom neutral in their effects—levying indeterminate costs on the liar, the deceived, and the society in which the lie was perpetrated.[22]

Bok's denunciation collided head on with the ritualistic forms of secrecy common in medicine, where full and open communication was rare—whether with respect to patients, profiteering researchers, the interests of trade secrecy, or double-blind studies with human subjects. And even granting the practicality of a hypothesis under investigation, circumstances often developed in the course of a study where the risks outweighed the benefits in continued concealment. Out of these concerns, Bok identified five principles required for the use of placebos:

1. Placebos should be used only after careful diagnoses.
2. No active placebos should be employed, only inert ones.
3. No outright lie should be told, and questions should be answered honestly.

4. Placebos should never be given to patients who have asked not to receive them.

5. Placebos should never be used when other treatment is clearly called for or all possible alternatives have not been weighed.[23]

As noted earlier, the use of the placebo was eventually dealt with in a research context through the principle of equipoise—namely, that a clinician is obligated to begin a trial on the hypothesis that no decisive evidence demonstrates that the existing treatment significantly outperforms the intervention being tested. In the clinical trial, therefore, the researcher employs a placebo in the hope that it will produce no therapeutic effect, thus supporting the safety and efficacy of a newer treatment. Whether the placebo is ethical in clinical practice, however, is an entirely different matter because, in contrast to the research context, the physician employs a nonspecific treatment in a clinical practice in the hope of producing a therapeutic effect. For many ethicists, an entirely different ethical standard is being used—that is, employing a lie to heal. Given that so often in matters of this sort the devil is in the details, the nonspecificity of the placebo becomes the point of contention. Is it considered a placebo only if it is in the form of a nonpharmacological sugar pill, or does it include psychological or psychophysiological factors such as bed rest, exercise, relaxation, conditioning, expectation, or even counseling? In the latter, there is no faulty dualism of body and mind at work, only a body–mind continuum that functions on the level of the patient's well-being.

For Beth Simmons, writing in the *Journal of Medical Ethics* in 1978, placebos should be used "only with full disclosure and consent whether in therapy or in research, and that this need not impede the success of either." Any intent to deceive the patient by providing too little or inaccurate information regarding any therapy or component of therapy constituted a breach of trust between the doctor and patient in that it denied "the moral autonomy of the patient or subject to make his own choice." The administration of a placebo represented an unethical deception that outweighed any positive benefits. The very nature of the act "tends to make it wrong, independent of its consequences," Simmons insisted. "Deceiving the patient or subject has serious implications on his right of self-determination, and therefore on his human dignity."[24]

Physicians do not typically offer patients a placebo as such. When they do, the ethical problem is not that the patient received an ineffective medicine, but that the doctor deliberately deceived the patient. On these grounds, some argue, the placebo treatment is unethical, violating the patient's right to be fully informed of his or her treatment. If, however, it is understood that a physician's intervention with patients occurs at multiple levels (i.e., suggestion, empathy, encouragement, resolution, personality, etc.), the deception would seem limited to only those who rationalize treatment in purely biomedical terms. Borrowing heavily from Sissela Bok's writings, Pesach Lichtenberg, Uriel Heresco-Levy, and Uriel Nitzan justified the use of placebos in clinical practice within a narrow set of rules:

- The intentions of the physician must be benevolent. . . . No economical, professional, or emotional interest should interfere with the decision.
- The placebo, when offered, must be given in the spirit of assuaging the patient's suffering, and not merely mollifying him, silencing him, or otherwise failing to address his distress.
- When proven ineffective the placebo should be immediately withdrawn.
- The placebo cannot be given in place of another medication that the physician reasonable expects to be more effective.
- The physician should not hesitate to respond honestly when asked about the nature and anticipated effects of the placebo treatment he is offering.
- If the patient is helped by the placebo, discontinuing the placebo, in the absence of a more effective treatment, would be unethical.[25]

In a 2006 national survey of placebo treatments prescribed by 679 practicing internists and rheumatologists in the United States who responded, approximately half admitted to prescribing placebo treatments on a regular basis, and some 62 percent considered the practice to be ethical. The treatments (using both active and inactive placebos) included over-the-counter analgesics (41 percent), vitamins (38 percent), antibiotics (13 percent), sedatives (13 percent), saline (3 percent), and sugar pills (2 percent). When asked how they explained the use of placebo treatment to their patients, a clear majority explained that although they saw the practice as ethically permissible, they preferred to use less than full transparency in their language (e.g., "a medicine not typically used for your condition but might benefit you").[26]

For Howard Brody, the placebo effect came not from the lie, but from the physician–patient relationship along with the patient's capacity for self-healing. "As the doctor-patient relationship is rediscovered as a worthy focus for medical research and medical education," he wrote in 1982, "the placebo effect assumes center stage as one approach to a more sophisticated understanding of this relationship."[27] Although Brody did not say the words, he certainly suggested that the placebo effect should be regarded as a nondeceptive and alternative form of healing stemming from the physician–patient encounter.

Provided that the ethical questions raised by the use of placebos are satisfactorily answered, researchers have urged an expanded use of the placebo for the benefit of patients. But this use raises other issues. Is there any assurance that the therapeutic effect that is presumably the result of a placebo is not due to some other overlooked factor? How does one determine causation if, by definition, a placebo produces no specific effects? How can one be certain as to the causation of any observed effects? The uncertainty that lurks behind the answers to these questions suggests a need to learn more about the placebo itself and how it may differ from the natural history of a disease, regression to the mean, and other factors that play out in a clinical trial. It will take a more scholarly imagination before the ritual of the medical visit and the richness of the psychological and social encounter between doctor, patient, and placebo are fully appreciated.[28]

When viewed from a more inclusive cultural perspective, however, the placebo becomes a nondeceptive technique, the whole of which is greater than the sum of its parts. It represents a pool of nonspecific elements working on the emotional states of apprehensiveness, anxiety, and so on and arriving at an expectant dimension of faith and trust in the physician and the outcome. It is this plane of multifactoral input and health dialogue that best explains the placebo phenomenon—the coming together of the body and the psyche that make the person feel whole. The placebo effect occurs at the indeterminate boundary between psychology and physiology where a pharmacologically inert substance (or prescribed medication) combines with the power of words and symbols, ritual and tradition, insight and transference, values and culture. This is why the term *placebo* is so inadequate and why, despite its many distractions, it should be regarded as an active therapy—or second therapy.

WHAT AND HOW

Beginning in the 1960s, the placebo became a recognized part of the psychological and physiological phenomena that played a role not only in the clinical trial, but as a positive health outcome that sometimes occurred outside the biomedical model. Research studies suggested that pain, depression, ulcers, blood pressure, cholesterol, warts, and heart rate could actually be influenced by placebos. In effect, the placebo became an object of interest in its own right with studies comparing suggestion with material causality, active treatment with both a placebo treatment and no treatment at all. Not surprisingly, in many of these studies the placebo group showed more positive results than the untreated group.[29] Given what was learned, researchers looked for a more comprehensive definition of the placebo. To be sure, some questioned ever finding an adequate definition; others invoked its nonspecific nature as the leading feature; and still others preferred to use "non-specific, psychological, or psychophysiological" as its defining features.[30] Behind the difficulty in definition lay the specter of Cartesian dualism, which views material medicine as working in the patient through some definable physiological process and the placebo as working through the mind in a psychological, nonspecific, and unquantifiable way.[31]

According to Arthur Shapiro and Elaine Shapiro, authors of *The Powerful Placebo: From Ancient Priest to Modern Physician* (1997), the placebo is "any therapy or component of therapy (or that component of any therapy) that is intentionally or knowingly used for its non-specific, psychological, or psychophysiological effect, or for its presumed therapeutic effect on a patient, symptom, or other illness but is without specific activity for the condition being treated."[32] Others have described the placebo as "a pharmacologically inactive substance that can have therapeutic effect if administered to a patient who believes that he or she is receiving an effective treatment"[33] and as "any genuine psychological or physiological response to an inert or irrelevant substance or procedure."[34] What makes these definitions important from an historical point of view is that they set the placebo apart from what society previously had denoted as divine intervention or some other form of paranormal behavior. This helps to explain why, until the era of postmodernism, the placebo effect, a classic example of the mind–body interaction, remained clinically undeveloped for so long.[35]

University of Michigan anthropologist Daniel Moerman and Wayne Jonas, director of the Samueli Institute at Georgetown University, have sought to bridge the Cartesian divide by arguing for the term *meaning response* because the placebo, an inert substance, cannot be the direct cause of anything. It is the "meaning" in "meaning response" that the brain associates with the placebo and that causes the effect, they reason.[36] The verbal and nonverbal psychological and behavioral exchanges between healer and patient—including confidence, level of interest, history taking, empathic listening, encouragement, concern for the patient, eye contact, touch, belief, trust, frequency of meetings, and even the level of fee—are all associated with positive therapeutic results. Conversely, failure in any of these essential areas is likely to limit the success of a treatment. In *Meaning, Medicine, and the "Placebo Effect"* (2002), Moerman describes the *meaning effect* or *meaning response* as "the psychological and physiological effects of meaning in the treatment of illness." For Moerman, these effects are no less important than a biologically efficacious treatment because both produce an outcome—the former through a medical treatment or procedure, the latter through mechanisms such as the endogenous opiates.[37]

"The more you believe you're going to benefit from a treatment," remarks Robert DeLap of the FDA's Office of Drug Evaluation, "the more likely it is that you will experience a benefit."[38] Similarly, the term *nocebo*, introduced by Walter Kennedy in 1961, suggests that not only positive therapeutic effects are demonstrated through the use of the placebo, but negative complications as well.[39] Since, then, the placebo response has been correlated to patient expectancy—that is, when patients come to believe their health will take a negative turn—the expectation becomes a powerful negative force and points once again to the importance of perceptions, expectations, and the brain's role in health.[40] Examples exist of subjects reporting symptoms such as dizziness, headache, fatigue, depression, hallucinations, diarrhea, vomiting, nausea, changes in blood pressure, skin rashes, palpitations, and hearing loss. In these instances, the suggestion of possible adverse effects sometimes causes subjects to experience them irrespective of the placebo's benign nature.[41] This explains why informed-consent procedures describing the general level of risk are judged both reasonable and essential in placebo-controlled trials.[42]

As research into the placebo gained traction, it was shown to be much more than simply mind over matter. Placebos could affect patients physiologically as well as psychologically. They could alter blood pressure, heart, respiratory rate, and even body temperature. Brain imaging suggested that placebo-induced expectations of analgesia increased activity in the prefrontal cortex—thus the conclusion that placebo treatments alter experience.[43] The catalyst that changed this thinking came with the discovery of endorphins, which, identified as having an endogenous pain-controlling system similar to an opium-based narcotic, were observed to act as an internal analgesic on the brain. When John Levin, Newton Gordon, and Howard Fields reported in 1978 that some forms of placebo analgesia were initiated by these endogenous (naturally occurring) opioids, a debate ensued within the scientific community over whether the placebo was truly as "inert" as its definition suggested or whether the placebo–endorphin connection purported something more substantive.[44] Was the placebo effect associated only with subjective complaints on various somatic and psychic functions, or did it include certain physiologic functions such as changes in blood chemistry, gastric acid secretion, and blood pressure?[45] If endorphins have opiate-like properties with the potential to alter pain perception, mood, and respiration, do they provide a nonaddictive source of pain relief?[46] According to Samuel Perry and George Heidrich, the emotional impact of an idea or suggestion upon the hypothalamus generates the release of endorphins—a factor that forced a rethinking of the mind–body relationship.[47] The intriguing possibility that the placebo effect might be caused by endogenous opiate-like substances in the brainstem, reticular formation, thalamus, and limbic system meant that the body's ability to control pain might be activated by some emotional excitement or psychogenic mechanism.[48]

DOCTOR AS DRUG

As the placebo itself became the focus of research, two specific factors were deemed essential for its action: a suitable disease and a mutually supportive relationship between physician and patient. Given that the placebo effect generally works in about one-third of the subjects, the question arose whether patients could be more accurately selected for placebo treatment? If true, how does experience affect the response? Are placebos more effective for clinical rather than experimental pain? Do they work better for mildly depressed patients than for severely depressed ones? Are there gender, suggestion, and intelligence aspects to be considered in responsiveness? In what diseases is the placebo response more likely to occur? For some researchers, the answers to these questions were already known because placebos had been judged to work in nausea, psychoneuroses, phobias, blood pressure, bronchial airflow, neuroses, mild depression, and chronic noncancer pain syndromes. For others, the answers remained more complex and indeterminate.[49]

The physician–patient relationship, once perceived and rationalized within a biomedical construct that attributed full credit to specific pharmacodynamic effects dispensed through the mediating role of a scientifically educated physician, dissolved with postmodernist medicine into an encounter where "illusion" earned equal value. Now substances (both active and inert) are seen to act out their effect with the help of a broad range of independent and interdependent variables. The positivist and authoritarian manner in which rational science once dominated the clinical encounter faces a postmodern society where mind and matter, subject and object are viewed as conditions no longer timeless or absolute. For postmodernist society, the world remains a construct of thoughts and experiences arranged into categories that will always be imperfect—the primacy of subjectivity over scientific certitude. Although the doctor–patient relationship plays a preponderant role in the "meaning" of the placebo—a ritual rich with implications that sociologists, anthropologists, and social historians have repeatedly shown—so, too, does the particular culture or human community within which the healer–patient encounter takes place.

Once this postmodernist perspective was acknowledged, researchers initially went off in a variety of directions looking at conditioning, expectation, healing rituals, and other factors that might explain the placebo response.[50] Considerable interest was raised in the late 1950s and early 1960s to ascertain whether personality were an important variable. This hypothesis was complicated by the fact that personality was affected by patient motivation, including the acceptance of self-management, which often lacks consistency. Self-management engages the patient, especially in chronic problems that are not well managed with conventional treatments. This investment of time and the patient's comprehension of the illness and its treatment are strong illustrations of physician–patient communication in the important areas of attitude, expectancy, and trust. In this environment, therapeutic interventions—whether active or inert—became symbols of the physician's ritualistic role as healer and an expression of expectant faith on the part of the patient. Nevertheless, with the possible exception of chronic anxiety, efforts to connect the placebo effect with a unitary personality type or cluster of traits failed to materialize.[51] "Despite long-standing beliefs to the contrary," wrote Richard Kradin, a medical researcher at the Massachusetts General Hospital in Boston and member of the Harvard Medical School faculty, "no specific personality traits distinguished placebo responders from nonresponders; rather, what was important was the context created by the caregivers."[52]

Having ruled out personality, researchers turned their attention to the ritualized environment of white coats and ceremonial expressions of skill, judgment, and belief in which both the doctor and patient participate. Shapiro noted that "placebo effects are produced or augmented when the physician is prestigious, dedicated to his theory or therapy, especially if it is his own innovation or if he is a recent convert; and when the therapies are elaborate, detailed, expensive, time-consuming, fashionable, esoteric, and dangerous." This "healing property" helped to explain the physician's power when much in his or her medical bag was objectively dangerous, if not actually harmful to the patient's well-being. How else could one rationalize the "cures" brought about by bleeding, blistering, and the heroic uses of calomel and tartar emetic in the past? How else was it possible to accept the success of interventions using animal and human excrement, hoof of ass, blood of lizards, grated human skulls, and tortoise shells?[53]

In *The Doctor, His Patient, and the Illness* (1957), Michael Balint (1896–1970), director of the Child Guidance Clinic in Manchester, England, suggested that the family doctor is a form of "drug" and that his role in the physician–patient encounter might be the most important catalyst for inducing a placebo effect.[54] To the extent that the physician shares or otherwise encourages a patient's belief that a given treatment is effective, both the drug and the placebo show positive results. If patients are told they will receive relief from a drug or placebo, the results are more positive than when they are informed that the benefits are unknown.[55]

When psychiatric resident Werner Mendel became part of a double-blind clinical study in 1957 testing the antihypertensive drug Reserpine on homicidal patients at St. Elizabeth's Hospital in Washington, DC, he concluded that the calming effect on his patients was an indication that they were receiving the active drug instead of a placebo sugar pill. When informed after the completion of the study that his patients had received only the placebo, he came to the conclusion that if the physician believes in a particular medication, his enthusiasm for the drug transfers belief to his patient, and the patient's condition thereby improves.[56]

In his 1959 article "The Influence of Personalities on Drug Therapy," Klaus Berblinger (1910–1982), associate clinical professor of psychiatry at the University of California School of Medicine, noted that the placebo effect applies to the nurse–patient relationship as well, particularly when it involves the administration of medications. The nurse's personality and the attitude she as a member of the medical team brings to the patient serve to augment the psychological factor in treatment, including those instances where a placebo is used. Berblinger's research reinforced the thesis that drug action takes place in a social milieu of doctor–nurse interaction—a relationship that is frequently misunderstood and undervalued. Nevertheless, some of the most effective responses occur when inert medications are administered in a hospital setting by a recognized authority figure.[57]

This relationship was again reinforced by Vanderbilt psychiatrist Charles Goshen (1917–1989), who explained that the placebo serves the physician and nurse as much, if not more, than it serves the patient's needs. "Chances are that very little use would be made of placebos in medical practice if they did not produce some real or apparent benefit to those who prescribe and administer them," he wrote. By that, he meant the satisfaction that the physician or nurse experiences in "outsmarting" the patient. Beginning with the use of antibiotics for the common cold, Goshen considered it no exaggeration to say that from two-thirds to three-fourths of all drugs prescribed by physicians and upward of 95 percent of over-the-counter medicines have only a placebo effect. Notwithstanding the fact that such medicines have little if any therapeutic properties to address the conditions for which they are used or prescribed, they provide a needed psychological effect by ameliorating anxiety, including that of the physician, who often fears the loss of his patient if the physician does nothing.[58] "A good doctor, like the shaman," observed Roger Squires of the University of St. Andrews, "will shield his specialist knowledge from those in his care." For the placebo to work for the physician means not only believing in the power of thought, but exercising that power.[59] The physician's ability to arouse and sustain faith in a particular treatment and reinforce the sufferer's faith in the effort introduces a psychotherapeutic role that has long been played by religious and lay healers over the centuries. Recognition of it has given the postmodern physician (and lay celebrity) another tool in his or her armamentarium.[60]

THE FACTOR OF TRUST

Psychiatrist and psychologist Jerome Frank (1909–2005), author of *Persuasion and Healing* (1961), utilized a combination of clinical experience and extensive knowledge of the literature to study the process of healing, which he described as a time-limited interaction between a healer and sufferer in which the healer tries to induce changes in the sufferer that results in either healing or an attitude change. In this exchange, the healer acts as a mediator between the sufferer and his or her conceptual framework of reality, providing empathy, hope, and a plan to regain mastery over life. Frank thus gave the placebo effect an even more positive value than Beecher had assigned to it. As he explained, "Placebo responsiveness was an indicator of the ability of these patients to trust their fellow men . . . and this had something to do with their capacity to adjust to the world outside the hospital."[61]

The interaction between the doctor and patient represents a form of nonspecific psychological treatment in which trust begins with the patient's willingness to seek care from a particular provider. From that point forward, trust affects the patient's submission to a particular form of treatment. Not surprisingly, trust is inseparable from any vulnerability stemming from an illness or invasive treatment and is a key element in the mind–body connection that underlies the placebo effect. The greater the vulnerability, the greater is the potential for trust. This explains why some patients have exaggerated expectations of their treatment, why their trust is directed to their physician's character, and why patients "seem to revere physicians as demigods, imbued with superhuman powers," explain researchers Mark Hall and his colleagues. Patients who exhibit high levels of trust in their physicians are more likely to experience more positive results that lead to statistically higher levels of expectations and satisfaction. The dimensions of trust include fidelity, competency, honesty, and confidentiality as well as holism in a global form.[62] This explains in large measure the concerns expressed by Sissela Bok, Tom Beauchamp and James Childress, Stanley Joel Reiser, Beth Simmons, and Robert Veatch that deception of the patient in the use of the placebo undermines patient autonomy and dignity.[63]

Long recognized, trust became the underlying element responsible for much of the placebo effect documented in the nonspecific and nonscientific aspects of healing.[64] "Trust is the core, defining characteristic of the doctor–patient relationship—the 'glue' that holds the relationship together and makes it possible," wrote Wake Forest's Medical School researcher Mark Hall in the *Stanford Law Review* in 2002. The healer is not merely an adjunct to treatment, but integral to the actual healing encounter—a placebo independent of the particular healing modality. "Deep-seated trust," explained Hall, "appears to activate a patient's own, internal healing mechanisms—mechanisms that are still largely undiscovered and unexplained." It represents a factor in the physician–patient encounter that extends "across all systems of medicine, including Western, Eastern, religious, herbal, and primitive." It is further enhanced by ritualistic actions such as laying on of hands, medications, and performances of various types. Freud described this enhancement as "transference" (i.e., redirection of feelings between healer and patient), whereas others have attributed it to "faith." In each, trust encompasses elements of fidelity, competence, honesty, and confidentiality.[65] In these instances, the outcome is arguably no different than it is for the faithful supplicant at the Shrine of Lourdes or for one of Dolores Krieger's nurse-healers making use of the therapeutic touch. Although Western medicine is committed to a biomedical-reductionist methodology, its doctor–patient interaction displays traits that are remarkably similar to religious and healing rituals that were present at the time of Galen and Hippocrates, that were exercised by mind-curists Emma Curtis Hopkins and Warren Felt Evans in the nineteenth century, and that constitute unconventional healing in the present day. Whether in reference to the doctor, priest, patient, or supplicant, the bridge between meaning, faith, and trust remains strongly incorporated in the experience that constitutes a patient's illness.[66]

This also explains why, in spite of dubious evidence-based results, the chiropractor–patient encounter continues to show strong patient satisfaction. Questions concerning the long-term efficacy of chiropractic treatment in areas other than low-back pain seem not to have affected its popularity as patients consistently express their satisfaction with its practitioners' sensitivity (i.e., touch and empathy), communication, and holism. Patients' willingness to accept their practitioner's belief system has undoubtedly contributed to the success of the treatment.[67] This factor alone, as supportive as it is of chiropractic treatment, puts in question the degree to which the modality is influenced by the placebo effect.[68] According to Richard Cooper and Heather McKee, "The fact that patients who choose to see chiropractors share chiropractors' belief system appears to contribute to the outcomes." Evidence of this placebo effect makes it difficult to evaluate the chiropractor's actual clinical effectiveness, a factor shared with naturopaths, acupuncturists, and other holistic healers.[69]

THE ASSUMPTIVE WORLD

On the basis of what is now known, it seems clear that the placebo phenomenon is common to all Western cultures and comes in guises that are both religious and secular, medical and nonmedical. Moreover, it is a variable with a wide range of elasticity and dependent in aggregate on any number of factors, not the least of which is a given population's history and culture. From a medical standpoint, it represents a combination of events, feelings, needs, revered literature, clinical insight, personal philosophy, traditional knowledge, and intentions that help to construct a personality that, in whole or in part, expresses confidence (or lack thereof) in the words, gestures, questions, empathy, and vision that resonates within the clinical encounter. This suggests that the degree of elasticity in the placebo effect may be quite different from one individual to another and from one culture or subgroup to another. What works in one may fail in another. Nevertheless, it is a factor that has long been unappreciated. Together with reductionist medicine, it offers the promise of a much more enriched clinical outcome.[70]

The question at hand is why the placebo effect continues to rattle cages in the camps of *both* biomedicine and CAM. It is fair to say that regular medicine has for the most part chosen to ignore the clinical significance of the placebo, choosing instead to make it simply a baseline against which to evaluate the clinical trial—that is, a means for reducing bias in the clinical trial. In doing so, it has dismissed the placebo as a worthy ally in the physician–patient encounter, devaluing it with such words as *inert, inactive, nuisance, dummy,* and *sham.* But CAM has similarly chosen to react defensively to the placebo, dismissing it as a polemical tool intended to marginalize its various therapies. In other words, both CAM and reductionist medicine prefer to ignore placebo intervention as a distinct entity, believing instead that their individual therapies are self-authenticating and equate fully to effects produced on the body. In doing so, they avoid explanations that incorporate such elements as regression to the mean; *vis medicatrix naturae;* cultural modifiers and rituals; the Hawthorne effect; compassion and empathy; relaxation, exercise, and diet regimens; imagination; the color of a pill; and the clinical encounter, to mention but a few. By ignoring the placebo as a distinct entity (i.e., an alternative therapy), they infer that their clinical outcomes would be effective regardless of any supportive nonspecific effects.

It should be understood, however, that touch, words, gestures, and myriad nonspecific aspects inherent in the physician–patient encounter play a role in conveying the power of the placebo. To date, we remain in the dark as to the importance of these nonspecific effects and their interaction with respect to specific treatments. The issues remain complex, which is to say that much more multidisciplinary research is needed, including how the use of the placebo effect actually differs between CAM and normative medicine. The concept of consciousness as a healing force and of the mind as a healing agent challenges both camps' healing paradigm. As we step briskly toward the third decade of the new millennium, it is important for reductionist medicine to lead postmodernism back to modernism with its belief in the existence of objectivity, impartial observation, and replication. Reductionist medicine must also find its compass in dealing with the placebo effect and the plethora of issues that it seems unable at this time to address. In answering the question "What is best evidence?" it remains a challenge for reductionist medicine to understand each patient's *uniqueness* as well as the statistical norms and to formulate a more inclusive foundation for medical knowledge. The challenge for biomedicine in the twenty-first century is to find a way to grow beyond the Enlightenment-based view of the mind–body dichotomy by acquiring a new scientific maturity that includes the postmodernist model of the unique patient acting out a role that incorporates the statistical or objective self.

The magnitude of the placebo effect cannot be ignored, any more than the power of suggestion can be dismissed as unimportant. As explained by infectious disease specialist Mark DiNubile in 2000, "The most important lesson is that placebo therapy with all its trappings (e.g., the time, attention, enthusiasm, and interest of the caregiver) is itself a viable but neglected therapeutic modality; it is rarely equivalent to no intervention at all."[71] Harald Walach and Wayne Jonas offer a similar interpretation, suggesting that rather than view the placebo effect as a nonspecific intrusion into the clinical trial, we should see it "as a ubiquitous healing response mediated by expectations and conditioning," which under proper handling can be utilized to foster optimal healing. In such circumstances, the placebo effect can become an "elegant, efficient and comparatively harmless way to harness healing processes."[72] Ted Kaptchuk at the Center for Alternative Medicine Research at Beth Israel Deaconess Medical Center and author of *The Web That Has No Weaver* (2000), a book on Chinese medicine, reinforces this view by describing the placebo effect as "an inherent capacity within a person to evoke renewed senses of well-being, intactness, and authenticity." Working through such mediums as belief, expectation, hope, imagination, will, intention, preference, and commitment, the placebo has become "one of the contradictions in modern medicine's conceptual structure."[73]

American psychiatrist Jerome Frank used the term *assumptive world* to conceptualize the combination of experiences, prejudices, culture, religion, age, and so on that affect the sufferer's view of the world as well as his or her emotional state, attitudes, and behavior. Into this world, Frank introduced the healer, who through persuasion, thought reform, and the placebo effect seeks to create the conditions of change needed to improve the sufferer's situation. The extent to which an individual thinks about a specific drug and its effect on how he or she feels, Frank explained, can arguably influence improvement more powerfully than the active substance itself. This is especially true in clinical trials of antidepressant drugs, wherein the placebo effect from an inert substance plays a disproportionate role in patient responses.[74]

There is also the issue regarding Beecher's conclusion that approximately 35 percent of the placebo control group shows gains or improvements. Subsequent analyses of his methods indicated that the so-called placebo effect masks a number of other elements.[75] According to Edzard Ernst and Karl Resch, the placebo in RCTs often confuses the *perceived* placebo effect with the *true* placebo effect. The perceived placebo effect is the "response observed in the placebo group of a randomized controlled trial." By contrast, the true placebo effect is much more variable in that it "equals this response [perceived placebo effect] minus other effects that often determine the outcome in all treatment groups of such studies." Included among the other nonspecific elements are the disease's natural history; false positives; attrition among patients who suspect they are receiving a placebo; regression toward the mean (i.e., patients often see their doctor when their complaint is at a peak); the Hawthorne effect (i.e., patients alter their behavior when participating in an experiment); other effects (i.e., investigator's skill, white-coat hypertension, seasonal changes); and unidentified parallel interventions (i.e., deliberate or unconscious modifications of lifestyle during a clinical trial). What the authors suggest is that the placebo response, which was thought to be a fixed constant, is misleading because the extent of the true placebo effect is different than the perceived effect. To be specific, certain aspects of the placebo effect may not always be present in clinical situations, a condition that will change the true placebo effect. This means that the true placebo response is "highly variable" and may be "substantially smaller" than the perceived effect.[76]

Some researchers doubt that a true placebo effect can be measured at all, suggesting instead that one should speak of "placebo maximizing" and "placebo minimizing."[77] For Rodney Coe in the Department of Community and Family Medicine at St. Louis University School of Medicine, sufficient variance exists in health and illness behaviors to justify that medical anthropologists and sociologists undertake more interdisciplinary efforts to conceptualize and design research findings that better explain the placebo's effects. Just as neurochemical and neuroanatomical evidence fails to explain acupuncture's modus operandi, so data from the field of psychoneuroimmunology have yet to demonstrate empirically the link between body and mind (i.e., "that beliefs and expectations in the psyche can and do have effects, for good or ill, on the soma"). Bridging the gap between the findings of biomedical reductionism and lay beliefs is as much an issue of culture as it is of scientific medicine. Within this paradigm are to be found different communication styles among physicians, the effectiveness of hope or faith as a placebo, and various treatments such as immunosuppression, relaxation training, and prayer.[78]

Daniel Moerman noted in 1983 that the differences among studies on the efficacy of drugs can be explained only if one views the placebo effect as a variable and not merely as a harmless control item. Perceptions and expectations are as important as microorganisms in that they can cure as well as render one ill. In other words, culturogenic illnesses have causal effects similar to those of biomedical diseases. This explains Moerman's higher placebo response rate (45 percent) compared to the more generally reported rate (35 percent) announced by Beecher in 1955.[79]

Howard Brody, a medical ethicist and family physician at the University of Texas Medical Branch at Galveston, dismissed Moerman's claim, suggesting instead that the range of variability between these two viewpoints might just as easily be due to three separate explanations that are not mutually exclusive—namely, that the patient got better due to the specific property of the drug; the natural history of the disease (*vis medicatrix naturae*); or a placebo response (healing power of the imagination).[80] Brody urged the adoption of the term *suggestion*—widely used by mind-curists in the late nineteenth and twentieth century—as an alternative to *placebo effect* because it carries less baggage.[81] As Brody explained, it was important to distinguish between the placebo, which served as an important research tool, and the placebo effect, which he urged doctors to include in their clinical practices.[82]

Rather than treat the placebo as a contaminating nuisance in the objective and scientific evaluation of therapies, investigators have come to consider it as having clinical and even theoretical significance of its own. For the Shapiros, its efficacy in both ancient and modern therapies is attributable to the patient's beliefs and expectations. The conclusion the Shapiros drew is that the nonspecific placebo effect can be made specific and used as an adjuvant to conventional medicine. Beecher, too, implied as much in the mid-1950s when he noted that placebos are effective in addressing increased stress. Decades later, author and physician Andrew Weil urged researchers to shift their theoretical focus from chemically based drugs to nonspecific placebo-based processes.[83]

Arthur Kleinman, Robert Ader, and Howard Brody have more recently suggested that biomedicine could benefit by adopting the placebo's power, however defined, into biomedicine's conventional therapies despite the placebo's lack of a Western-style explanation. The placebo effect has been around for a sufficient amount of time, they argue, that it is no longer a curiosity in the medical world. It exemplifies, explains Marcia Meldrum, "the meaningful interaction of healer and patient within the physical and cultural body, whether mediated or not by an endogenous tool or intervention."[84] Writing in the *British Medical Journal* in 1994, V. M. S. Oh described the placebo as "the most effective medication known to science, subjected to more clinical trials than any other medication, yet [it] generally always does better than anticipated. The range of susceptible conditions appears to be limitless."[85] Its range of effectiveness has been applied not only to subjective conditions such as pain and anxiety, but also to objective aspects of health such as blood pressure, angina pectoris, and even epilepsy and cancer.[86]

The positive role of the placebo is of particular interest to naturopaths, who insist that confidence surrounds every aspect of their therapeutic encounter. For the naturopath, the placebo effect involves a complicated web of conscious and unconscious associations that, when combined with active pharmacological substances, work with the body's natural defense mechanisms to trigger positive changes in a patient's health. This description implies the patient's confidence in the naturopath, the naturopath's confidence in the specific therapy, and a relationship between the two parties that is "mutually conducive of respect, trust, and compassion." This relationship includes verbal and nonverbal communication involving education, listening, interview skills, touch, conditioning, and cultivating hope through imagery and visualization. Supporting these skill sets are the active components of plant medicines intended to provide strength to the body when the placebo effect weakens (i.e., a process known as "placebo sag") over time.[87]

For Anne Harrington at Harvard, the placebo phenomenon is the "ghost" that haunts the house of biomedical objectivity. Its creatures "rise up from the dark and expose the paradoxes and fissures in our own self-created definitions of the real and active factors in treatment." Although acknowledging the role of placebos in the testing of new drugs, she explains that the placebo response is all too often regarded as "non-specific noise" to which little attention is paid.[88] For Harrington, there is sufficient evidence to assert that the placebo effect is something more than a "psychologic prop." Focusing on conditioning stimuli, including such variables as expectations, beliefs, culture, and physician–patient interactions, she argues that under the right circumstances any one of these factors can instill a positive placebo response. In studies of treatments for ulcers, for example, Germans experienced a 63 percent placebo response, whereas the average for other countries was about 36 percent. Other examples were to be found in the phenomenon known as voodoo and the so-called stigmata. In other words, "our understanding of the placebo effect must be put on a far richer empirical and theoretical basis than it is now," Harrington argues. "Only then will it be possible to return to a dialogue with the gatekeepers of mainstream modern medicine and to look again at their demand that all alternative treatments demonstrate their efficacy by passing the rigors imposed by a placebo-controlled trial."[89]

In essence, Harrington has challenged the basic premise behind the RCT that a treatment, to be deemed effective, "must demonstrate efficacy beyond the placebo effect because it is understood that the effect is a mere additive, with no relevance to understanding the working of the real treatment being tested." Instead, she suggests that the placebo may have "a direct modulating effect on the treatment itself." If proven, this argument would mean "that a specific biologic or skill-based treatment that has taken pains to eliminate the placebo effect is not purifying itself of all psychological noise, but actually altering the magnitude and specific nature of its own efficacy." If so, Harrington reasons, one might argue that the RCT no longer determines the true efficacy of a specific drug or treatment and that, instead, researchers should collaborate to determine "to what extent these factors are not simply incidental additives to a treatment, but integral modulators of it."[90]

Blind assessment, or the testing of human subjects under conditions of intentional ignorance, has long been considered an essential component of medical research. However, the very intent to eliminate the role of imagination, bias, or even trickery in the assessment creates an artificial environment that is itself a false representation of the physician–patient encounter. Each placebo-controlled RCT undermines the misplaced hubris found in biomedical reductionism because the objective reality used to explain the disease or illness hides an unmapped world of the patient's subjective self. As Ted Kaptchuk explains, "Relying on objectivity in medicine is putting a veneer over an ocean of subjective perception. . . . The simplistic placebo effect just points a finger at an ocean of healing that resides in self relationship and utter subjectivity."[91]

■ ■ ■

The placebo, a product of Cartesian dualism, is found almost exclusively in the biomedical world of reductionist science. By contrast, in the healing modalities of non-Western therapies, almost all medicinal substances are thought to contain some degree of intentionality whose causality is nonphysical. The placebo, which has a clinical and theoretical significance of its own and is responsible for most ancient and modern therapies, should be regarded as a second therapy rather than as the absence of a therapy. The placebo highlights the nonspecific (i.e., nonbiological) aspect of medicine, a condition that creates a distracting ambiguity for the medical scientist who finds it difficult to build a bridge between the material and the psychosomatic and behavioral side of healing. To ignore or otherwise discount this phenomenon is to deny the multifactoral nature of disease causation. There is much that is still unknown about the placebo that requires further investigation, including the social and cultural aspects of illness. Although Western societies have allied themselves with reductionist science, their placebo-healing rate varies from one society to another and is suggestive of variables that are lodged deeply in their respective cultures. As we look to the future, it seems especially important for scholars to examine more closely the variations that exist from one culture to another.[92]

There is sufficient information to state that the placebo plays an important role in assessing the safety and efficacy of both conventional and unconventional medicine. What is not sufficiently established is the degree to which this effect varies from one healer–patient encounter to the next, from one culture or subculture to another, and whether other processes (i.e., regression to the mean or the natural progression of the illness, life changes, color of the pill, etc.) are at work. That said, there remains much that the placebo can teach in that it influences the behavior of both patients and doctors and relates to body–mind modalities that have long been used in Western societies as alternatives to pharmacologically active drugs and other interventions.

Constructed in the shadow of EBM and used as an instrument to prove the power and function of the RCT, the placebo has been overlooked as an active intervention strategy. Nevertheless, its contributions to healing are shown to affect both healer and patient through expectation, imagination, conditioning, and other contributing elements. To be sure, its nonspecific variables lead down trails strewn with provocative but confusing evidence of its effectiveness—that is, outcome measures that are subjective rather than objective in nature. These nonspecific effects must be progressively combined to produce statistically and clinically significant outcomes if we are to determine their distinct contributions to clinical care. This must be done and done convincingly in order for the placebo to be considered a legitimate therapy in its own right and to be factored positively into both CAM and reductionist medicine.

4

POLITICS OF HEALING

Although democracy has its evident social virtues, majority opinion does not necessarily rule OK in science and medicine.

—Patrick D. Wall, "Trials of Homeopathy," *British Medical Journal* (1991)

With medical costs growing exponentially from the 1970s on, there was mounting evidence that Americans were turning in increased numbers to unconventional therapies, spending billions each year on interventions ranging from dietary supplements to homeopathy, crystal healing, anthroposophy, therapeutic touch, high-energy perception, and meditation. Thus, it came as no surprise that political pressure would be levied on the NIH to find and justify the substitution of alternative therapies for orthodox medicine's more costly treatments. In 1991, Senator Thomas R. Harkin (D–IA), chair of the appropriations subcommittee with oversight of the NIH and a strong advocate of bee pollen for allergies, captured this sentiment when he added a clause in the NIH 1992 appropriation creating a twenty-person advisory panel and charging it to recommend a research program that would "fully test the most promising unconventional medical practices."[1] Elements within the NIH seethed with resentment that the testing of fringe therapies, some of which had already been barred by the FDA, would undermine the NIH's credibility; others, less distraught, believed that if the panel members did their job, many of these unconventional practices could be disproved and buried once and for all.[2]

OFFICE OF ALTERNATIVE MEDICINE

Within a year of the committee's deliberations, the NIH created the Office for the Study of Unconventional Medical Practices, later the Office of Alternative Medicine (OAM), and sought a director. During the years that followed, the advisory panel was dominated by a group of so-called Harkinites that included former congressman Berkley Bedell, Frank Wiewel, Ralph Moss, Gar Hildenbrand, and Royden Brown—all outspoken advocates of unconventional medicine. Bedell, a longtime friend of Harkin, supported colostrum, derived from cow's milk, as a cure for Lyme disease and 714-X, a derivative of camphor, for prostate cancer. Wiewel was a longtime enthusiast of immuno-augmentative therapy for cancer and operated a travel service called Patients Against Cancer for patients seeking unconventional therapies. Brown promoted high-desert bee pollen capsules for allergies; Hildenbrand was the executive director of the diet-oriented Gerson Institute for alternative cancer treatments; and Moss, a PhD in the classics, was an adviser on alternative cancer therapies and publisher of *The Moss Reports*, which provided extensive information on CAM modalities worldwide in the treatment of cancer.[3]

From the very beginning of the OAM, Harkin and his supporters used political clout to agitate, threaten, and bully NIH's leadership. At issue was whether conventional research methods were appropriate in testing unconventional practices or, alternatively, whether there should be a reexamination and perhaps even a reconstruction of conventional medicine's evidence-based pyramid. The latter position had been encouraged by several new CAM journals, including *Cancer Chronicles* (1989), *Subtle Energies and Energy Medicine Journal* (1990), and *Alternative Therapies in Health and Medicine* (1995), precipitating a flurry of competing opinions and causing one observer to remark that devising the appropriate plan to study CAM was like "orchestrating a roomful of cats . . . or setting the agenda for a convention of anarchists."[4]

With each CAM therapy confident that its results, however managed, were "proof" enough of its claims, the NIH struggled under pressure from the Congress to find and implement an appropriate validation process. Because the RCT represented the gold standard of scientific validation within NIH, there was genuine apprehension among the institutes' staff that practices such as mind–body interventions, bioelectromagnetic applications, yoga, acupuncture, homeopathy, and a host of nutritional supplements would be judged on standards different from conventional medicine.[5] Evidence of this apprehension was the report prepared for NIH titled *Alternative Medicine: Expanding Medical Horizons* (1995), also known as the *Chantilly Report*, which one skeptic called "an uncritical catalog of virtually every dubious and unproven treatment method of the past 100 years."[6]

With the appointment in October 1992 of Joseph Jacobs, a Yale-educated physician with a deep love for Native American healing, to head the OAM, all parties hoped that calm would ease the fevered opinions bantered on both sides. Recognizing that many of the CAM modalities had been around for hundreds, if not thousands, of years, Jacobs reasoned that simply because a particular treatment's modus operandi was counterintuitive to prevailing theories, its success should not be ruled out. This position, however disconcerting to conventional researchers, gave hope to CAM proponents that their particular modalities could gain approval as part of a new *integrative* medicine.[7]

Jacobs initially seemed to please the Harkinites as someone who, having Native American ancestry (son of a Cherokee father and a Mohawk mother), was willing to view CAM as compatible with conventional medicine. He began by looking for new approaches to clinical analysis, including the establishment of research centers within academe to test the validity of CAM therapies. He quickly realized after a congressional review undertaken by Harkin in 1993, however, that he was being held hostage by a not insignificant lobby whose advocates were using political muscle to force validation of their interest in bee pollen, shark cartilage, antineoplastons, Revici cancer treatment, and other dubious therapies.[8] As one observer commented, the proponents of CAM were eager to have the "imprimatur" of the NIH on their particular therapies but were not interested in acquiring that status based on the rigor of the RCT. Jacobs, however, refused to capitulate. "As a taxpayer," he explained, "I wouldn't trust what comes out of my office under a system like that." He insisted, therefore, that the prevailing methodology of the RCT remain the standard for evaluation and that all CAM therapies be evaluated in university-operated research centers.[9] In keeping with this intent, he approved thirty proposals (out of 450 submissions) for funding and allocated $1.8 million to establish two research centers (at Bastyr University in Seattle and at the University of Minnesota Medical School) modeled on a recommendation from Harvard internist and professor David Eisenberg, a member of the OAM's policy committee.[10]

Exemplary of naturopathy's importance within CAM has been Bastyr's recognition as a center for research on HIV and acquired immunodeficiency syndrome (AIDS) funded by the federal government. Founded by naturopathic physicians Les Griffith, William Mitchell Jr., and Joseph Pizzorno Jr., Bastyr University is a nonallopathic institution whose goal is to bring scientific legitimacy to natural medicine. Through the establishment of the Naturopathic Medical Research Alliance funded by the NIH, there has been a dramatic increase in peer-reviewed scientific literature assessing the efficacy of naturopathic therapies. In addition, cross-training in research now takes place in cooperation with the University of Washington School of Medicine and the Oregon Health Sciences University. Within the ranks of naturopathy are homeopaths, herbalists, and hygienists who are graduates of correspondence schools and practice without any formal training, certification, or licensing and so are often forced to operate under acupuncture and chiropractic licenses.[11] Much of naturopathic practice consists of principles and practices incompatible with EBM, including many unproven (i.e., homeopathy and reflexology) or disproven (i.e., rolfing and iridology) treatments. Hans Baer thus observes that "despite considerable rhetoric on the part of both the graduates of the four-year naturopathic schools and the partially professionalized naturopaths, it is virtually impossible in the absence of considerable ethnographic research to determine how their respective philosophies are implemented in their scopes of practice."[12]

WAYNE JONAS

The combination of pressure from Harkin and the litany of complaints originating from OAM's advisory panel accusing the director and his staffers of being too pro-establishment led to Jacobs's resignation in September 1994 after only two years.[13] His replacement was Wayne Jonas, a graduate of Bowman Gray School of Medicine in Winston-Salem, North Carolina, and former NIH deputy director. What appealed to CAM's proponents was Jonas's medical experience in Germany, where as a lieutenant colonel in the US Army and clinic director of the 130th General Hospital in Dexheim he had observed the widespread practice of homeopathy and had trained in bioenergy therapy, diet and nutritional therapy, mind–body methods, spiritual healing, acupuncture, and clinical pastoral education. Upon his return to the states, he had accepted a faculty position at the Uniformed Services University of the Health Sciences, where he codirected a seminar on alternative medicine and later chaired a conference on research methodology in alternative medicine. Jonas was also a student at the Esalen Institute in California, where he was introduced to Chinese, Tibetan, and Ayurvedic medicine as well as homeopathy, herbalism, rolfing, gestalt therapy, journaling, imagery, and bioenergetics.[14]

Convinced that CAM was a good thing and willing to entertain variants to the RCT, Jonas appeared to be an excellent choice to lead the OAM into a new era of consensus building. He included in his reorganization plans the establishment of research centers outside regular medical schools; the expansion of databases in the National Library of Medicine to capture a broader array of treatments and modalities; the sponsoring of assessment conferences; and an increase in sponsored research programs to test new CAM products. Considered by many as a "closet" homeopath, Jonas would eventually coauthor with Jennifer Jacobs, a member of his advisory committee, *Healing with Homeopathy: The Complete Guide* (1996) and *Healing with Homeopathy: The Doctor's Guide* (1998).[15] Under Jonas's leadership and with the support of a Republican-dominated Congress, OAM benefited from yearly increases in funding. Harkin managed to double OAM's budget from $3.5 million in 1994 to $6.0 million in 1995 and then to nearly $12 million in 1997, making it a focus of attention.[16]

The need to accommodate the diversity of CAM systems did not come easily to clinical researchers, basic scientists, and policymakers. Nevertheless, the demand for accommodation continued to grow. In his effort to find a satisfactory starting point, Jonas suggested three methods for determining relevance (qualitative methods, epidemiological and outcomes research, and health service research) and three for explanation and verification (laboratory research, RCTs, consensus conferences, systematic reviews, and meta-analyses). Depending on the purpose and goals for which the information was needed, he believed there was justification for a variable set of standards. To accelerate this process, Jonas organized the OAM into six service units (Public Affairs and Clearinghouse; Database and Evaluation; Research Development and Investigation; Extramural Affairs; Intramural Research Training; and International and Professional Liaison) and doubled the staff.[17]

According to Jonas, there were ten reasons to classify a proposed practice as CAM:

1. The explanatory model of the practice is not generally accepted, and so additional criteria are required for proof (e.g., homeopathy, prayer).
2. The origin of the practice is outside of the dominant system (e.g., acupuncture).
3. The amount of data or type of data is considered insufficient or otherwise inadequate (e.g., herbalism, megavitamin therapy).
4. The use of the practice is marginalized in that it is not available within conventional hospitals (e.g., relaxation techniques).
5. The teaching of the practice is marginalized in that it is not generally taught within medical, nursing, or graduate schools of the dominant institutions (e.g., nutritional therapy).
6. The amount of research funding, infrastructure, and capacity for investigating the practice is low (e.g., cancer, chiropractic).
7. The practice is not reimbursed by insurance companies and third-party payers.
8. The practice is not readily used for feasibility, acceptability, or other reasons (e.g., clinical ecology, complex lifestyle programs).
9. The practice is not regulated or licensed in most states (e.g., naturopathy).
10. An aspect of the therapy is marginalized under other names or subdivisions (e.g., antineoplastons, shark cartilage).[18]

The director's goal was to bring together the worlds of science and spirituality, bridging a divide that had occurred during the Enlightenment and that effectively separated the rational, analytical, and objective from the intuitive, spiritual, and subjective. This division, which he and others viewed as artificial, had created a "face" on conventional medicine that turned toward the material and technical side of healing and away from the more human side of disease and suffering.[19] However, bridging this divide proved difficult at best. Most CAM systems had remained unchanged over time, and their proponents had chosen to ignore hypothesis-driven testing and peer review for practices justified solely on the basis of their being holistic and anecdotal. Because most complementary systems ascribed to a unitary view of the body, which meant treating the body as a whole rather than as isolated organs, they preferred to disregard anatomy and physiology for subtle energies (chakras, auras, chi, etc.) that allegedly operated on the whole body.[20] For Jonas, this position was untenable. "To accept such views," he reasoned, was "to falsely label conventional medicine as nonholistic and reject the hard-fought gains made in the use of basic biological knowledge, the randomized, controlled clinical trial, and evidence-based medicine for health care decision making." Conventional medicine was the world's leader in disease management, pathology, biotechnology, and drug development. To throw these developments over for practices that hid behind ratiocinations that denied the efficacy or applicability of RCTs endangered the whole of medicine.[21]

By October 1995, grants were allocated to establish eight more research centers in alternative medicine. OAM would eventually fund twenty-four research centers, most at biomedical institutions whose research methodology involved the double-blinded RCT. Each of these centers sponsored clinical trials and offered opportunities for training researchers in such topics as acupuncture, antioxidants, botanicals, phytotherapy, chiropractic, millimeter wave theory, mind–body medicine, meditation, osteopathic medicine, and traditional Chinese medicine (for a list of these centers, see the appendix).

QUANTITATIVE METHODS WORKING GROUP

In an attempt to resolve the question whether alternative therapies could or should be evaluated using conventional research methods, the NIH organized eight working groups (focusing on types of evidence, definitions, placebos, summarizing evidence, practice and policy guidelines, outcomes and measurement and research networks, qualitative research, and quantitative methods) around the NIH Conference on Complementary and Alternative Medicine Research Methodology, which met April 26–28, 1995. Among the eight groups, the Quantitative Methods Working Group was charged with providing a set of guidelines to serve as a framework in the design and conduct of empirical research on alternative therapies. Its membership, representing the fields of social epidemiology, medical sociology, chronic disease epidemiology, psychology, human ecology, and family practice, included chair Jeffrey Levin from the NIH; Thomas Glass from the Department of Health and Social Behavior, Harvard School of Public Health; Lawrence Kushi from the Division of Epidemiology at the University of Minnesota School of Public Health; John Schuck from the Department of Psychology at Bowling Green State University; Lea Steele from the Kansas Commission on Veterans Affairs; and Wayne Jonas from OAM.[22]

Given the proliferation of alternative therapies in the US health-care system, some of which had already been integrated with conventional therapies, the members of the Quantitative Methods Working Group were divided on whether the RCT, amplified by the Cochrane Collaboration, should remain the gold standard. Not surprisingly, the advocates of CAM therapies urged a redesign of research methodologies, arguing that the distinctions between and among patients created situations inappropriate for comparison. There were distinctions not just between patients, but also in the same patient if evaluated at different stages in the history of an illness. Differences also existed between those complementary systems such as chiropractic that often use complex forms of intervention (i.e. spinal adjustment, ultrasound, heat and cold therapy, lifestyle coaching, and herbals), and others that rely on a single protocol with an expected sequence of outcomes.[23] Just two years earlier, in 1993, an entire book had been devoted to a scholarly analysis of alternative research methodologies for unconventional therapies.[24] That same year the *New England Journal of Medicine* published a study on the patterns of unconventional medicine that became one of the most influential publications on the subject.[25]

Following considerable discussion, the working group agreed that even though all research projects did not lend themselves to the double-blind, placebo-controlled RCT, it was important to reaffirm the RCT's place at the top of the evidence-based pyramid. All research projects required a clear statement of purpose in their study design, careful data collection through clinical trials, and meaningful data analysis. Nevertheless, the working group agreed that other designs capable of producing "valid and interpretable comparisons" should be admissible for addressing specific study questions. It recognized, however, several methodological challenges that had been raised by CAM supporters who argued against sole reliance on the RCT. These challenges included *complex individualized interventions* (i.e., CAM therapies treating AIDS might use a combination of dietary change, herbal medicine, counseling, and massage, making it hard to create comparisons); *individualization of therapeutic effects* (i.e., recognizing that the same protocol might elicit a different response in different individuals or in the same individual at a different time); *focalized effects versus systemic perturbations* (i.e., the delivery of a single intervention such as Bach's water violet to bring serenity to the mind/body); *systemic correspondences and correlations* (i.e., the naturopathic assumption that pathological phenomena may be expressed on multiple levels of the system); *long-term effects* (i.e., believing that CAM therapies are intended primarily for prevention or the management of chronic problems); *reconceptualization of the human body* (viewing the individual as a unitary whole whose operation contravenes known physical laws); and *multifactorial etiologies* (i.e., chakras, disruptions in the bioenergy, impeded chi, and spiritual disturbances that offer alternative worldviews or paradigms).[26]

Recognizing that most CAM modalities have had a history of practice without any systematic form of scientific testing using established rules of evidence, the working group sought to document the effects of specific unconventional therapies along with the methodological and analytic options available, including those social research methods outside of medicine. Soon after the group began its deliberations, it concluded that it was impossible to develop "practice guidelines" for CAM therapies.[27] Instead, it produced a "methodological manifesto" that listed seven principles intended to help frame approaches by clinical and basic science researches to CAM research (the material in italics is added summary):

1. Different study questions require different methodological and analytic approaches.

Every research project is contingent upon a clear statement of the purpose and objectives before the selection of the study design. Without such a statement, there is nothing to direct the collection of usable data. The question being asked determines the type of method or approach taken by the researcher.

2. Researchers should use the strongest possible design and most appropriate statistical procedures for a given study question.

Only a strong study design can produce valid information and interpretable comparisons between treatment groups. Here again, different types of questions require the use of different knowledge domains, designs, and methodologies.

3. Clinical trials are not the only game in town.

Numerous options are available to researchers, including epidemiological and social research methodologies (i.e., systematic surveys, probability sampling, multiwave panel studies, etc.) where large and expensive clinical trials would be inappropriate.

4. Results of observational studies can inform the design of intervention trials.

These results are an important source of medical knowledge, especially where experimental designs are unethical, unfeasible, or impossible—for example, the relationship between cigarette smoking and lung cancer.

5. Alternative therapies, yes; alternative outcomes, no.

Provided there is a consistent set of rules for assigning values, reliability is possible for any type of unconventional therapy regardless of its peculiarities. By itself, unorthodoxy does not preclude validation.

6. Existing quantitative procedures are generally robust for researching alternative therapies and complementary medical systems.

There is no basis for arguing that CAM research using existing methods and rules of positivism is hindered on grounds of its different or alternative epistemology. Each and every observable phenomena of unconventional therapy, including those that claim to represent an alternative paradigm or worldview, can be measured and assessed.

7. Complex complementary medical systems can be studied as "gestalts."

It is possible to study the effects of a CAM therapy as a system rather than through its component parts, which could distort the treatment by deconstructing the overall intervention.[28]

The issues challenging CAM research, explained the members of the working group, were not uncommon to research generally in that differences sometimes created difficult conceptual and measurement challenges. To offset these issues, acceptable options included large and small RCTs; nonrandomized trials with contemporaneous controls; nonrandomized trials with historical controls; cohort studies; case–control studies; cross-sectional studies; surveillance studies; consecutive case series; and single-case reports. In other words, established methodologies (i.e., experimental trials, observational epidemiology, and social survey research) and data procedures (i.e., analysis of variance, logistic regression, multivariate modeling techniques) were "quite satisfactory for addressing the majority of study questions related to alternative medicine—from research on therapeutic efficacy to basic science research on mechanisms of pathogenesis and recovery."[29]

Out of its deliberations, the working group concluded that if an unconventional therapy had an "identifiable, systematic, and consistent set of rules," reliability could be ascertained even though its etiology was based on "unknown, mysterious, or novel mechanisms of action." This meant that the unconventional nature of a given system would not, of itself, create an impediment to its validation through the use of appropriate research strategies.[30] Accordingly, there was no justification for an unconventional therapy to refuse testing based on the argument that the particular technical challenges posed by characteristics inherent to CAM made it impossible to assess. The working group also refused to countenance the argument that the rules of biomedical reductionism could not be applied to CAM because it represented "an alternative paradigm with its own standards." With both propositions, the working group "emphatically disagreed," arguing that new methodologies using nonlinear modeling (i.e., chaos theory, neural net theory, fuzzy sets theory) were potential substitutes.[31]

The working group cautioned against claims of special circumstances to delay or avoid evaluation. Unless or until unconventional therapies agreed to enter into research studies, they had only themselves to blame for any negative judgment leveled against them by conventional medicine. Besides, patients deserved to know if the therapies were "safe and effective." Thus, although showing its willingness to compromise at the edges, the working group drew a line beyond which CAM therapies would lose their standing, however strong the political pressure to keep them in the public's eye. Patients needed to feel safe when they sought treatment from unconventional systems. For that reason, CAM could not fail to accept closer scrutiny in the form of reasoned, well-executed research. Until this was done, cautioned Levin and his colleagues, CAM had to undergo the same degree of scientific scrutiny expected of conventional therapies.

> If practitioners, researchers, and advocates of CAM fail to accept this fundamental premise, then the advent of reasoned, well-executed research and the credibility that this will bring will be further delayed. Likewise for complementary systems of medicine: whether or not their purported mechanisms of action can be revealed tangibly to everyone's satisfaction, therapeutic effects for now must be demonstrated in relation to accepted outcome measures. As others have noted, a prospective patient ought to be able to begin a course of treatment with a reasonable idea of its success rate beyond just the practitioner's opinion. Without these modest caveats, CAM will not, and should not, become accepted by the larger medical community.[32]

The very fact that the *Journal of the American Medical Association* and the nine archive journals of the American Medical Association chose in 1998 to coordinate a thematic publication of CAM therapies served as a marker of CAM's coming of age. That a majority of the nation's medical schools now included discussion of CAM therapies in their curricula, that hospitals were operating integrated-medicine programs, and that managed care was brokering packages that included CAM practitioners suggested that mainstream medicine had to be more forthcoming in its accommodation. "We are in a culture with only a weak consensus on much of what passes for CAM," wrote Fred Frohock, professor and chair of the Political Science Department at the University of Miami, "and maybe this culture is in a state of welcome transition to more reliable understandings of health and healing. Sometimes, it is possible to believe that we are on the verge of a new paradigm in medicine that will abandon the false polarities, and even distinctions, between mind and body." Such an integrated model, however, required careful negotiation.[33]

Notwithstanding the pressures coming from Senator Harkin and CAM proponents generally, conventional scientists remained unpersuaded by the arguments to change or replace the RCT. Evidence of this refusal was conveyed in a 1998 article in the *Journal of the American Medical Association*, whose editors were unequivocal in their assessment of what constituted acceptable research.

> Priority for research funding for alternative medicine should be given to investigations of relevant clinical problems for which well-designed studies have shown encouraging results for alternative therapies, especially for conditions that are common and those for which conventional medicine has not been effective. Attention should be given to evaluation of safety and efficacy, but also to examining the effectiveness of a treatment strategy, with consideration of community practice settings, patient expectations and compliance, and cost-effectiveness. Collaborative research, especially among the federally funded centers for alternative medicine research in the U.S. and with international alternative medicine research centers, may improve efficiency in answering important research questions. We encourage high-quality, rigorous research on alternative medicine and invite authors to submit their best papers for objective evaluation and consideration for publication.[34]

Equally important had been the joint editorial in the *New England Journal of Medicine* in 1998 by editors Marcia Angell and Jerome Kassirer, both of whom were longtime critics of the American health-care system and, in particular, of the pharmaceutical industry and who came down resoundingly against the category *alternative medicine*, which they viewed as little more than "junk science." "There cannot be two kinds of medicine," they insisted. "There is only medicine that has been adequately tested and medicine that has not, medicine that works and medicine that may or may not work."[35] For them, there were not multiple levels of medical legitimacy, only one level: that which could be tested and shown to work. The postmodern crisis of medicine was in finance and delivery—not in the standard of scientific medicine. CAM medicine should be subjected to the same rigorous standards for safety and efficacy as biomedicine. "What we've learned, painfully and slowly over the last century, has been the necessity to test," Angell explained elsewhere. "We've learned that the testimonial, the anecdote, even through very powerful, is not enough to say a particular drug works."

> We are applying a double standard, and there are lots of reasons why we're doing that. The very term "alternative medicine" means there are two kinds of medicine, conventional and alternative. And we say conventional medicines needs to undergo rigorous scientific testing, but somehow we're excusing alternative medicine from that same requirement. That was made quite explicit when Congress exempted the dietary supplement industry from the usual regulations on drugs that require the manufacturers to show that a drug is safe and effective before it can be marketed. Alternative medicine is now outside the FDA purview. So that's what I mean by a free ride. Makers of dietary supplements can put anything they want in their bottles, as long as they label it a dietary supplement and don't claim that it cures a particular disease. Nobody knows what's in those bottles, and whether it works or not.[36]

NCCAM

Notwithstanding the precautions taken by the Quantitative Methods Working Group, conventional researchers were alarmed that so many unsubstantiated CAM therapies were practiced across the United States and, even worse, that they were being covered by third-party payers. They were also in disbelief that OAM's budget had expanded from $20 million in 1998 to $50 million in 1999 and $68.7 million in 2000. This realization had no doubt influenced Congress's decision to elevate the OAM to the status of a center within the NIH—the National Center of Complementary and Alternative Medicine (NCCAM)—and with an expanded mandate "to explore complementary and alternative healing practices in the context of rigorous science; to educate and train CAM researchers; and to disseminate authoritative information to the public and professionals."[37] Two key words in the mission mandate, *rigorous* and *science*, gave skeptics hope that CAM research would continue to be defined within a biomedical structure. This meant that alternative systems based on vitalistic or spiritual principles had to be framed within a reductionist set of assumptions. In other words, no research dollars were to be expended to evaluate paranormal epistemologies (i.e., psychic healing) unless done in a reductionist context. In an era of managed care, clinical researchers, basic scientists, and policymakers insisted upon practices that not only were safe and effective, but could stand upon a high degree of proof.[38]

Supported by Representative John Porter (R–IL), who chaired the subcommittee that provided oversight of the NIH's budget, as well as by Senator Arlen Specter (R–PA) and Senator Harkin, NCCAM became a reality despite the concerns voiced by scientists across the country. "Clearly the political push for expanding [OAM] into a center didn't want to wait for any critical review," complained Nobel Prize biologist Paul Berg of Stanford University.[39]

Representative of this hardening of feelings, Harold Varmus, former director of the NIH and president of the Memorial Sloan-Kettering Cancer Center in New York, warned that "new facets" were being added to the NIH "without much thought to overall design." Before the NIH became even more fragmented, he urged, supporters needed to give greater care to its structure. Prior to World War II, there existed only the National Institute of Health and the National Cancer Institute. In 1960, there were seven institutes. By 2001, the number had grown to twenty-four centers and institutes, along with the National Library of Medicine. At issue, explained Varmus, was the unnecessary duplication of responsibilities that would eventually affect the institutes' respective budgets and grant-making authority. To make matters worse, other prospective institutes were waiting in the wings to be authorized. "Having more institutes also means less flexibility, less managerial capacity, less coordination, and more administrative burden," he warned.[40]

Stephen Straus, a virologist with strong research credentials, including twenty-three years at the National Institute of Allergy and Infectious Diseases, was appointed NCCAM's first director and put his reputation on the line as he sought to assuage Harkin and his allies while insisting on continued scientific rigor for NCCAM's funded research support. Given the breadth of alternative medicine's treatments and practices, most of which had been unexamined for either safety or efficacy, Straus hoped to identify those therapies worthy of incorporation into conventional medicine and to inform the public of those that lacked credibility.[41] To achieve both goals, he had to convince critics that the NCAAM was not simply "a countercul-ture enclave for pseudoscience."[42]

In 2000, NCCAM's advisory board approved the investigation of so-called frontier therapies such as the use of magnets, energy healing, acupuncture, and homeopathy, which operated outside known biologi-cal mechanisms. Although acupuncture and homeopathy were relatively well known, therapies such as the Gonzalez Protocol were less known and poorly understood.[43] For critics from the scientific community, trials to examine these aberrant "sciences" constituted a waste of money and a disgrace to the scientific method. For Straus and his management team at NCCAM, whose intramural research programs had expanded each year due to CAM's muscular lobbying, the pressure to test these fringe thera-pies remained an ongoing challenge.[44]

An advocate of good science, Straus walked a careful path between the proponents of CAM and the scientific community hostile to CAM. His aim was to offer an opportunity to those frontier modalities whose modus operandi derived from forces outside scientific sensibility to seek legal status and protection that would legitimize their cures. To achieve this opportunity, he recommended validity through RCTs, preferably double-blind, to ensure a level playing field. Most alternative systems, however, considered the offer specious, if not irrelevant, arguing that Straus was seductively offering approval *only* by using reductionist medicine's "house rules." True to his word, Strauss supported large double-blind, placebo-controlled RCTs testing acupuncture for knee arthritis (University of Maryland); ginko biloba for dementia (University of Pittsburgh); glucos-amine and chondroitin sulfate for knee arthritis (University of Utah); St. John's wort for depression (Duke University); shark cartilage for lung can-cer (M. D. Anderson Cancer Center); the Gonzalez Protocol for pancre-atic cancer (Columbia-Presbyterian); and saw palmetto extract for benign prostatic hyperplasia (Veterans Affairs Medical Center, San Francisco).[45]

At the National Cancer Institute, scientists drew up plans in 1998 for a $2.5 million clinical trial to test the effectiveness of the product Neovastat manufactured by Aeterna Zentaris, a pharmaceutical company located in Quebec. Unlike the more crude dietary supplements consisting of dried shark cartilage of dubious preparation and used for various cancers that were unresponsive to conventional therapies, Neovastat was derived from shark cartilage liquid extract. The product was tested on eight hundred lung cancer patients on the assumption that it stabilized tumor progression. The study, cosponsored by the newly created NCCAM, resulted from pressures stemming from both Congress and the CAM community to sponsor such a trial for shark cartilage, combining it with a placebo and with the standard regimen of chemotherapy or radiation or both. Other studies were carried out by the Mayo Clinic and the M. D. Anderson Cancer Clinic in Houston, testing both Neovastat and the product Bene-Fin against the placebo. The BeneFin experiment was halted early after enrolling only eighty patients in an initially planned six-hundred-cohort study of breast and colon cancers. The results, albeit limited, showed no evidence of an improved quality of life. An additional clinical trial was carried out on the orally administered Cartilade (powdered preparation of shark cartilage). To date, the cumulative evidence is either insufficient or inconclusive or both.[46]

NCCAM also funded trials of chelation therapy for coronary artery disease at more than one hundred sites and at a cost of $30 million in spite of earlier controlled trials that had already found this therapy ineffective. The same was true of the Gonzalez Protocol for patients with stages II to IV pancreatic cancer.[47] In each of these trials, as well as those on St. John's wort, echinacea, and saw palmetto, none of these treatments was found to be more effective than the placebo.[48] An NCCAM-sponsored clinical trial focusing on St. John's wort and published in the *Journal of the American Medical Association* in 2002, found the herb to be "no better than placebo for the treatment of major depression."[49] Despite a steady stream of criticism lodged by the herbal industry claiming that the tests had been flawed, Straus stood behind the clinical results.[50]

For EBM critic Vincanne Adams, professor of anthropology at the University of California in San Francisco, Straus's "house rules" had been predicated on the proposition that all alternative healing systems operated on the same "epistemological playing field." This proposition, Adams noted, assumed a one-to-one correspondence between biomedical reductionist thinking and alternative medicine. "There is more at stake here than the question of whether we are talking about different names for the same diseases (or that the empirical foundation is the same even though the names we assign to them vary cross-culturally)," she complained. There were very real epistemological issues at stake. Disease categories did more than identify biological symptoms. They not only identified "unique approaches to bodily suffering, radically different models of anatomy, and logics of treatment protocols" but also defined "different empirical realities."[51]

In the case of Tibetan medicine, for example, Adams felt that biomedical equivalents were conspicuously absent. Tibetan medicine classified diseases in terms of old and new cases and looked for patterns of imbalance in the body that related to the patient's humoral constitution. Given this approach, patients with the same biomedically diagnosed disease would be seen in Tibetan terms as having different diseases with different etiological pathways requiring different treatments. Tibetan medicine included such diagnostic factors as spirit causation, karma (moral and immoral behavior) from past lives, and so-called inner winds that resulted from environmental and political influences, all of which were beyond the purview of biomedical reductionism. This approach undermined the logic of treating alternative medicine with RCTs and reduced the possibility of a "statistically successful outcome." That a well-designed clinical trial with outcomes defined biologically, molecularly, cellularly, and biochemically would provide reliable empirical data on the comparative strengths and weaknesses of Tibetan medicine was an assumption that Adams considered untenable, particularly when both drugs and treatment changed over the course of a disease, preventing the use of studies designed to assess the efficacy of a single active ingredient. Moreover, because some Tibetan medicines were compounded of sixty or more different ingredients, outcome-based RCTs of them were difficult if not impossible to develop. Even more complicating was the claim that the active ingredients in a particular medicine were the result of a "spiritual" or "magical" empowerment brought about through karma, winds, chakras, auras, and so on.[52]

Critics aside, NCCAM found collaborators in several federal agencies to promote conferences, workshops, and symposia on the importance of CAM research. These agencies included the Agency for Health Care Research and Quality, the FDA, the Centers for Disease Control and Prevention, the Health Research and Services Administration, the Substance Abuse and Mental Health Services Administration, the Department of Veterans Affairs, and the Department of Defense. While funding for NCCAM had increased from $50 million in 1999 to $68.7 in 2000 to an estimated $104.6 million in 2002, the total amount of funding through other agencies increased from $116.0 million in fiscal year 1999 to approximately $247.6 million in fiscal year 2002.[53] The NCCAM budget appropriation for 2005 was $123 million—an amount that actually understated the expenditures on CAM research, which totaled almost $305 million.[54]

WHITE HOUSE COMMISSION

On March 7, 2000, President Bill Clinton signed Executive Order Number 13147, creating the twenty-person White House Commission on Complementary and Alternative Medicine Policy. The commission was directed to develop legislative and administrative recommendations that would "help public policy maximize potential benefits, to consumers and American health care, of complementary and alternative medicine (CAM) therapies—chiropractic, acupuncture, massage, herbs, and nutritional and mind–body therapies, as well as a host of other therapies."[55] Appointments to the commission included conventional physicians, conventional health professionals who had integrated CAM into their practices, several interested health professionals, business executives, and patient advocates. To fulfill its charge, the commission held town-hall meetings in four cities, invited expert testimony during ten regular meetings held in Washington, and conducted site visits at institutions that were integrating CAM into their mainstream practice.

In "The Chairman's Vision" in the commission's final report, James Gordon, a Harvard-educated psychiatrist and founder of the Center for Mind–Body Medicine at Saybrook University in San Francisco, noted that most Americans had not turned their back on conventional medicine, knowing full well the benefits of modern scientific medicine. However, there was a general consensus regarding conventional medicine's "limitations and side effects." This consensus explained why so many individuals had turned to CAM therapies "without valid scientific information to guide them." Because people were choosing a variety of approaches—reflecting both biomedical and CAM perspectives—it was in the interest of public safety to provide solid information with which the public could make sound health-care decisions.[56]

Among the assumptions shared by the commissioners was the belief that in the absence of good information many Americans were making poor choices regarding CAM modalities; that science could help sort good CAM from the bad; that some CAM modalities would be proven safe and effective; and that ultimately there was only one type of medicine—namely, that which tested safe and efficacious. Given these assumptions, it was essential to understand the benefits and liabilities of CAM approaches because all systems of health and healing should be held to the same standards of good science.[57]

The White House Commission's final report, released in 2002, advocated a *holistic* orientation to future health care as a supplement to a strictly biomedical approach to health. "Health involves all aspects of life–mind, body, spirit and environment—and high quality health care must support care of the whole person," stated its authors.[58] The term *holistic medicine* generally implies giving the individual patient an instrumental role—both conscious and unconscious—in building and maintaining his or her medical landscape, involving physical, social, and mental well-being through health promotion, treatment, healing, and disease prevention. In contrast to the positivistic framework of mainstream or regular medicine, holism looks beyond the formalized canon of reductionist science to the interrelationship of mind, body, and spirit as contributing factors in human wellness. It assumes, therefore, that each individual represents a complexity of interdependent functions that are affected by physical, mental, spiritual, and environmental factors, any one of which might negatively or positively influence the whole body as well as the individual part.[59]

The commission listed ten principles intended to guide its recommendations:

1. Health involves all aspects of life—mind, body, spirit, and environment[,] and high-quality health care must support care of the whole person.
2. The Commission is committed to promoting the use of science and appropriate scientific methods to help identify safe and effective CAM services and products and to generate evidence that will protect and promote the public health.

3. People have a remarkable capacity for recovery and self-healing, and a major focus of health care is to support and promote this capacity.

4. Each person is unique and has the right to health care that is appropriately responsive to him or her, respecting preferences and preserving dignity.

5. Each person has the right to choose freely among safe and effective care or approaches as well as among qualified practitioners who are accountable for their claims and actions and responsive to the person's needs.

6. Good health care emphasizes self-care and early intervention for maintaining and promoting health.

7. Good health care requires teamwork among patients, health-care practitioners (conventional and CAM), and researchers committed to creating optimal healing environments and to respecting the diversity of all health-care traditions.

8. Education about prevention, healthy lifestyles, and the power of self-healing should be made an integral part of the curricula of all health-care professionals and should be made available to the public of all ages.

9. The quality of health care can be enhanced by promoting efforts that thoroughly and thoughtfully examine the evidence on which CAM systems, practices, and products are based and make this evidence widely, rapidly, and easily available.

10. The input of informed consumers and other members of the public must be incorporated in setting priorities for health care and health-care research and in reaching policy decisions, including those related to CAM, within the public and private sectors.[60]

Holistic medicine is by no means new to the Western world. From Native healing practices first glimpsed by Europe's earliest explorers of the Americas to the healing practices of the botanics, Thomsonians, homeopaths, hydropaths, eclectics, physiomedicals, and mind-curists of the eighteenth and nineteenth centuries, it has been an integral part of any number of representative groups who have shown a greater interest in the connection between mind and body in the treatment of disease and illness than so-called medical orthodoxy. In other words, these groups have willingly accepted and integrated beliefs that have one or more physiological, environmental, psychological, or even spiritual components. This multidimensional approach, which is most evident in the postmodernist age, had roots well nourished by practitioners from antiquity into the modern age. As a consequence, the American landscape has been dotted with holistic practices dealing with health and health care that defy the more focused field of reductionist medicine.[61]

Premised, therefore, on the holistic belief that the mind, body, and spirit are integral elements in the healing process, the White House Commission recommended well-designed demonstration projects grounded in first-class scientific research to ensure the safety of products, appropriate levels of training of health-care practitioners, and dialogue between and among the different types of health-care providers. "The American people want their conventional healthcare practitioners to help them make wise decisions about whether to use complementary and alternative therapies—and which ones to use—and they want their CAM practitioners to be responsive and informed partners with their mainstream medical caregivers," remarked Chairman Gordon. For this reason, he insisted that conventional health-care providers serve as "gatekeepers" by offering guidance to those seeking safe and effective CAM therapies.[62]

Due to the lack of what it perceived as substantive domestic clinical trials of CAM interventions, the commission recommended that the nation's future research agenda include not only comparisons of CAM therapies with conventional treatments, but the utilization of integrative and collaborative models as well. It also recommended a national coding system that would support standardized data collection. As a prerequisite to these recommendations, the commission urged the states to regulate and license those unconventional practitioners whose practices and products could be shown to be beneficial using standardized evaluative procedures. It also recognized the importance of CAM in the promotion of good health habits and attitudes in such areas as community and school-based programs addressing poor dietary habits, smoking, substance abuse, lack of exercise, depression, and other wellness issues affecting underserved and special populations. Finally, it urged the secretary of the Department of Health and Human Services to seek the cooperation of private, state, and federal agencies (e.g., Veterans

Affairs, Defense, Indian Health Service) in partnering with CAM well-ness and prevention programs to integrate safe and effective practices and products into the health-care system.[63]

Given that the American public was relying on anecdotes, beliefs, testimonials, theories, and opinions to justify the safety and efficacious nature of CAM products and that most CAM research had been con-ducted beyond the research arm of academe, the commission urged com-parability and replication in all future testing. It also understood the need for pharmaceutical and herbal manufacturers to agree on some level of standardized practice to ensure consistency in product purity and safety.[64] Although dietary supplements, for example, represented $17 billion in sales in 2000, reaching 158 million consumers, these products lacked the same level of testing and oversight demanded of prescription drugs. Understandably, the public should expect the same level of safety for these supplements that is guaranteed for prescription drugs. The commission therefore recommended that dietary supplement manufacturers register their products and suppliers with the FDA and maintain records of any adverse effects. To ensure a responsible level of safety, it urged Congress to "periodically evaluate the effectiveness, limitations, and enforcement of the Dietary Supplement Health and Education Act of 1994 and take appropriate action when needed."[65]

Because federal backing to assess the legitimacy of CAM modalities required an acceptable evidence-based methodology that would sat-isfy critics and proponents alike, the commission recommended that NCCAM collaborate with conventional medicine and its researchers to identify guidelines, research priorities, methodologies, and resources to examine those CAM therapies whose epistemological foundations lay outside the biomedical paradigm. It also encouraged alternate forms of evaluation, including basic research, nonrandomized studies, empirical observation, case studies, evaluations of practice-based data, and prac-tice-based outcomes research. An understanding existed among the com-mission's members that some of CAM modalities would be proven safe and effective, whereas others would fail in the process. Because research on unpatentable products was not likely to attract private research dol-lars, the commission's report urged the government to offer incentives to stimulate private-sector investment.[66]

The report insisted that both CAM and conventional medical researchers have rigorous training in the fundamentals of clinical, basic, and
health services research. This training would include a proper ground-
ing in "research process and methodology," the "collection and record-
ing of unbiased data," "protocol or study design and execution," and an
"understanding of the expertise needed to form a research team." The
commission urged cooperation and even joint applications by CAM and
biomedical researchers and their accredited institutions to realize these
training elements. The results of this research, the commission urged,
should be published in "recognized, rigorously peer-reviewed research
journals" and collected in databases available through NCCAM, the
Cochrane Collaboration, the Agency for Health Care Research and
Quality, and both the PubMed and MedlinePlus databases in the
National Library of Medicine.[67]

Finally, the White House Commission urged that CAM be included in
medical school curricula to ensure that it is taught in combination with
reductionist medicine. With this inclusion, CAM students, practitioners,
institutions, and organizations could benefit from loan and scholarship
programs, gain greater appreciation for the fundamental elements of biomedical science, improve their competency as practitioners, and improve
relationships with their biomedical counterparts. Moreover, CAM should
partner with conventional medicine to provide service to medically
underserved populations, facilitate better quality and accuracy of CAM
information available to the public, and ensure consumer safety through
improved training, licensing, and certification. With a better understanding of each other's expertise and both group's willingness to compromise,
the commission hoped that CAM and conventional medicine would
eventually build mutual respect, understanding, and an environment of
improved health care for all.[68]

Notwithstanding these objectives, the commission's hopes were not
always shared by the parties involved. Spokespersons for conventional
medicine felt themselves dragged into an unholy relationship (i.e., a double standard) whose outcome had negatively impacted their share of the
health-care market. Similarly, many CAM proponents remained fearful of
being judged by the standards set by conventional research, causing them
to be overly defensive to the point of denying comparable standards of

quality and rigor.[69] Two of the commission's members, Tieraona Low Dog and Joseph Fins, wrote a dissenting letter, recommending that funding for CAM therapies should be evaluated against all other proposals and disbursed on the basis of merit and not simply because they were CAM. "Asking for more research money to investigate an approach, practice or product simply because it is 'CAM' is an ideological, not evidence-based approach to science," they complained.[70]

According to Dónal O'Manthúna, professor of bioethics and chemistry at the Mount Carmel College of Nursing in Columbus, Ohio, the initial flaw in the commission's report was its approval of a definition of CAM that was far too encompassing. The definition adopted included the following statement: "Complementary and alternative medicine, or CAM, can be defined as a group of medical, health care, and healing systems other than those included in mainstream health care in the United States. CAM includes the worldviews, theories, modalities, products, and practices associated with these systems and their use to treat illness and promote health and well-being." This definition, O'Manthúna explained, included everything from religious and philosophical systems to physical manipulation and therefore led to serious issues of public policy. It made no distinction, he claimed, between those protocols that were complementary (some of which were evidence based and used by regular physicians); those that were scientifically unproven; those that were scientifically questionable (i.e., homeopathy); those that were so-called energy medicines; and, finally, those that were clearly fraud. Implied in these differences was the fact that the report ought to have adjusted its recommendations to the substantive differences between and among the categories. Moreover, he insisted that the inclusion of spirituality as a CAM therapy was patently wrong. Those practices that invoked spirituality (e.g., prayer, Reiki) should be treated conceptually different than protocols using acupuncture or St. John's wort. Such inclusion violated the very evidence-based principles endorsed by the commission. More to the point, it transcended the assumptive premises of both conventional and unconventional medicine. [71]

Subsequent attempts to accommodate medical pluralism, or what Wayne Jonas, the second director of the OAM, once described as the "democratization" of medicine, has not been a peaceful process. Despite the popularity of CAM therapies across all levels of American society, clinicians have continued to find serious methodological issues in them. Having placed so much importance on the RCT, and having made it the gold standard for the testing and assimilation of new medicines and treatments, conventional researchers have found it difficult to substitute alternative analyses or what Kenneth Schaffner at George Washington University calls "methodological pluralism."[72]

Even with their fixation on the RCT, biomedical researchers seem open to exploring ways to address at least some of the issues. "Mind and body are . . . so closely connected in most healing practices," explained Fred Frohock of Miami, "that there are good reasons to abandon the distinction altogether." Examples abound of body-to-mind and mind-to-body responses to different stimuli. Unfortunately, the ability to "disentangle the placebo effect from the medicinal effect" continues to plague clinical researchers. Frohock suggested that "the binary self may be an inadequate model for the human person."

> The belief, not the clinical trials, may be the decisive variable in the efficacy of the product. The problem for determining efficacy is that a joining of mind and body makes it exceedingly difficult to identify the true antecedent variable bringing on the effect, whether beliefs or the substance taken. Put in terms of the deeper issue, mind and body may constitute a complex framework, perhaps a kind of layered unitary self, able to influence and undermine clinical trials with findings in the larger world of human experiences.[73]

In his edited volume *The Role of Complementary and Alternative Medicine: Accommodating Pluralism* (2002), Daniel Callahan, senior research scholar and president emeritus of the Hastings Center, examined both the culture and practices of CAM and the challenges it has raised for mainstream medicine.[74] The essays in the book spoke of a new diversity in contemporary American culture that acts as a potential change agent to conventional medicine's biomedical model, including the possibility of unintended consequences for the values and assumptions attached to biomedical research. The various authors stressed the need to respect the value preferences evident among different healing groups along with the need for clinical outcomes-based research that includes both CAM and conventional medicine. Callahan and his contributors encouraged the creation of a new paradigm dedicated to carrying on a more enlightened conversation about health and disease instead of following a path that distorts and devalues both orthodox and heterodox healing systems. Exemplary of this view, physician and anthropologist Marc Micozzi, author of *Fundamentals of Complementary and Alternative Medicine* (1996), executive director for the College of Physicians of Philadelphia, and former editor of the *Journal of Alternative and Complementary Medicine*, argued for greater tolerance and medical pluralism, with increasing focus directed to self-care and self-cure. Recognizing the power shift from physician to patient, he urged combining psychoneuroimmunology with concepts of vitalism, bioenergy, and holism, believing that these three elements offer a more comprehensive understanding of health and healing than strict biomedical reductionism. He suggested that quantum physics and biology/ecology are better evaluators of alternative therapies than the existing double-blind approach of the RCT. In looking at the varieties of alternative medicine, he seemed to favor naturopathy, which he called the "new eclectic medicine" in that it uses the best of everything regardless of source, theory, or methodology. To be sure, Micozzi stretched far beyond the opportunities and avenues of assessment offered by the Quantitative Methods Working Group in 1995. [75]

INSTITUTE OF MEDICINE REPORT

A more paradigmatic change came from the Institute of Medicine (IOM), an independent, nonprofit organized in 1970 under the aegis of the National Academy of Sciences to provide unbiased advice to the public and to decision makers regarding issues of medical care, research, and education. The IOM's sixteen-member committee to study CAM, which began meeting in 2003, published its report two years later.[76] The report, *Complementary and Alternative Medicine in the United States*, some three hundred pages in length, gave generous recognition to the fact that nearly a third of the US population was using CAM therapies routinely and often in a manner complementary or parallel with conventional therapies. It identified the major scientific, policy, and practice issues; reviewed the existing methods and approaches used in CAM research; made recommendations concerning the challenges of conducting CAM research; and stressed the need to translate CAM research findings into practice.[77]

In his comments on the IOM report, David Eisenberg, director of the Osher Institute at Harvard and one of the sixteen committee members who shared in its authorship, stressed the need to ensure "that health-care professionals are providing evidence-based, comprehensive care that encourages a focus on healing, recognizes the importance of compassion and caring, emphasizes the centrality of relationship-based care, encourages patients to share in decision making about therapeutic options, and promotes choices in care that can include complementary and alternative medical therapies where appropriate." This statement by itself represented a watershed change in thinking in that it demonstrated the degree to which evidence-based patient care had been affected by more holistic elements. To the committee's credit, wrote Eisenberg, its members sought to create a "level playing field" on which all therapies could be judged. This meant that the same rules of evidence that weighed so heavily in conventional medical trials should apply as well to CAM treatments. Each and all, regardless of modality, should be put to the test of safety, efficacy, and cost effectiveness. What once applied only to conventional medicine now applied equally to CAM.[78]

Eisenberg recognized that much remained unknown about CAM and the modus operandi behind its many therapies. Given this conundrum, the IOM committee encouraged research that would examine the complex social and cultural components of illness; the degree to which CAM users adhered to treatment protocols; the effects of CAM as a preventative; the manner in which the public accessed and processed CAM information; and an examination into the positive and negative interactions between CAM and conventional treatments.[79] Implied in this expanded viewpoint was a recommendation for considering a range of methodological approaches in addition to the RCT. These approaches included single-patient trials; testing bundles of therapies; qualitative research strategies; and the evaluation of nonspecific (placebo) effects. The committee also urged research into the use of multiple treatments, including the integration of CAM and conventional treatments, particularly because such combinations more accurately approached the actual use of CAM therapies by the adult population. Finally, the committee recommended the inclusion of CAM therapies in the curricula (at all levels) of the nation's health profession schools—namely, medicine, pharmacy, nursing, and allied health.[80]

THE NEXT DECADE

In 2009, NCAAM began its second decade with the appointment of Josephine Briggs as its director. Educated at Harvard and trained at the Mount Sinai School of Medicine, Briggs pursued a career in research at Yale and later at the University of Michigan. From 1997 to 2006, she directed the Division of Kidney, Urologic, and Hematologic Diseases at the National Institute of Diabetes and Digestive and Kidney Diseases. In looking forward to NCCAM's second decade, Briggs expressed her intention to reinforce the importance of EBM by giving increased emphasis to translational research, meaning an accelerated process for applying research outcomes to clinical and community practice. Noting that the boundaries between CAM and conventional medicine had narrowed in recent years, with numerous CAM interventions amalgamated into integrative medicine, and noting as well that approximately 40 percent of Americans were spending more than $33 billion for out-of-pocket CAM interventions, the time had come to ensure more accurate and timely evidence-based information on CAM for the public.[81]

NCCAM's second decade is intended to advance the research priorities of its first decade with a leveraged focus on three long-range goals: (1) focusing on the science and practice of symptom management; (2) developing effective, practical, personalized strategies for promoting health and well-being; and (3) enabling better evidence-based decision making regarding CAM and its integration into health care and health promotion. Pointing to the reduced sale of St. John's wort and echinacea following the publication of several NCCAM-supported clinical studies that identified issues of safety and efficacy, the agency took claim of its mission to promote a science-neutral approach to CAM practices and interventions.

Significant differences still remain. After NCCAM's ten years of existence and more than $200 million spent testing the effectiveness of alternative therapies in more than 2,500 research projects, critic Wallace Sampson, editor of the *Scientific Review of Alternative Medicine* and emeritus clinical professor of medicine at Stanford University, remarked: "It is time for Congress to defund the National Center for Complementary and Alternative Medicine (NCCAM) . . . [because] . . . it has not proved effectiveness for any 'alternative' method. It has added evidence of ineffectiveness of some methods that we knew did not work before NCCAM was formed."[82] Gerald Weissman, editor of the *Journal of the Federation of American Societies for Experimental Biology*, added to the criticism: "If the trend persists, perhaps MIT or Cal Tech will march in step with the medical schools and offer prizes for integrative alchemy or alternative engineering."[83] According to Donald Marcus of Baylor and Arthur Grollman of Stony Brook, the issue is not whether the NIH should support research into alternative therapies—their popularity has made it imperative from a public-policy point of view to properly evaluate their efficacy and safety. Rather, the issue is whether NCCAM is the appropriate agency to do the evaluations. For both Marcus and Grollman, NCCAM has fallen below the threshold standards of other NIH institutes in that it "funds proposals of dubious merit; its research agenda is shaped more by politics than by science; and it is structured by its charter in a manner that precludes and independent review of its performance." Over and over again, funding was granted for clinical trials of therapies (i.e., echinacea, saw palmetto) already long identified as having no more effective outcomes than the placebo controls. Equally disturbing, NCCAM's review groups included individuals with both limited scientific credentials and potential conflicts of interest due to their association with the botanical industry. Finally, according to these authors, oversight of the NCCAM's extramural programs had "escaped critical evaluation because its charter required a preponderance of proponents of alternative medicine on its council." For these reasons, they conclude that the evaluation of alternative therapies would be better performed by other NIH centers and institutes.[84]

Issues and controversies continue to trouble the relationship between the supporters of CAM and the supporters of normative science. The Internet has numerous sites that track NCCAM's newsletters for misinformation; check the accuracy of comments Briggs gives in lectures and to the press; comment on NCCAM's hesitancy to address CAM objections to vaccinations; take frequent note of its indecisiveness toward homeopathy; and criticize its tendency to promote CAM in general as well as specific CAM modalities prior to evidence-based studies. "It seems to us that the NCCAM (at least so far) has never closed the door on any modality, no matter how implausible and no matter how much evidence for lack of efficacy there is," complains Yale clinical neurologist Steven Novella. NCCAM's public statements show "strict adherence to evidence-based medicine and science being neutral, but interspersed with this is an uncritical presentation of ancient superstition as if it were science, and endorsement of treatments that are not backed by science." This pattern, Novella concludes bitterly, has only confirmed his worst fears—that NCCAM's "very existence, and the generally positive and uncritical information it provides to the public, is used to promote and endorse unscientific medical modalities."[85]

■ ■ ■

For the moment, it would appear that biomedicine has tamed postmodernism's enthusiasm for CAM by finding ways to integrate those therapies proven successful and containing the remainder through rigorous clinical trials. Rather than fight the forces of history with all its potential risks, conventional medicine chose a seductive and pragmatic approach, one that it has used time and again to co-opt the power of its adversaries: adopting those elements that can be incorporated into itself. Terri Winnick describes this strategy as "co-optation,"[86] meaning that those remedies and treatments shown to be safe and efficacious have been absorbed into conventional medical practice and those that remain on the outside face a judgmental condemnation relegating them to existence as unproven, unaccredited, and unlicensed. Thus, although conceding to pressure from Congress for the establishment of OAM and NCCAM, conventional medicine has been able to ensure that the program's activities would be guided in a publicly responsible manner through the strict application of an evidence-based pyramid using the normative methods of science. The fact that so few outcomes have been judged successful suggests that most CAM modalities are faith-based practices, placebos, the detritus of psychosomatic medicine, entrepreneurial expedie worse, outright quackery.

5

COMPLEMENTARY AND ALTERNATIVE MEDICINE'S CHALLENGE

A Case Study

It is not as if our homeopathic brothers are asleep; far from it,
they are awake—many of them at any rate—to the importance
of the scientific study of disease.

–Sir William Osler, "Unity, Peace, and Concord—a Farewell Address to the
American Medical Profession" (1905)

G iven the political and ideological pressures that mounted in the 1960s and continued into subsequent decades urging the NIH and its affiliate centers and institutes either to accept the historical validity of CAM therapies or to produce evidence that they were capable of positive health outcomes, it was not surprising that the RCT's status at the top of the evidence-based pyramid would come under attack. As noted in previous chapters, the proponents of unconventional therapies offered a smorgasbord of arguments that the RCT contained within it a plethora of biases that diminished its objectivity. The most serious indictment grew from the very heart of postmodernism, questioning the equivalency of the terms *objectivity* and *scientific knowledge*. Before one accepts the validity of an RCT, postmodernists reasoned, it is important to understand the environment in which the researcher has formulated his or her knowledge as well as the subjective world of the patient who is part of any research cohort. For both, perception is a contributing component to the outcome; indeed, it is an essential part of reality itself.[1]

This criticism, which might have acted as an Achilles heel for bio-medicine and its RCT, was offset by Henry Beecher's announcement that approximately 35 percent of patients in RCT control groups respond positively to the placebo. Not only did this claim launch a paradigmatic change in RCT research, but along with it came the following stunningly simple challenge: Is the effect attributed to an active drug or to a CAM therapy equivalent to or exceeding what otherwise could be attributed to the placebo effect? Knowing that drugs with active substances can also produce a placebo effect meant that biomedical therapies were not immune from the question. This admission resulted in a leveling of the playing field for researchers who insisted that CAM therapies be subjected to the same standards of evidence as those required in the biomedical world.

Clearly, testing this hypothesis has not been an easy task because CAM therapies are legion, including not only the more popular treatments (i.e., acupuncture, homeopathy, chiropractic, massage, naturopathy, and psychotherapy), but also indigenous medical systems (e.g., traditional Chinese, Ayurvedic, and Native American), spiritual or energy healings (i.e., therapeutic touch, distant healing, intuitive diagnostics), relaxation therapies (i.e., yoga, meditation); natural products (i.e., herbs), and various nondescript therapies (i.e., magnets, rolfing).

In North and South America, western Europe, and Australia, postmodernist medicine has drawn heavily from shamanic traditions as well as from ancient Eastern healing systems and practices. In public-opinion polls outside of the United States, surveyors have found CAM therapies popular in Canada (15 percent) and Australia (49 percent). Similar percentages apply to countries in Europe.[2] Among the most popular types of CAM treatments, homeopathy is a favorite in Belgium and France; reflexology is most often used in Denmark and Finland; and anthroposophical medicine is especially favored in Germany.[3] Across Europe, regulation varies widely, with CAM therapies tightly regulated in France, Spain, and Italy, largely unregulated in the United Kingdom, and only moderately regulated in Germany and the Scandinavian countries.[4]

In the United Kingdom, the most popular forms of alternative medicine are herbal remedies, osteopathy, homeopathy, acupuncture, chiropractic, healing, hypnotherapy, reflexology, naturopathy, and aromatherapy.[5] In support of the professionalization of alternate forms of medicines, the universities of Exeter and Southampton offer degrees in chiropractic, osteopathy, acupuncture, and herbal medicine.[6] By the mid-1990s, nearly 40 percent of physicians in general practice were providing patients with access to some level of CAM.[7] This percentage remained steady through 1999, with the majority of treatments utilizing either chiropractic or osteopathy for low back pain. Other popular modalities include acupuncture, relaxation classes, massage, and yoga.[8]

Britain's homeopathic hospitals were accepted into the National Health Service at its inception in 1947 and were followed several years later by the medical Faculty of Homeopathy. Thus, even with resistance from conventional doctors, homeopathy exercised a high degree of legitimacy within British medicine. As of 1999 in the United Kingdom, there were five homeopathic hospitals, the largest of which were located in Glasgow and London. Besides these National Health Service providers, numerous independent centers offer complementary medical services.[9] Together, they include a range of both conventional and complementary treatments. In addition, conventionally trained physicians have the opportunity to take postgraduate education for a primary-care homeopathic certificate. There are also training courses for those without a medical background. The main regulatory body is the Faculty of Homeopathy for medically trained homeopaths and the Society of Homeopaths for non–medically qualified homeopaths.[10]

MORE OF LESS IS MORE: HOMEOPATHY

Of all the different schools of healing that have emerged in postmodernist society, homeopathy offers a casebook example of CAM's challenge to the reductionist paradigm. By insisting upon a reconstructed reality, it supports two mutually exclusive worldviews. For the homeopath, the experience is the moment of truth; it is the moment in conscious life that outweighs science, rationality, and historical memory. Regardless of what society views as normal science, the homeopath gives priority to the subjective over the objective, claiming a perspective that connects to the fundamental elements of the universe. Such pure experiences give objectivity a back seat to intuition. Relying on experience, the homeopath tests and refines belief. From the homeopath's metaphysic of experience comes the challenge to biomedicine's reductionist methods, including the RCT. For the homeopath, there is no bedrock outside experience on which to construct one's claim to knowledge. The experience derived from taking a homeopathic remedy determines what one is willing to accept or reject.

Founded in the late eighteenth century by German physician Samuel Christian Friedrich Hahnemann (1755–1843) as an alternative to medicine's proto-orthodoxy, homeopathy consists of several eternal principles or laws: (1) *similia similibus curantur*, or "like cures like"; (2) the prescription of medicines for symptoms alone; (3) the use of infinitesimal doses; (4) the potentization of medicines by trituration with sugar of milk or by succussion in alcohol and water; (5) the prescription of a single simple medicine at a time; (6) use of "provings" (i.e., the testing of a potentized substance on healthy volunteers to determine which symptoms a given substance is capable of producing and hence curing); (7) administration of medicines by placing pellets on the tongue or by olfaction; (8) and belief in psora, sycosis, and the syphilitic doctrines.[11]

During its peak years in the nineteenth century, homeopathy seemed to have shaken allopathic medicine to its very roots, having drawn many of its nearly ten thousand practitioners from the ranks of old-school medicine. During this time, orthodox doctors, disillusioned with their tidy categories of rationalistic thinking, offered weak ratiocinations to explain their abandonment of such time-honored practices as bleeding, blistering, purging, salivation, and heroic doses of harsh drugs.[12] These halcyon years for homeopathy coincided with proto-orthodoxy's rising self-doubt; its gradual migration to the concept of self-limited diseases; the use of the microscope in clinical pathology; and the adoption of a more expectant system of treatment. In their interpretation of the unfolding changes, homeopaths enthusiastically reported that allopathy was "on the brink of homeopathy."[13] But as historian Naomi Rogers correctly noted, "American medicine was changing, but it had not necessarily drawn closer to the homeopathic ideal."[14]

Although some homeopaths touted their system's strengths, those who had been academically trained in regular medical schools began distancing themselves from Hahnemann's principles in the second half of the nineteenth century. Two groups of homeopaths emerged: those who held to the universality of the law of *similia*, the importance of single doses, the efficacy of serial dilutions, and a belief that Hahnemann had provided the keys to a distinct school of medicine; and those, a clear majority, who accepted the law of *similia* but chose to be more selective in accepting Hahnemann's other principles. The latter group, many of whom had migrated to homeopathy from regular medicine, represented the liberal arm of homeopathy. Having witnessed positive changes in regular medicine, they pushed for a more adjuvant form of homeopathy, perhaps even becoming a specialty within conventional medicine. This meant the acceptance of bacteriology, the new serum therapies, and laboratory science—all of which diluted homeopathic identity.[15]

By the closing decades of the nineteenth century, the familiar features that once defined homeopathy were barely alive in its medical schools. In 1900, only twenty-two of its sixty-nine colleges were still in existence, and with the American Medical Association's revision in its Code of Ethics in 1903 permitting academically trained homeopaths to return to the fold, there followed a precipitous decline in their numbers and a decline in the number of homeopathy schools, with many of them closing or merging. In 1938, the two remaining schools (Hahnemann Medical College of Philadelphia and the New York Homeopathic Medical College and Flower Hospital) relinquished their homeopathic status and became regular medical schools. Academic homeopathy's efforts to accommodate to scientific medicine ended with its virtual disappearance from the medical landscape. By 1945, only five states continued to operate homeopathic examining boards.[16]

Emerging from this unpleasant conflagration was the American Foundation for Homeopathy, organized in 1924 by a group of high-dilutionist physicians (i.e., those choosing highly attenuated medicines 30C and higher) and devotees affiliated with the equally conservative International Hahnemannian Association. From this time forward, homeopathy's power base shifted dramatically from academic to lay professionals. By the 1960s, homeopathy had come to represent a nonhierarchical and grassroots practitioner–patient phenomenon closely associated with personal and spiritual transformation, self-study groups, feminism, and New Age culture. Today, homeopathy constitutes a sizable portion of the health-care system in the United States, with the number of adherents quadrupling from 1990 to 1997.[17]

In the postmodernist era, what remains of academic homeopathy finds itself stymied by those lay professionals who reject a licensed identity, educationally trained experts, and standardized programs using a core curriculum. With this rejection, homeopathy has become a cottage industry led by celebrity lay teachers commanding center stage and offering lessons through short courses, videos, workshops, and social networking via the Internet. Out of this phenomenon has emerged a largely unregulated healing system that can best be described as open, pluralistic, lay dominated, antiestablishment and antiregulation, prone to deviant theories, opposed to scientific scrutiny, having a preference for metaphysical rather than empirically based practices, and divided into groups defined by its teachers. Most postmodernist homeopaths seek to distance themselves from the scientific paradigm and to rely instead on a philosophy-based system of energy forces that continues to defy conventional medicine's standards of proof.[18]

Thus, academically trained homeopaths' quest for authority, expertise, and status in the field has been checked by those lay enthusiasts who, despite their many contradictions, are content with their independence from standardized training, rules, licensing, and codes of ethics. For the most part, lay homeopaths have accepted an alternative—not complementary—status as their mantra and have no desire to submit their therapies to the evidence-based pyramid. Having prided themselves on the absence of rules and boundaries, these homeopaths have shown little indication of wanting to professionalize. As a consequence, they will probably fail to secure status or the financial rewards accruing to those who choose to move toward some level of professionalization.[19]

With no established schools or standardized curricula, the theories and practices of American homeopaths deviate considerably.[20] Not only do they isolate themselves from each other, but they choose to remain silent concerning more controversial issues. This silence applies to such topics as immunization, in which practitioners tend to delegate the decision to children's parents rather than to take full responsibility for objecting to its use; their denial of the RCT as the best means for evaluating the efficacy of its medicines; and their division over the exact mechanism to explain the potentizing or dynamizing aspects of their serially attenuated remedies. These issues constitute serious obstacles to homeopathy's acceptance as a complementary or integrative partner with conventional medicine. In fact, the line between homeopathy's scientific claims and its nonscientific deviancy appears to be ever widening, forcing advocates and critics alike to conclude that its efficacy is due to an interior placebo effect, a paranormal process grounded in belief, or some distant scientific principle yet to be discovered. In this drama, conventional medicine remains an imposing factor, serving as the representative of normative science whose standards define the manner in which research is conducted and determine the line between acceptability and rejection.[21]

Notwithstanding these impediments, the empathy established in homeopathy's physician–patient encounter has been well documented. The literature suggests that in the health-appraisal interview, patients treated homeopathically experience a more comforting cognitive and emotional mental state—a more positive engagement and resonance with the patient's personal problems and biopsychosocial history. Based on a "whole-person" approach to the patient as well as on a vitalistic philosophy of organism, homeopathy approaches the treatment of disease and illness using variously triturated and succussed single medicines to provoke a self-regulatory response intended to resolve conditions in the body that are intrinsically reversible and to serve as a palliative where the problems or conditions are irreversible. As one of CAM's more popular modalities, homeopathy offers options in those areas where conventional medicine has failed, where no conventional treatment exists, where the side effects from conventional medicine are problematic, and where patients are fearful of conventional treatment. It is viewed as supportive rather than curative, demonstrating positive patient responses in nonspecific areas where nonvalidated treatment exists. By emphasizing hygiene, avoiding dangerous measures, and administering medicines in minuscule doses that are typically below the level of biological activity, homeopaths are seldom accused of doing harm. As a result, homeopathy remains one of the most widespread, heterogeneous, and controversial therapies in modern times.[22]

HOMEOPATHIC PRACTICE

Homeopathy rightly claims to have a long-admired doctor–patient relationship. Perceived as differentiated, symptom driven, individualistic, and free from the potential of adverse drug and other conventional therapeutic effects, it benefits from positive patient expectations, experiences, and unconscious conditionings. Part of homeopathy's strength also lies in its location within the private health sector, in which it treats illness as a variable within the patient's control. Believing that illness is caused by deleterious social and environmental stresses on the individual's vital force, homeopaths seek to match the remedy with the patient's particular body–mind construct. Homeopathic remedies represent a symptomatically based knitting together of a subjective discourse with biological functioning to activate the body's internal healing agent. In interpreting the true pattern of the individual's vital force, the homeopath claims to create a somatic and bodily reaction that returns the body's energy field to its rightful balance. Through its nonconventional holism best embodied in the biopsychosocial consultative encounter, homeopathy offers a connection between the patient's somatic and organic components. This holism represents a clear contextual difference between homeopathy and conventional medicine's clinical diagnostic methods.[23]

Inasmuch as homeopathy originated at a time when illnesses were long and drawn out, its physician–patient encounter reinforces this healing profile with a lengthy gathering of symptoms, an equally lengthy process of correlating those symptoms with the long lists of symptom complexes cataloged by "provers" in published repertories, and the careful testing of appropriately triturated and succussed medicines. By any standard, the homeopathic consultation is time-consuming and remains significantly at variance with conventional medicine, where the doctor–patient history-taking encounter is relatively shorter, though it is often augmented by preliminary workups by a nurse, physician assistant, or lab technician. Modern homeopathy has eased some of this time-consuming process with the help of computers, but it remains a much lengthier process than that of conventional medicine. It involves asking a long list of questions and constructing the information in a manner that establishes an empirically based and individualized case history. Because homeopathic remedies number several thousand, the computer has become for the homeopathic healer what the laboratory and imaging technology are for molecular biology as it quickly matches the symptom complex with several possible remedies from which the homeopath makes an appropriate choice. Along with computers and intuition in the selection of remedies, some practitioners employ electronic instruments such as biophoton analyzers, radionic equipment, and Sulis remedy makers to create energetic remedies.

A homeopath's typical caseload includes patients with rheumatoid arthritis, fatigue, asthma, migraine, eczema, hay fever, irritable bowel syndrome, and mood disorders as well as children whose complaints often defy conventional diagnosis. The caseload also includes patients with more serious pain-management needs, including those being treated for cancer and other life-threatening illnesses. Homeopaths explain that their medicines lack the potential for destructive side effects and therefore can be used in pregnancy as well as at the extremes of life without doing harm. What this suggests is that homeopathy is intended principally for those "fringe" areas where medically trained physicians often fail with their pharmacotherapeutic methods. Yet homeopaths also argue that their high dilutions have to be carefully prescribed lest they prove too powerful for the body to absorb.[24]

The term *classical homeopathy*, which implies close adherence to Hahnemann's doctrines, is used when practitioners identify a single, individualized, and potentized medicine prepared according to the law of *similia*. This means the selection of a medicine whose provings correspond with the patient's symptom complex—that is, the patient's current symptoms, medical history, personality, behavior, and so on. Implied in this individualized encounter is the supposition that two patients with very similar biomedical diagnoses may nevertheless require two very different homeopathic approaches. For the most part, classical homeopaths follow a fairly standardized approach to treatment, with infrequent doses every few days or weeks of a single remedy. Once a diagnosis is made, patient response is measured for patterns of improvement, though not necessarily cure. Individual treatments tend to be less costly; however, because they extend beyond the natural history of an illness, the overall cost is often higher than that of conventional medicine, which begins and ends with the disease or illness.[25]

In keeping with the principle of *similia*, homeopathic patients are treated with an active or inert substance thought to trigger symptoms similar to the illness. These remedies are even deemed helpful when diluted to the point where none of the original substance exists in the solute. Here, homeopathic theory runs counter to the laws of normative science. Anomalies remain an important, if not an essential, aspect of modern paradigmatic science, but the novelty of homeopathy's ultramolecular medicines extends far beyond being simply a conflict with normative science's expectations, models, and theories. It suggests that the issue is not only one of scientific anomaly, but one of belief—not in the sense of methodological value, but of epistemological judgment.[26]

Whereas the proponents of homeopathy insist on the validity of their ultramolecular medicines, science critics continue to find it a waste of time and effort. At issue is something very basic—namely, whether biomedical reductionism can or should be the method to test the claims of ultramolecular potencies. If homeopathy's ultramolecular potencies are impossible to detect in a laboratory, can one conclude that the hypothesis falls outside the rigors of the scientific method? Is it an issue with no currently supportive evidence or some level of unjustified opinion? If homeopathy were the dominant medical treatment today and conventional medicine were attempting to gain a foothold, the question asked of the latter would be the same that is currently being asked of homeopathy today: *How does your medicine work, and does it do more good than harm?* Unable to explain itself in a plausible way and unable to organize its proofs in a manner other than in the individualized case history, which emphasizes the stand-alone nature of each patient, homeopathy finds itself facing the full brunt of conventional medicine's scientific reductionism, objectification, and replication.

MATTER AND ENERGY

Homeopathy has historically given matter a small role in the healing process. Nevertheless, matter does factor into its therapeutics. Until 1829, Hahnemann disapproved dynamizing medicines higher than the thirtieth dilution, believing that at some point there was no longer any medicine present in the medium. "There must be some end to the thing," he admitted, "it cannot go on to infinity."[27] By the time of the 1833 edition of *Organon of Homeopathic Medicine*, however, Hahnemann had begun speaking favorably of the dynamic capabilities of medicines taken to the three hundredth attenuation. This view of potentization directed homeopathy in an increasingly metaphysical direction, articulating a philosophy that encouraged a decidedly nonmaterial dimension to its healing process. These attenuations would eventually become the basis of pure *Hahnemannianism*, a term that would acquire special meaning in the years that followed. The cautions exercised by Hahnemann, however, were ignored by his disciples, many of whom chose to take their medicines to the fifteen hundredth attenuation and more.[28] Today, homeopathic medicines are serially triturated and succussed to levels of one hundred millesimal and higher.[29]

Homeopaths frequently refer to the dynamic capability of their medicines as they undergo succussion or trituration, warning that excessive shaking or rubbing of a medicinal substance can make it too dangerous to use. That said, the modus operandi for the process remains as elusive as ever. To explain the way it works, homeopaths have variously suggested physical, chemical, electromagnetic, and spiritual modifications to the solute. Such suggestions help clarify Hahnemann's initial fascination with Franz Anton Mesmer's science of animal magnetism and his theory regarding the distribution of cosmic healing energies to the afflicted parts of the body. Hahnemann clearly saw a relationship between his own principle of dynamization and the energy field discovered by Mesmer.[30]

Later explanations for homeopathy's high-potency medicines came about through the influence of Dr. James John Garth Wilkinson (1812–1899), a homeopath and biographer of the Swedish scientist, philosopher, and religious writer Emanuel Swedenborg, whose law of correspondences purported that individuals who have a living relationship with the visible and invisible world allow them to see the causes behind actions that are usually taken for granted. Disease, according to Swedenborg, had a spiritual causation that manifested itself in the material body. For Wilkinson, the principle of Hahnemann's infinitesimals reminded him of a descending order from the soul to the vital force and then to the material body.[31]

Through the work of Wilkinson and the writings of the Reverend Frank Sewell (1837–1915) and physician James Tyler Kent (1849–1916), a combination of Hahnemannian and Swedenborgian thought became the centerpiece for American high dilutionists in the waning years of the nineteenth century and early decades of the twentieth. Kent chose to mix Hahnemann's basic laws of *similia*, the single remedy, and the minimum dose with Swedenborg's notions of body, mind, and soul. In doing so, he stressed the correlation between the principles of miasm and vitalism, rejected modern scientific and pathological knowledge as a guide to diagnosis, and emphasized psychological symptoms in prescribing his high potencies. Kent and his followers looked to mental healing and the correspondence between man's affections and the vital force of the soul.[32]

Kent adopted Swedenborg's concepts of internals and externals, meaning that in the correspondence between all things spiritual and physical, the key to curing physical disease was to address its spiritual manifestations. But Kent was selective in his application of Swedenborgian concepts in that he chose not to include the world of angels, spirits, and devils in his metaphysical thinking. Instead, he attuned himself to the theory of signatures (i.e., herbs that resemble parts of the body also take on medicinal typologies) and to the primacy of the patient's inner state.[33]

Responding to derision from conventional medicine, including the signature critique by Oliver Wendell Holmes, in 1842 lectures titled "Homeopathy and Its Kindred Delusions," classical homeopaths were challenged to find alternative explanations for the modus operandi of their dynamized solutions.[34] Some who found Kent's theories wanting were drawn to the so-called OD Theory (pronounced "ode") of German chemist and philosopher Dr. Karl von Reichenbach (1788–1869), who explained that highly sensitive patients could feel and respond to subtle forms of cosmic energy.[35] Others looked to the work of Albert Abrams (1863–1924), whose *New Concepts of Diagnosis and Treatment* (1916) explained the power of homeopathy's drug attenuations as the result of traceable energy forms or vibrations discovered in high-potency remedies by means of his invention known as the "Dynomizer."[36] Still others viewed the X-ray as a potential explanation for the special properties of dynamized drugs. Both Henry C. Allen (1836–1909) in 1910 and Federico Anaya-Reyes in the 1960s endorsed the X-ray as an "awakener" of the potential power of inert substances and a subsequent stimulant to the body's resistance to disease.[37]

With the development of quantum theory, homeopaths were quick to adopt terms such as *atoms, vibrations, force fields, resonance,* and *electromagnetic fields* in their discussions. Borrowing from the work of German physicist Max Planck (1858–1947), they suggested that the energy from serialized dilutions "interlocked" with the world of atoms, electrons, and protons, releasing bundles known as *quanta* that varied by frequency and that had the power to evoke symptoms (*similia*) that restored health to the sick.[38] This change in terminology was helped along by the influence of German-born physicist Albert Einstein (1879–1955), whose theory of relativity explained that mass could be converted into energy ($E = mc^2$). For speculative thinkers such as K. C. Hiteshi, whose healing modality was anchored in energy, matter was simply one form of its manifestation. This meant that a little inert matter, perhaps even something beyond *Avogadro's limit*, could be converted into a healing agency. Named after the nineteenth-century Italian scientist Amedeo Avogadro (1776–1856), Avogadro's limit represents the quantity of atoms or molecules (6.022×10^{23}) in a cubic centimeter of water. Hiteshi reasoned that the atomic bomb verified the law of dynamization in that it explained how, through succussion, an infinitesimal inert substance was "smashed" and converted into energy—a transformation from its physical form into pure energy. This same energy, according to Hiteshi, could penetrate the body and restore the patient's recuperative powers.[39]

In June 1988, John Maddox, editor of *Nature*, published a paper by French chemist Jacques Benveniste (1935–2004) concerning a series of experiments that measured the response of human white blood cells to an antibody that had been diluted in distilled water to a point where the solute contained no remaining molecules of active substance. In explaining the response of the white blood cells to the solute, Benveniste and his colleagues theorized that the antibodies had left their "imprint" on the water molecules and that this imprint was sufficient to cause a reaction from the white blood cells. The antibody remained active even when diluted to one in 10^{20} parts of water because the water, following serial dilution and succussion, "remembered" the antibody's chemical properties and rearranged its hydrogen atoms in a manner (i.e., vibrations, resonance, force fields) that mimicked the antibody's action. As a condition of publication, Benveniste agreed to have his experiment replicated by laboratories in Israel, Italy, and Canada. Choosing not to wait for this confirmation, Maddox published the article on the condition that an investigative team of his own be permitted to observe Benveniste and his researchers replicate their experiment.[40]

A month later, in the July 1988 issue of *Nature*, Maddox, along with Walter Stewart (an expert on fraud) and James Randi (an investigator of the paranormal), published the results of their investigation, condemning the work of Benveniste and his team as "statistically ill-controlled, from which no substantial effort has been made to exclude systematic error, including observer bias, and whose interpretation has been clouded by the exclusion of measurements in conflict with the claims." Benveniste was unable to reproduce his original results, and the three other labs reported similar failures. Maddox and his coauthors found no evidence of fraud but, reminiscent of the French commissions appointed in 1789 to assess the merits of mesmerism, ascribed the results as the product of "autosuggestion."[41]

The incident refused to die as Benveniste denounced Maddox for gross ignorance of immunology and for carrying out a witch hunt against him and his colleagues. To add to the mix, questions arose almost immediately from the scientific community over the editor's decision to publish such questionable research. Why had not the journal waited for confirmation from one or more of the laboratories? Why publish the paper and then condemn it? If editor Maddox did not believe in the results or questioned its methodology in the first place, why publish the article at all?[42]

A year later the *British Medical Journal* published a paper by Peter Fisher and his colleagues on the effect of homeopathic treatment on fibrositis using a tincture of the leaves of poison oak diluted to 10^{12}. The team's inability to provide a plausible rationale to explain the drug's modus operandi, aside from postulating an indeterminate form of energy unknown to science, was met with similar hostility by conventional medical researchers, who felt the claim conflicted with the normative laws of chemistry and physics.[43] Todd Hoover, president of the American Institute of Homeopathy, later argued that such impediments "should not prevent a true scientist or open-minded physician" from looking at the evidence because homeopathy had two hundred years of documented clinical experience.[44]

Homeopathy's academically educated physicians as well its non-medically trained healers and consultants insist that their ultramolecular medicines, whose modus operandi remains as yet hidden from view, have a scientific basis that somehow stimulates and provokes the body's defense mechanism. Having tried unsuccessfully to predicate the universality of their principle using mesmerism, radiation, atomic fusion, thought energy, and water memory, they now believe that by decoding the subatomic world of energy matter, they can bring closure to their ongoing debate with reductionist medicine. Having adopted the language of quantum physics, homeopaths claim it as the newest modus operandi behind the mystery of dynamization.

One example of this adoption came from celebrity teacher and lecturer George Vithoulkas (b. 1932), who saw the dynamization process as the product of the body's electromagnetic field. Borrowing from Fritjof Capra's *The Tao of Physics* (1977),[45] he asserted the basic unity of the universe—namely, that all material objects are "inseparably linked" with the cosmos, whose quanta field of subatomic particles are present everywhere. Thus, matter and energy are interchangeable. Drawing from studies carried out by Yale neuroanatomist Harold S. Burr, who discovered that changes in an organism's electromagnetic field ("aura") precipitated specific pathologies, and from Kirlian photography, which hypothesizes the ability to visually identify an electrodynamic field surrounding all living and nonliving objects, Vithoulkas concluded that a correlation exists between the emanations from the body's electrodynamic field (i.e., vital force) and its physical and emotional state in health and disease.[46]

With this starting point, Vithoulkas reasoned that homeopathy's dynamized dilutions are a form of "energy medicine" whose vibrations affect the patient's electrodynamic field at the atomic and subatomic levels. In other words, changes in a person's vibrational level affect the body's equilibrium and make it susceptible to disease. Because disease is the result of a weakened defense mechanism, true therapies are those that "strengthen the resonant frequency of the entire organism." The use of acupuncture, the laying on of hands, and homeopathy's potentized remedies allow for the patient to be stimulated "at precisely the resonant frequency . . . which then allows the strengthened defense mechanism to complete its work in proper order." All three of these therapies work, he explained, but homeopathy requires less training than the other two and therefore offers the greatest hope in reaching the most people. Vithoulkas concluded:

> To affect directly the dynamic plane, we must find a substance similar enough to the resultant frequency of the dynamic plane to produce resonance. Since the defense mechanism's only manifestation perceptible to

our senses is the symptoms and signs of the person, it follows that we must seek a substance which can produce in the human organism a similar totality of symptoms and signs. If a substance is capable of producing a similar symptom picture in a healthy organism, then the likelihood of its vibration rate being very close to the resultant frequency of the diseased organism is good, and therefore a powerful strengthening of the defense mechanism can occur—through the principle of resonance.[47]

For David Feinstein and Donna Eden of the Energy Medicine Institute in Ashland, Oregon, energy medicine is challenging the dominance of the biochemical paradigm. On the premise that illness "results from disturbances in the body's energies and energy fields," they predict that energy medicine will soon supersede conventional medical practices by affecting gene expression and gene activity. Based on Burr's *The Fields of Life* (1972),[48] Feinstein and Eden hypothesize that electromagnetic fields not only work in concert with the fundamental biological processes but can significantly influence the healing process. Thus, interventions to the body's electrical energies, electromagnetic energies, and so-called subtle energies can affect the pathways (chakras, meridians, etc.) to the body and the health of the organs. Whereas conventional medicine is focused on the biochemistry of cells, tissues, and organs, energy medicine addresses the energy fields that organize and control them. These authors identify six characteristics of energy medicine: (1) *reach*, or optimization of the energies that surround, permeate, and support the body; (2) *efficiency* in regulating the biological processes; (3) *practicality*, or the use of non-invasive and readily available methods; (4) *patient empowerment* in the building of resilient energy patterns; (5) *quantum compatibility*, or the influence of imagery and focused thought to engage the healing power; and (6) *holistic orientation* by successfully integrating body, mind, and spirit. Together, these characteristics form the pillars upon which energy medicine makes its claim.[49]

These attractive explanations aside, dynamization remains the most controversial and elusive aspect of homeopathy and serves as the "unguarded flank" most frequently attacked by critics. Given the absence of a clear and replicable modus operandi for their ultramolecular solutions to become energized through trituration or succussion, homeopaths are faced with finding a plausible scientific explanation or, alternatively, of accepting dynamization as a faith-based principle or as a placebo. That said, those who desire homeopathy to become a scientifically based adjunct to conventional medicine are forced to deviate from the classical principles enunciated by Hahnemann and to allow for variations that bring into question homeopathy's very homeopathicity.[50] Unless conventional medicine is willing to compromise its assumptions concerning the parameters of normative science, it is doubtful that homeopathic dilutions beyond the Avogadro number will be considered as anything more than water. To date, volunteers in homeopathic trials have failed to distinguish between homeopathic remedies and water.[51]

SHIPS IN THE NIGHT

In 1994, the *British Medical Journal* published an exchange of opinions between Robert Buckman, a medical oncologist, and George T. Lewith, senior research fellow in the Complementary Medicine Research Unit at Royal South Hants Hospital in Southampton. Buckman congratulated Lewith for having superb interpersonal skills, commenting that a video of his physician–patient encounter "should be shown to every medical student in the world as an example of what good doctoring looks like." That said, he felt that Lewith's most powerful medication was himself, which led to two questions: First, is there a "verifiable physical mechanism" in homeopathic remedies that actually affects a disease? And second, do homeopathic remedies make patients feel better? Buckman was convinced that the latter question could be answered affirmatively because it was in large part due to the emphatic and supportive manner in which Lewith treated his patients. Believing, however, that the first question could not be answered affirmatively, he wondered if homeopaths would be satisfied with an "end point" that simply targeted the patient's "sense of wellbeing [*sic*]."[52]

In his reply, Lewith admitted that the mechanism of homeopathy remained unknown but felt that it was less important than concentrating on the effectiveness of the treatment. He pointed to "convincing evidence" of homeopathy's effectiveness in hay fever, migraine, and fibromyalgia in clinical trials. Given this evidence, Lewith insisted that homeopathy provided more than a placebo effect and, because of its success, brought into question "the pharmaceutical and biochemically dominated world of conventional medicine." Although he appreciated Buckman's compliments on his consultative techniques, which most certainly had a therapeutic effect on his patients, he nevertheless insisted that homeopathy had "proved therapeutic benefits (in some instances) greater than those expected from a placebo."[53]

Buckman challenged Lewith on each of the three clinical trials offered as evidence of homeopathy's success. The trial by Bruno Brigo and Giovanni Serpelloni in 1991 for migraine headache showed that homeopathic remedies were "exceptionally active" in migraine, but when the trial was repeated, the results were not reproducible. Similarly, neither the study by David Taylor Reilly and his colleagues on hay fever nor the study by Peter Fisher and his colleagues on fibromyalgia provided "reproducible objective evidence."[54] Future studies might show a reproducible effect, but none as yet had been forthcoming. Given that in all three studies the placebo produced "a considerable decrease in symptoms," Buckman suggested that both regular practitioners and homeopaths provide a sign in their waiting room that would state the following: "As part of your treatment your doctor may prescribe certain drugs which have not—so far—been proved to have a specific action against diseases. Nevertheless, these drugs are completely safe and many patients find them beneficial. If your doctor thinks they may help you, she or he may recommend them to you."[55]

Lewith replied that he and his colleagues were developing replicable clinical trials that he hoped would settle the questions Buckman raised. Admitting that "not enough good research has been done to prove the clinical effectiveness of homeopathy," he countered by noting that 85 percent of conventional medicine had yet to be properly evaluated. Admitting that the placebo effect was an "enormously positive" factor in the doctor–patient equation, he urged that it be taught to medical students "so that they understand the limits of scientific medicine and the importance of their intervention."[56]

Beckman responded to Lewith's comments by pointing out that there was "no reproducible evidence that homeopathy differs from placebo." This caused him to conclude that homeopathy had no clinical effect over and above that of placebo. He decided that homeopathy was no more than a form of chaplaincy that often brought symptomatic relief to patients through prayer. "Perhaps that is the right model for cooperation between people who do not have the same beliefs but acknowledge thoughtfulness of what the other person does," he concluded.[57]

TO RCT OR NOT TO RCT

As explained earlier, the RCT eventually became the gold standard for the verification of safe and efficacious pharmaceutical medicines. Among scientists and practitioners, it is the undisputed method for identifying useful medicines in a bias-free environment. Underlying the RCT is the principle of replicability and the supposition that all the participants are taking the same remedy for the same problem, suggesting that whatever contaminants remain are few and inconsequential. Thus, before conventional physicians are willing to refer patients to homeopathic healers, there is an expectation that the RCT would need to provide evidence-based justification for these healers' serially succussed and triturated medicines.

From the mid-1980s until roughly 2000, numerous reviews and meta-analyses provided only half-hearted support for the supposition that homeopathic remedies were more efficacious than a placebo.[58] In a comprehensive review published in 1991 by the *British Medical Journal,* a research team commissioned by the Dutch government reviewed 107 trials of homeopathy. Out of those trials, many of which were of low quality, they found 81 that showed positive results for homeopathy. "The evidence presented in this review would probably be sufficient for establishing homeopathy as a regular treatment for certain conditions," the team reported. "Based on this evidence we would be ready to accept that homeopathy can be efficacious, if only the mechanism of action were more plausible."[59] A similar analysis managed by the European Commission in 1996 concluded that "it is likely that among the tested homeopathic approaches some had an added effect over nothing or placebo."[60] However, the failure to explain homeopathy's modus operandi made the results uninterpretable—a "game of chance" between an inert solvent and an infinite dilution.[61]

In a 1997 criteria-based meta-analysis of eighty-nine clinical trials looking at author, sample size, condition, intervention, and outcome, Klaus Linde and his colleagues assessed whether the effect observed with homeopathic remedies was equivalent to that of the placebo. "If the hypothesis that all clinical effects of homeopathy are due to placebo is correct," they reasoned, "it would mean that in all properly conducted placebo-controlled trials on homeopathy, one placebo had been compared with another." Implied in such a result would be that the pooled effects of the homeopathic group would show zero difference with the placebo group. After extracting the data, the researchers found that 73 percent of the results failed to confirm their hypothesis that the clinical effects of homeopathy were no different from those due to placebo. However, because many of the low-budget clinical trials were small, they could not rule out publication bias as an explanation for the results. That said, their study found "little evidence of effectiveness of any single homeopathic approach on any single clinical condition." On the basis of their findings, the researchers concluded that further research was "clearly warranted despite [homeopathy's] implausibility."[62]

In 2000, testing the hypothesis regarding whether homeopathy is a placebo, Mortag Taylor and his colleagues designed a randomized, double-blind, placebo-controlled, parallel-group, multicenter study of fifty patients with allergic rhinitis who were assigned an oral 33C homeopathic preparation of allergen whose dilutions reputedly contained no molecules of the original substance from which it was prepared, or a placebo. The patients were tested for changes from the baseline over a period of four weeks. Although both groups reported improvement in their symptoms, the homeopathic group showed "a clear, significant, and clinically relevant improvement in nasal inspiratory peak flow" compared to the placebo group. The researchers concluded that homeopathic treatment differed from the placebo but cautioned that their one study was insufficient and urged further testing. For the present, however, they were satisfied that their study had failed to confirm their original hypothesis—namely, that homeopathy was a placebo.[63]

Given the uncertain results of these clinical trials, few conventional researchers were willing to give credence to additional studies. Meta-analyses suggesting a "modest effect" of homeopathy over placebo included so many small and methodologically questionable trials that researchers tended to discount them due to publication bias or financial interest or both. The challenge remained to replicate these trials' results in much larger trials.[64] "If you cannot conceive of highly diluted solutions with undetectable drug concentrations having a biological effect, then no matter how well designed the trial or robust the meta-analysis, a positive result will not change your views," concluded Gene Feder and Tessa Katz. Forcing a leap of something more than faith, the biomedical world was being asked to accept the proposition that a solute containing no detectable drug could have a biological effect. Considering that homeopathy was biologically implausible because of the Avogadro limit, acceptance meant that the biomedical world had to abide by a very different model of the universe. It is doubtful that any finding from such trials would convince biomedical clinicians that ultramolecular dilutions can have a measurable physiological effect on a patient. "We believe that new trials of homeopathic medicines against placebo are no longer a research priority," argued Feder and Katz in 2002. "Randomized controlled trials may be efficient arbiters of clinical effectiveness," they reasoned, "but they are not particularly good for resolving philosophical disputes."[65]

In 2002, Lewith and his colleagues administered either an oral ultramolecular potency of homeopathic immunotherapy or placebo to participants in an RCT involving thirty-eight general practices in Hampshire and Dorset and using 242 asthma patients (186 of whom completed the test). At the end of the sixteen-week trial, he and his researchers observed no clinical difference in lung function or quality of life between those treated with an ultradiluted allergen and those receiving a placebo, concluding that "homeopathic immunotherapy is not effective in the treatment of patients with asthma" and that the "different patterns of change between homeopathic immunotherapy and placebo over the course of the study are unexplained." They explained more fully, "There was no evidence of significant change in bronchodilator use in either group, although participants in the homeopathy group were using less bronchodilator than the placebo group in the last four weeks of the study. There was no evidence that homeopathic immunotherapy was better at treating asthma than placebo. There was no significant correlation between attitudes to complementary and alternative medicine and improvement on any of the outcome variables."[66]

The conclusions that Lewith and his researchers came to resulted in a "dust-up" among homeopathic readers of the *British Medical Journal*, who harshly criticized the editors for publishing the article. "Does the *BMJ* have any homeopaths as reviewers, or was the paper looked at by people who are as ignorant of homeopathy as the authors obviously are?" asked Meryl Dorey, national president of the Australian Vaccination Network. Dorey insisted that the homeopathically prepared allergen had actually been a test of isopathy (a schismatic element within homeopathy) and not of classical homeopathy, thus invalidating the results.[67]

In a 2003 examination of four comprehensive meta-analyses, Wayne Jonas, Ted Kaptchuk, and Klaus Linde noticed positive evidence for homeopathy's effectiveness for the treatment of influenza, allergies, postoperative ileus, and childhood diarrhea but cautioned that the limited size and number of trials made it impossible to judge homeopathy's overall effectiveness. "Homeopathy deserves an open-minded opportunity to demonstrate its value by using evidence-based principles," the authors reasoned, "but it should not be substituted for proven therapies." Unfortunately, they concluded, "even the best systematic reviews cannot disentangle components of bias that may exist in small trials, nor can they rule out that true effects may be obscured with pooling of heterogeneous studies, thereby making it impossible to draw definitive conclusions."[68]

In a study originally published in 2001 and revised in 2004, Danish epidemiologists Asbjørn Hróbjartsson and Peter Gøtzsche performed two meta-analyses involving 156 clinical trials in which an active substance was compared to both a placebo group and an untreated group. The question they sought to answer was whether the placebo group showed any significant difference in outcome from the untreated group. In both studies, the researchers found no statistically significant difference between the placebo group and the untreated group when an objective outcome was measured by an independent observer. Only when the outcome was reported by the subjects themselves were small differences noted. The authors concluded that there is "little evidence that placebos in general have powerful clinical effects."[69]

This study was followed in 2005 by a five-year study by researchers at the University of Berne in Switzerland of more than 110 trials using homeopathic remedies and 100 trials (eventually reduced to 8 and 6 larger clinical trials of higher quality) using conventional medicine for matching conditions. The authors concluded that "the effects seen in placebo-controlled trials of homeopathy are compatible with the placebo-hypothesis." As a result of the group's findings, the Swiss government moved to withhold insurance coverage for homeopathy because it no longer met efficacy and cost-effectiveness criteria.[70]

In response to these multiple trials and demands for some formal position, the *Lancet* published a series of articles in 2005 critical of homeopathy, concluding what many had already decided—namely, that the effects of homeopathy were no better than those of a placebo. In fact, the editors argued, there was no further need to perpetuate research in homeopathy. "Now doctors need to be bold and honest with their patients about homeopathy's lack of benefit, and with themselves about the failings of modern medicine to address patients' needs for personalized care."[71] As David Ramey, a prominent voice in EBM, was quick to point out, meta-analyses had "failed to identify a single condition for which [homeopathic] remedies are efficacious and, more recently have noted that the best studies show no effect." Given that homeopathy remained at odds with the fundamental laws and principles of physics, chemistry, and pharmacology, he wondered at what point the true believers in homeopathy were likely to admit that their medications lacked standing. "Most likely it will be never," he concluded, "as evidence does not seem to be able to consistently change beliefs."[72]

The *Lancet* editors' decision to oppose further research into homeopathy created a storm of protest from homeopaths, who claimed bias, political intrigue, misuse of data, lack of transparency, and mismatched trials.[73] Peter Fisher, director of research at the Royal London Homeopathic Hospital in London, was among those who took exception to the *Lancet's* conclusions, arguing that "the way forward is open, transparent science, not opaque, biased analysis and rhetoric."[74]

A year later, in a 2006 trial designed to determine statistical differences, if any, between homeopathic treatment and nonspecific placebo effects on seventy-five patients diagnosed with dermatitis, researchers divided the patients into four groups: a waiting-list control group; a homeopathy group treated with verum; a double-blind group treated homeopathically with verum; and a double-blind group treated with placebo. The results of the trial showed no statistically significant differences among the groups.[75]

In RCTs carried out in 2008 with patients diagnosed with irritable bowel syndrome, researchers found that the percentage of patients reporting relief (62 percent at three weeks and 61 percent at six weeks) from a placebo-based regimen was comparable with the rate of those patients receiving active drug treatment. The researchers concluded that "factors contributing to the placebo effect can be progressively combined in a manner resembling a graded dose escalation of component parts and non-specific effects that can produce statistically and clinically significant outcomes, with the patient-practitioner relationship being the most robust component."[76] Despite this hopeful, if not optimistic, language suggesting the creative bundling of the placebo to improve a clinical outcome, the result did not change the conclusion that homeopathy provided little or no efficacy beyond that of the placebo effect.[77]

The assertions that homeopathic treatment demonstrates favorable results is uneven at best, suggesting a clear distinction between large trials, which are generally negative, and smaller, lower-quality trials that tend to favor its efficacy over the placebo. The evidence does not unequivocally prove that the clinical effects of homeopathy are that of a placebo, but it does suggest the need for better controlled trials that factor in the levels of potentization and a better handling of dropouts (i.e., those who leave the clinical trial before it is completed). This does not, however, address the judgment made by critics that the expense of such trials cannot be justified given homeopathy's lack of a modus operandi. Researchers generally agree that both homeopathy and the placebo have a positive effect on an illness, and in these interventions the effectiveness of the former can exceed the effectiveness of the latter. But when both are examined against an active treatment, little difference is found between them. In instances of mild illness, where an active treatment provides marginal benefit, both the placebo and homeopathy have proven useful.[78]

Given the overall vagueness of homeopathy's efficacy other than as a complex placebo, conventional researchers in Britain's National Health Service and in the United States have balked at future trials, claiming that such trials would indicate little more than wishful thinking or publication bias. In the absence of any significant evidence to the contrary, the only reasons to pursue additional trials are homeopathy's political clout, its availability, and the cost of conventional medicine—none of which makes for a convincing rationale. "Why should homeopathy be allowed to hide behind a smokescreen that is denied to conventional medicine and why should the National Health Service fund such treatment in the absence of any evidence of useful effect?" asked Michael Foley at James Cook University Hospital in Middlesbrough.[79]

Then again, conventional researchers question how homeopathy can prove its efficacy within the biomedical model of the RCT using medicines that lack a molecule of active substance. If a homeopathic drug can "cure" without even one molecule of active substance in the solute and do so without a plausible mechanism, how can it satisfy the prevailing demands of scientific research? How does it differ from faith healing? How can one judge homeopathy if its underlying theory runs counter to the epistemological foundations of normative science? Are there alternative ways to bring homeopathy into an efficacy trial that would satisfy the concerns of an independent set of investigators? Most conventional researchers—both in the United States and in the United Kingdom—have answered these questions in the negative, arguing that homeopathy, because of its serial dilutions, requires even stronger evidence of its efficacy before being taken seriously by regular medicine.[80]

THE REBUTTAL

In light of findings from RCTs, the paucity of evidence growing out of meta-analyses, and the damning judgment leveled by the *Lancet*, homeopaths have looked for ways to discount altogether the demand for EBM, reasoning that what counts as evidence for homeopaths differs from that required for the testing of conventional medicines. For homeopathy's staunch defenders, the centerpiece of its science is individualization—a fact they argue works at odds with conventional medicine and the RCT's empirical components.

In examinations of the efficacy of naturopathy, homeopathy, acupuncture, chiropractic, therapeutic touch, and other interventions using evidence-based clinical trials, individualization remains a major issue. Licensed acupuncturists, for example, have been known to include cupping, dietary changes, exercise therapy, moxibustion, massage, and botanicals as part of their intervention. Then, too, there are differences that include the number and length of treatments, selection points, and depth of needle insertion. Thus, examining the efficacy of acupuncture in a standard RCT creates a clinical encounter that seriously misrepresents the actual treatment. Credible trials to evaluate auricular acupuncture treatment remain highly complex. How, for example, does one provide a placebo control for the ritual of needle insertion? How does one account for relaxation preparatory to needle insertion? How does one determine a biomedical marker that differentiates an active from an "inert" control treatment? Does the difference involve how and where the needles are inserted? Interestingly, RCTs have demonstrated that true acupuncture is more effective when applied along the channels of the meridian than in sham points.[81]

In comparing a sham acupuncture needle with an inert pill in patients with persistent upper-arm pain due to repetitive use (repetitive strain injury), Ted Kaptchuk and his colleagues concluded that the placebo effects from the sham acupuncture device had greater effect on subjective outcomes than the pill. This suggested to these researchers that placebo effects "seem to be malleable and depend on the behaviors embedded in medical rituals."[82] More recent developments in sham acupuncture have been of assistance in clinical trials, indicating positive results with respect to myofascial pain syndrome. Among proponents, there is a feeling that future studies of sufficient size will prove the efficacy of the acupuncture needle beyond that of placebo.[83]

All this helps to explain why the proponents of CAM have urged a reexamination of their claim that the RCT ought not to be the only standard for evaluating alternative therapies.[84] "The reductionist approach of the randomized controlled trial," Iain Smith explained in the *British Medical Journal* in 1995, "may fail to allow for the holistic effect that is central to the philosophy of most complementary therapies." The RCT should compare "whole treatments" rather than individualized components, he reasoned. Doing so "would allow inclusion of the things that matter to patients rather than just those that matter to the investigators."[85]

In support of this position, CAM proponents point to the human genome project as proof that medicine needs to be more patient centered and personalized. "The age of the 'medicine for the average' and the block-buster 'one size fits all' drug is starting to change to a new age of the individual," wrote Jeffrey Bland, a member of the editorial board of *Alternative Therapies in Health and Medicine*. This paradigm change, he explained, has moved "the primacy of diagnosis to a focus on understanding the antecedents, and triggers or precipitating events that give rise to the release of specific mediators that are then associated with the frequency, intensity, and duration of the signs and symptoms of the patient." The shift has been away from monotherapies and toward multiple therapies in a healing environment where many variables are at play. This alone, he argued, demonstrates the inherent weakness of the RCT.[86]

Thus, despite initial efforts at accommodation, homeopaths currently reason that there is little common ground to be found between homeopathy and conventional medicine because decisive points of reference are missing. In conventional medicine, clinicians view therapeutic interventions as patterns to be studied and quantified. The RCT relies on an impersonal set of statistical and clinical procedures applied to a generalized population. Homeopathy, in contrast, relies on a personal form of intervention involving a wide number of sociopsychological factors that affect the illness. In interviews with homeopathic practitioners, Robert Frank of the University of Bielefeld discovered an almost unanimous opposition to evaluating their therapeutic treatments using the RCT. A hundred patients with a given diagnosis might receive the same remedy in conventional medicine, but each one of that same hundred might receive a different homeopathic remedy. In essence, the "common diagnostic category" is considered irrelevant in homeopathy.[87]

Operating from this holistic understanding, Frank and other defenders of homeopathy have insisted that individualization serves as a deterrent to the statistical methodology of the RCT and, in effect, places the two healing modalities in different and arguably incompatible contextual settings. Homeopathy and biomedicine represent two fundamentally different approaches to the individual malady. The repertories developed by Hahnemann and his successors focus on both physical and psychic effects of their drug provings in the days and weeks following a single dose of medicine. For homeopaths, drug provings serve as the equivalent of the RCT, representing the clinical trials of classical homeopathy and thereby justifying their empirical identity. Given that most trials of homeopathic medicines do not individualize treatment, a characteristic that serves as the hallmark of homeopathic practice, the question remains as to the possibility of carrying out a real trial comparing homeopathic medicine with conventional medicine or with the placebo.[88]

Notwithstanding the position taken by Frank and others, those practitioners known as "complex homeopaths" view the RCT as a path to scientific respectability and have accepted the RCT under conditions, a situation that has led classical homeopaths to decry the complex homeopaths' adaptive efforts to imitate scientific standardization in their clinical trials. As noted earlier, the classical homeopath might choose a single drug from several dozen possibilities to provide an individualized therapy, whereas those seeking a more adjuvant path are willing to accept a "complex" remedy (containing several synergistic ingredients), thinking that the spectrum of coverage justifies its being tested along lines established by the RCT. Among the advocates of complex homeopathy are some who are painstakingly detailed in their studies, including Farokh J. Master of India, editor of *Homeopathic Heritage International,* and Luc De Schepper of California, author of *Hahnemann Revisited* (1999), who provides professional training in classical homeopathy. Both are unapologetic advocates of applied homeopathy, endeavoring to place homeopathy on a parallel course with conventional medicine.[89]

For classical homeopaths who claim to follow "eternal laws" as distinct from the open-knowledge system of normative science, the use of complex remedies is neither fish nor fowl—and is certainly not the homeopathy taught by Hahnemann.[90] Complex homeopathy represents too heavy a price to pay to gain scientific respectability. Whereas elements within the pharmaceutical industry support complex homeopathy and hope to benefit by adapting to the rules of normative science, classical homeopaths continue to keep their distance, believing that the efficacy of homeopathy requires no further justification. Nevertheless, the temptation to "do" science weighs heavily on homeopathic practitioners because it offers perhaps the only possibility of building any credibility within the medical community.

One disincentive even for complex homeopathy is the fact that its medicines are natural products and provide little economic incentive to spur corporate sponsorship. Since 1938, the complex herbal remedies used in homeopathy, naturopathy, chiropractic, and other alternative therapies have been exempt from FDA regulations and, since 1994, have been further protected from FDA interference by the Dietary Supplement Health and Education Act. The act's reclassification of herbal products, vitamins, and minerals as dietary supplements has left them in a "limbo" somewhere between food and over-the-counter drugs. Without monitoring for standardized quality control, issues of contamination and safety remain unattended.[91] This leaves manufacturers free to make "structure–function" claims if supported by scientific evidence and to stay free of regulation unless their compounds are shown to pose a danger. In 1996, the FDA's new labeling rules mimicked that of nutritional information required of processed foods. In essence, the FDA is empowered to intervene only when the product is shown to be harmful.[92]

After examining seven authoritative books on the topic of herbal therapies and extracting more than a hundred different treatments for asthma, Edzard Ernst noted in 1998 that opinions that "often contradict the existing evidence seem to dominate complementary and alternative medicine and this highlights the necessity of bringing opinion into line with evidence." Resolving this contradiction means well-designed clinical trials—nothing more, nothing less. To those who insist on "generalizations" or a "softer" process for legitimizing CAM, Ernst replied that the days of the double standard are numbered. The real challenge for researchers is to better understand the power of the placebo. In this regard, "the research question then shifts to how non-specific effects might be optimized so that more patients . . . can profit from them."[93]

THE DILEMMA

In the area of normative science, homeopathy has yet to be persuasive. This handicap remains an annoyance for many homeopathic practitioners and lay consultants who feel that two hundred years of history more than justifies their place in the nation's health-care system. This claim has fallen on deaf ears within the scientific community, which argues that homeopathy has demonstrated neither its theoretical persuasiveness nor the scientific evidence to justify its practice. Unwilling to accept homeopathy as a legitimate form of medical science, the scientific community has forced homeopathy to find an alternate identity in a form of psychotherapy, chaplaincy, or other faith-based systems of healing—all of which could arguably fall under the rubric of the placebo effect. Exemplary of this attitude is NCCAM's recent reluctance to fund further homeopathic studies.

That there is considerable interest in homeopathy cannot be denied as more and more people exercise their right to choose its treatment. Nevertheless, the question of recognizing its legitimacy without some theory and evidence justifying that it can indeed provide a "cure" for specific diseases and illnesses remains unanswered. How can the principle of *similia* and the use of ultramolecular potencies bring about an improvement in a person's health? How can homeopathic remedies retain biological effectiveness in the absence of an active pharmaceutical substance? Can the attributes of homeopathy's attenuated solute be explained in any other way? How can homeopathy's closed-knowledge system find compatibility within the open-knowledge-seeking world of reductionist science? How can homeopathy demand scientific acceptance when its knowledge base differs so radically from biomedicine? How is homeopathy any different from psychotherapy? Should homeopathy, admittedly popular in both Western and non-Western societies, be treated as a belief system or as some yet unknown system operating in an epistemological field distinct from reductionist medicine? Should homeopathy be expected to show a scientific basis and undergo an examination process using a scientific style of explanation involving currently accepted scientific standards, or should it be treated as a belief system operating under a wholly different set of epistemological premises? One has only to search the Internet for conversations between homeopaths and their skeptics to know that neither side is willing to concede its position. Skeptics fall back on the methods of normative science, and homeopaths defend their position with the fervor of true believers.

Homeopathy flourishes in part because it is appreciated by a segment of society that believes strongly in the values of the postmodernist world. Although the skeptic can point out the anomalies that underlie homeopathy's theory or application, the fact that homeopathy is socially regarded as successful within the broader community trumps the skeptic's charge. Knowing that currently accepted scientific knowledge can expect to be replaced at some future time in favor of an alternative conceptualization, the homeopathic community assumes that its claims will eventually be legitimized. But at what point will the supporters of homeopathy no longer be categorically rejected by scientific consensus and viewed merely part of an "exchange" of opinions within the sphere of scientific legitimacy? What factors cause those two different responses? When and how is deviant science normalized? For the homeopath, current science is a temporary artifact that over time will construct and deconstruct its practices based on the interests and forensic evidence accepted by the scientific community. Science is thus little more than a temporary conceptual ordering of nature's caprices.[94]

The feud—both scientific and ideological—between conventional medicine and homeopathy goes back to the early decades of the nineteenth century and continues uninterrupted into the present day in the debate over the relevancy of placebo-controlled trials. For those conventional physicians and researchers for whom homeopathy's ultramolecular dilutions defy the laws of physics, little that homeopaths say or do will be taken seriously. For proponents of reductionist medical science, homeopathy requires not only a replicable example of their success, but a theory that can explain its results. Otherwise, homeopathy remains a therapy in search of scientific legitimacy. Are there convincing electromagnetic, physical, or chemical explanations to explain the success of its medicines and treatments? Homeopathy's proponents contend that its legitimacy derives from two hundred years of provings that verify the law of *similia*, a similar period of observational data and anecdotal information, and generations of appreciative patients who have "voted" with their feet and pocketbooks. Its knowledge base, they argue, is not less accurate—only different.

■ ■ ■

The tension between conventional medicine and homeopathy represents a war of cultures between those for whom the mechanism of disease constitutes the ideal type of evidence and those who consider outcomes more important. From conventional medicine's point of view, the causation of disease begins at the cellular level and follows a complex course whose outcomes must be carefully analyzed to separate out bias and chance. In contrast, homeopathy views disease causation as highly individualized, meaning different things in different settings. This has allowed homeopathy to disregard a substantial body of scientific data, including Avogadro's law, as irrelevant to the credibility of its claims. Conventional medicine argues that the best estimate of an individual's response to a given therapy is the average response of a group, whereas the homeopath insists on a more individualized therapy that may or may not fit evidence-based practices. The "may or may not" option allows homeopaths to accept those findings that support their position and to reject those that challenge their claims. The contrast is between conventional medicine's rationalist-empiricist roots and homeopathy's empiricist lineage, which falls back ultimately on context or the particulars of a disease or symptom complex.

The question to be posed is whether homeopathy—and, by implication, the rest of CAM—has become a substitute religion, supplying patients with a paranormal view of reality, celebrity teachers and healers, authoritative laws and principles, and an eschatological view of healthy-mindedness. As with numerous forms of spirituality, homeopathy's strength remains anchored in its impressive array of cross-cultural data, including a banquet of anecdotal examples drawn from all corners of the globe. Nevertheless, its belief in eventually discovering the modus operandi for its principle of dynamization keeps it at a point somewhere between a pseudo-materialistic concept of disease and the absolute idealism of Christian Science. Dependent on the patient's subjective mental and emotional responses, homeopathy emphasizes health and wholeness in which the mind, in conjunction with the body, searches for coherence, clarity, and creativity amid the subtle energies of the universe. Because of the particular patient-centered environment surrounding homeopathic treatment, it can be argued that there is a remarkable similarity between homeopathy and psychotherapy. If psychotherapy represents myriad nonspecific theories that prove beneficial to many patients, might it be that psychotherapy is little different from homeopathy, prayer, faith, desire, expectancy, and even the placebo response? Should this be the direction homeopathy and other CAM therapies need to pursue in the coming decades?

6

REASSESSMENT

Belief kills; belief heals. The beliefs held by persons in a society play a significant part in both disease causation and its remedy.

–Robert A. Hahn and Arthur Kleinman, "Belief as a Pathogen" (1983)

Given what has been presented in this study, several observations are worth noting. First and foremost is the fact that conventional biomedical research and practice fail to account for the full measure of human experience in health and disease. With approximately 80 percent of the world's population, including half the US population, using some form of CAM, the scientific community can no longer view these therapies as simply a fringe interest among consumers. However, because CAM therapies diverge sharply from reductionist science, the nature of their evidence and the subjective manner of their production create substantive problems for evidence-based medical knowledge. This suggests a remarkable similarity between CAM therapies and numerous nonspecific theories and practices such as psychotherapy that, although difficult to explain in terms of their modus operandi, have proven beneficial to patients. The current tension between conventional therapies and unconventional therapies represents a collision of epistemologies. For the former, disease causation constitutes the ideal form of evidence; for the latter, outcomes are of equal or greater importance. In our postmodern world, multifactorial causation has become more accepted as doctors and medical researchers adopt a more integrative role for unconventional therapies—a road that neither is straight nor accompanied by clear markers.

As the usage of homeopathy, acupuncture, herbals, chiropractic, and other CAM modalities amply demonstrate, their poor performance in clinical trials have caused little or no diminution in their popularity. They remain robust in their claims and ever anxious to expand their therapeutic applications.[1] Even with increased consumer interest, however, only a small number of CAM therapies are expected to achieve legitimacy alongside conventional medicine. Unlike biomedicine, which is constantly justifying its existence through replication and evidence-based research, most CAM modalities have yet to prove their efficacy or replicability, standing firmly on a static set of principles and practices that appear to "work," albeit only marginally better than the placebo. To date, only a few have been able to build a scientific explanation for their efficacy. And for those that have achieved this status, the outcome has not always been to their benefit. The fact that the management of chronic disease constitutes 78 percent of medical expenditures in the United States explains why conventional medicine has been so aggressive in fighting CAM and, where possible, co-opting its more effective therapies.[2]

To the extent that CAM therapies choose to seek third-party approval, they can be expected to institute some degree of standardized training and professionalization. This translates into a need to demonstrate not only a sense of stability, but one of replication—the ultimate test of their working truths. But the issues don't end there. How is it, ask skeptics, that millions of Americans can still believe in meridians, crystals, auras, chakras, and water memory to cure disease? Worse still, how can those same individuals demand that the federal government spend taxpayer dollars to investigate modalities that defy the normative laws of science? Should there be a clear dividing line between biomedical and nonreductionist systems, or is this distinction determined by time, place, and attitude? How do CAM modalities use and abuse science? When is enough known to conclude that a practice is worthless? Do individuals have the right to demand that their health-care plans supply them with the therapy they desire? Should society be burdened with paying for treatments that are neither safe nor proven effective? Should druggists advise or caution purchasers concerning their choice of alternative medications? Is it really medicine if it has not been tested by the RCT? Will integration of EBM with alternative medicine enhance health care or simply appease patients or both? Should an evidence-based approval process be required for all CAM systems? Is there any substitute for science-based evaluation?

Overall, most CAM therapies have failed to meet the standards demanded of the evidence-based pyramid. Those few that have succeeded in achieving some degree of efficacy have done so with results that beg the question of whether they are equal to or more than what might be expected from the placebo effect alone. Most high-quality RCTs and meta-analyses of CAM therapies use such operative phrases as "safe but without clear evidence of benefit," "not enough evidence," "inadequate to allow any conclusion," "insufficient evidence," "the data do not allow firm conclusions," "further studies are recommended," "there is some evidence . . . but the results are not consistent," "can make no definitive statement," "currently no reliable evidence of benefit," and "more trials are required." In an environment where expense is no object, further research would perhaps be justified. In today's world, that luxury is less of an option.

Given that poor evidence is often worse than no evidence at all, CAM continues to fight a perennial uphill battle due to weak methodologies, small trials, and the lack of predetermined criteria for evaluating claims. It counters criticism by claiming to be a holistic, consumer-driven phenomenon whose therapeutic benefits occur at levels not always quantitatively measurable, setting it directly opposite EBM with its quantifiable, reproducible outcomes. Nevertheless, only those CAM therapies that reach beyond their rhetorical defenses are likely to achieve the same degree of legitimacy as conventional practice. Aside from issues with the evidence-based pyramid, the challenge remains for systems such as homeopathy, naturopathy, therapeutic touch, anthroposophy, and other unconventional therapies to show that their outcomes for patients are more than the result of words, symbols, ritual, tradition, insight, or transference.[3]

As noted in earlier chapters, most CAM proponents question the suitability of the RCT, but they do not uniformly rule out other forms of qualitative analysis using observational studies, ethnography, phenomenology, and interviewing techniques to bring forth information worthy of survey research and other data manipulation.[4] Some have suggested a biopsychosocial model rather than a strictly biomedical model of medicine to research the physical and psychical aspects of healing.[5] Nevertheless, until more replicable evidence is demonstrated utilizing these forms of modeling, CAM therapies will continue to be criticized for lack of scientific rigor.[6]

All of this begs the question whether CAM therapies should be considered a form of psychotherapy, chaplaincy, or other faith-based (paranormal) system of healing. There is good reason to suggest that most fall under the umbrella of the placebo effect and that their strength lies in symptom management and in personalized strategies for health promotion. In the area of normative science, however, most CAM therapies have yet to be persuasive. To the extent that they are intent on seeking greater legitimacy, they must as a matter of good public policy submit to evaluation. There is an obligation to balance the patient's right to medical pluralism with the public's right to safe and efficacious therapies.

By contrast, EBM continues to provide the most credible information for justifying a clinical practice. Nevertheless, its ultimate value remains uncertain because so much of what happens in a clinical trial fails to capture the various independent and related variables that intrude into the encounter. Beyond the shadow it casts from atop the evidence-based pyramid, the RCT remains an imperfect tool, lacking a touchstone on which its intentionality ultimately rests. Representative of so many possible variables, it lacks a core to give it solid identification. Calibrating the outcome of a medical procedure, including the efficacy of a pharmacologic treatment, defies prediction or certitude insofar as the organic side of the medicine tends to be infused with so many psychotherapeutic interventions, some of which are intended and others are hidden. This suggests that there has been an overestimation of the value of the RCT in resolving the challenges presented in clinical medicine. For this reason, more creative efforts are needed that compare "whole treatments" rather than just individualized components with which conventional medicine is most acquainted.

Given the complexity of the human organism, the question naturally arises whether evidence from the RCT can or should be the sole judge of the safety or efficacy of an intervention when other factors might intrude.[7] In other words, issues of clinical effectiveness and inference, causation and correlation, clinical judgment, and collective knowledge continue to challenge the RCT's claims. Outside the range of acceptable data-based evidence are numerous subjective factors (e.g., beliefs, ethics, language, education, training, politics, cultural biases, etc.) that demand sensitivity to a particular contextual environment operating parallel to the empirical model. The neglect of this environment undermines the logical deductions extracted from the data.[8] As Ted Kaptchuk explained, "Human subjectivity can undermine objectivity even under double-blind conditions."[9]

CAM's general failure to conform to the biomedical model does not necessitate its retreat from the field. The mind–body dualism has long overstayed its visit. Western science needs to advance beyond the current reductionist model to some blending of the subjective and social aspects of healing that includes the placebo. This will require conventional medicine to end its either–or reliance on the RCT. Equally important, both CAM and conventional medicine must spend less time generating arguments of mutual disparagement and look for new and different tools with which to understand the causal links to explain and treat disease and illness. Such a task is not easy, and getting there will probably be fraught with considerable error before it can provide a better approach for medical research.

In the interest of both reductionist science and CAM, the next decade must include the challenge of bringing together the polar entities of objectivity and subjectivity in some viable, observable, and replicable evidence-based system that will separate those belief systems that remain wedded to a priori laws and principles from those that can stand with biomedicine as partners in the nation's health-care system. The clinical encounter represents the nexus of biology, medicine, and meaning. Integral to this encounter will be the placebo in all its current and future guises. Franklin Miller and Ted Kaptchuk said it best in referring to the need to reconceptualize the placebo effect as "contextual healing," a phrase that emphasizes the connection between the clinical encounter and improvement in the patient's condition. "That aspect of healing that is produced, activated or enhanced by the context of the clinical encounter, as distinct from the specific efficacy of treatment interventions," they wrote, "is contextual healing."[10]

Making this argument for the integration of subjectivity and objectivity into the evidence-based pyramid does not negate past findings, nor does it rule out the role and purpose of the RCT and meta-analysis in the absence of a viable alternative. Until such integration is successfully accomplished, it remains in the skeptic's purview to question. Skepticism represents an ingrained agnosticism within the biomedical world. If the statistical outcome of an RCT demonstrates the efficacy of a CAM intervention, or if the difference between the intervention and the placebo shows little statistical variation, the skeptic sees the opportunity for making a reasoned judgment. Yet even with this information the skeptic understands the risk of the influence of expectation on findings, which can in turn lead to biased results. Blinding (concealment) is intended to eliminate bias, but its relevance varies with the circumstances, and it is not always possible because of different styles of patient management or the nature of the alternative therapies. If blinding is inadequate, results fail to be credible. Until now, reductionist medicine has remained the most trustworthy form of therapy due to its willingness to be subjected to the constant challenge of verifiability and replicability—an intense process of error detection in pursuit of some unifying (even if temporary) "truth" or "meaning." For sociologist Robert King Merton, author of the classic paper "Science and Technology in a Democratic Order" (1942), replication is the "norm of universality."[11] The authority behind reductionist medicine is in its persistent search for evidence of what is being asserted over periods of time. Nevertheless, biomedicine remains an uncertain science; for all its benefits, it carries a degree of unpredictability. Nietzsche once commented, "But science, spurred by its powerful illusion, speeds irresistibly towards its limits where its optimism, concealed in the essence of logic, suffers shipwreck."[12] Certainty remains illusive, and so practices, systems, assumptions, and research methods require continued verification and explanation.

Biomedicine, which is both theoretically and empirically based, justifies its legitimacy on the most current science and the healing effects of its therapies. It applies the methodological rigor of evidence-based testing as the basis of its admission into the world of reductionist science. This, its proponents argue, is what distinguishes science from nonscience. But science remains conceptually unsettled—and always will be. CAM therapies, in contrast, rely on their healing effects alone under the belief that, in the fullness of time, future science will ultimately explain what is now inexplicable. How different is this from religion, which explains the contradictions of life as issues answerable only in the afterlife? Both CAM therapies and religion have used this ratiocination to define their role as well as to close off debate. CAM's strength lies exactly where the torch of science fades, and that remains the conundrum facing the scientific world.

From the many contributors to this discussion, one learns to appreciate—as did William James, from whom we still have much to learn—that epistemologies that seem illogical and irreconcilable with normative science may nonetheless *work*. The question at hand is not only whether conventional and unconventional therapies can stand on their own self-authenticating authority, but whether it is possible to modify the context of these two opposing camps into something both can benefit from sharing. To date, there is no hard-wired connection, but the bridge between them is nowhere as long nor the chasm beneath them as deep as they once appeared.

APPENDIX: U.S. CENTERS FOR THE STUDY OF COMPLEMENTARY AND ALTERNATIVE MEDICINE

STATE	CENTER NAME	ADDRESS	SPECIALTY
Massachusetts	Center of Excellence for the Neuroimaging of Acupuncture Effects on Human Brain Activity	Massachusetts General Hospital	acupuncture
Oregon	Center of Excellence for Research on CAM Antioxidant Therapies	Linus Pauling Institute, Oregon State University	antioxidants
Louisiana	Botanicals and Metabolic Syndrome	Pennington Biomedical Research Center, Louisiana State University	botanicals
Illinois	Botanical Dietary Supplements for Women's Health	University of Illinois at Chicago	botanicals
Illinois	Botanical Estrogens: Mechanisms, Dose, and Target Tissues	University of Urbana Champaign	botanicals
Montana	CAM as Countermeasures Against Infectious and Inflammatory Disease	Montana State University	botanical and bacterial products

STATE	CENTER NAME	ADDRESS	SPECIALTY
Missouri	Center for Botanical Interaction Studies	University of Missouri	botonicals
South Carolina	Center for CAM Research on Autoimmune and Inflammatory Diseases	University of South Carolina	botanicals
Illinois	Center for Herbal Research on Colorectal Cancer	University of Chicago	botanicals
Arizona	Center for Phytomedicine Research	University of Arizona College of Pharmacy	botanicals
Missouri	International Center for Indigenous Phytotherapy Studies: HIV/AIDS, Secondary Infections, and Immune Modulation	University of Missouri at Columbia School of Medicine	phytotherapy
New York	Protective Roles of Grape-Derived Polyphenols in Alzheimer's Disease	Mount Sinai School of Medicine	botanicals
Minnesota	Trametes Versicolor-Induced Immunopotentiation	University of Minnesota	botanicals
California	UCLA Center for Excellence in Pancreatic Diseases	University of California at Los Angeles	botanicals
North Carolina	Wake Forest and Harvard Center for Botanical Lipids	Wake Forest University Health Sciences	botanicals
Iowa	Developmental Center for Clinical and Translational Science	Palmer College of Chiropractic	chiropractic

STATE	CENTER NAME	ADDRESS	SPECIALTY
Iowa, Kansas, New York	Mechanisms and Effects of Chiropractic Manipulation	Palmer College of Chiropractic	chiropractic
Pennsylvania	Center for Mechanisms Underlying Millimeter Wave Therapy	Temple University Commonwealth	millimeter wave theory
Oregon	Complementary/ Alternative Medicine: Expectancy and Outcome	Oregon Health and Science University	mind-body medicine
California	Metabolic and Immunologic Effects of Meditation	University of California at San Francisco	meditation
Wisconsin	Wisconsin Center for the Neuroscience and Psychophysiology of Meditation	University of Wisconsin at Madison	meditation
Texas, Arizona	Mechanisms of Osteopathic Manipulative Medicine	University of North Texas Health Science Center	osteopathic medicine
Maryland	Center for Arthritis and Traditional Chinese Medicine	Kernan Hospital	traditional Chinese medicine
Maryland	Functional Bowel Disorders in Chinese Medicine	Kernan Hospital	traditional Chinese medicine

NOTES

INTRODUCTION

1. Dean I. Radin, *The Conscious Universe: The Scientific Truth of Psychic Phenomena* (San Francisco: Harper Edge, 1997), 13–21. See also Thomas S. Hall, *Ideas of Life and Matter: Studies in the History of General Physiology, 600 B.C.–1900 A.D.*, 2 vols. (Chicago: University of Chicago Press, 1969); Christopher U. M. Smith, *The Problem of Life: An Essay in the Origins of Biological Thought* (New York: Wiley, 1976); Norman Kemp Smith, *New Studies in the Philosophy of Descartes* (London: Macmillan, 1952).

2. D. Stempel, "Angels of Reason: Science and Myth in the Enlightenment," *Journal of the History of Ideas* 36 (1975): 63–78; J. Roger, "The Mechanistic Conception of Life," in David C. Lindberg and Ronald L. Numbers, eds., *God and Nature: Historical Essays on the Encounter Between Christianity and Science* (Berkeley: University of California Press, 1986), 277–95; J. S. Haller Jr., "The Great Biological Problem: Vitalism, Materialism, and the Philosophy of Organism," *New York State Journal of Medicine* 86 (1986): 81–88. According to Anne Harrington, Descartes was not so much the raison d'être for the insensibilities of mind–body medicine as "more or less a symbol of modern errors, a foil against which modern champions of one or another story of mind–body integration express their nostalgia for a fantasized premodern past when we all were whole and integrated, mind and body." Anne Harrington, *The Cure Within: A History of Mind–Body Medicine* (New York: Norton, 2008), 21.

3. M. S. Goldstein et al., "Holistic Physicians: Implications for the Study of the Medical Profession," *Journal of Health and Social Behavior* 28 (1987): 103–19; M. S. Goldstein et al., "Holistic Doctors: Becoming a Non-traditional Medical Practitioner," *Urban Life* 14 (1986): 17–44.

4. Read John S. Haller Jr., *Swedenborg, Mesmer, and the Mind/Body Connection: The Roots of Complementary Medicine* (West Chester, PA: Swedenborg Foundation, 2010); Catherine L. Albanese, *A Republic of Mind and Spirit: A Cultural History of American Metaphysical Religion* (New Haven, CT: Yale University Press, 2007).

5. Haller, *Swedenborg, Mesmer, and the Mind/Body Connection*, 158–87. See also John S. Haller Jr., *American Medicine in Transition, 1840–1910* (Urbana: University of Illinois Press, 1981), *Medical Protestants: The Eclectics in American Medicine, 1825–1939* (Carbondale: Southern Illinois University Press, 1994), and *The People's Doctors: Samuel Thomson and the American Botanical Movement, 1790–1860* (Carbondale: Southern Illinois University Press, 2000).

6. Horatio W. Dresser, *The Spirit of the New Thought* (London: Harrap, 1917), 4–6; Robert Peel, *Health and Medicine in the Christian Science Tradition* (New York: Crossroad, 1988), 23–31, 45–54. Read also John S. Haller Jr., *The History of New Thought: From Mind-Cure to Positive-Thinking and the Prosperity Gospel* (West Chester, PA: Swedenborg Foundation, 2012); Albanese, *A Republic of Mind and Spirit*; C. Alan Anderson and Deborah G. Whitehouse, *New Thought: A Practical American Spirituality* (Bloomington, IN: self-published, 2002).

7. William James, *The Varieties of Religious Experience: A Study in Human Nature* (New York: Modern Library, 1902), 77–124.

8. Harrington, *The Cure Within*, 122–25. See also Herbert Benson, *The Relaxation Response* (New York: HarperTorch, 1975) and *The Mind/Body Effect* (New York: Berkley, 1979); Larry Dossey, *The Extraordinary Healing Power of Ordinary Things* (New York: Three Rivers Press, 2006) and *The Power of Premonitions* (New York: Dutton, 2009); and Bernie Siegel, *Love, Medicine, and Miracles: Lessons Learned About Self-Healing from a Surgeon's Experience with Exceptional Patients* (New York: HarperCollins, 1986).

9. A. K. Shapiro, "A Contribution to a History of the Placebo Effect," *Behavioral Science* 5 (1960): 109–35; J. W. Estes, "Medical Skills in Colonial New England," *New England Historical and Genealogical Register* 134 (1980): 259–75.

10. H. K. Beecher, "The Powerful Placebo," *Journal of the American Medical Association* (*JAMA*) 159 (1955), 1602–6.

11. J. A. Turner et al., "The Importance of Placebo Effects in Pain Treatment and Research," *JAMA* 271 (1994): 1609–14; C. R. B Joyce, "Placebos and Complementary Medicine," *Lancet* 334 (1994): 1279–81; V. M. S. Oh, "The Placebo Effect: Can We Use It Better?" *British Medical Journal* 309 (1994): 69–70.

12. James C. Whorton, *Nature Cures: The History of Alternative Medicine in America* (Oxford: Oxford University Press, 2002).

13. Norman Gevitz, ed., *Other Healers: Unorthodox in America* (Baltimore: Johns Hopkins University Press, 1988).

14. William Rothstein, *American Physicians of the Nineteenth Century: From Sects to Science* (Baltimore: Johns Hopkins University Press, 1972); Paul Starr, *The Social Transformation of American Medicine* (New York: Basic Books, 1982); John Harley Warner, *The Therapeutic Perspective: Medical Practice, Knowledge, and Identity in America, 1820–1885* (Cambridge, MA: Harvard University Press, 1986); Charles E. Rosenberg, ed., *No Other Gods: On Science and American Social Thought* (Baltimore: Johns Hopkins University Press, 1997).

15. Jeanne Daly, *Evidence-Based Medicine and the Search for a Science of Clinical Care* (Berkeley: University of California Press, 2005).

16. J. Rosser Matthews, *Quantification and the Quest for Medical Certainty* (Princeton, NJ: Princeton University Press, 1995).

17. Harry Marks, *Progress of Experiment: Science and Therapeutic Reform in the United States, 1900–1990* (New York: Cambridge University Press, 1997).

18. Read Marcia Angell, *The Truth About the Drug Companies: How They Deceive Us and What to Do About It* (New York: Random House, 2005); Jerome P. Kassirer, *On the Take: How Medicine's Complicity with Big Business Can Endanger Your Health* (New York: Oxford University Press, 2005); R. Smith, "Medical Journals and the Pharmaceutical Companies: Uneasy Bedfellows," *British Medical Journal* 326 (2003): 1202, and "Medical Journals Are an Extension of the Marketing Arm of Pharmaceutical Companies," *PLOS Med* 2 (2005): 1371; Fiona Godlee and Tom Jefferson, *Peer Review in Health Sciences* (London: BMJ Books, 2003); Ray Moynihan and Alan Cassels, *Selling Sickness: How the World's Biggest Pharmaceutical Companies Are Turning Us All Into Patients* (New York: Nation Books, 2005); Nortin M. Hadler, *Worried Sick: A Prescription for Health in an Overtreated America* (Chapel Hill: University of North Carolina Press, 2008); Ben Goldacre, *Bad Science* (London: Harper Perennial, 2009).

19. J. H. Warner, "'The Nature-Trusting Heresy': American Physicians and the Concept of the Healing Power of Nature in the 1850's and 1860's," *Perspectives in American History* 11 (1977–1978): 291–324; Arthur K. Shapiro and Elaine Shapiro, *The Powerful Placebo: From Ancient Priest to Modern Physician* (Baltimore: Johns Hopkins University Press, 1997) and *Ethical Controversies About the Use of Placebos, the Double-Blind, and Controlled Clinical Trials* (Cambridge, MA: Harvard University Press, 1997); Sissela Bok, *Lying: Moral Choice in Public and Private Life* (New York: Vintage, 1978).

20. Anne Harrington, ed., *The Placebo Effect: An Interdisciplinary Exploration* (Cambridge, MA: Harvard University Press, 1997).

21. Howard Spiro, *The Power of Hope: A Doctor's Perspective* (New Haven, CT: Yale University Press, 1998); W. Grant Thompson, *The Placebo Effect and Health: Combining Science with Compassionate Care* (Amherst, MA: Prometheus Books, 2005); Richard Kradin, *The Placebo Response and the Power of Unconscious Healing* (New York: Routledge, 2008); Ted J. Kaptchuk and Michael Croucher, *The Healing Arts: A Journey Through the Faces of Medicine* (London: Guild, 1986); Ted J. Kaptchuk, *The Web That Has No Weaver: Understanding Chinese Medicine* (Chicago: Contemporary Press, 2000).

22. Robert Burton, *The Anatomy of Melancholy* (1621), http://ebooks.adelaide.edu.au/b/burton/robert/melancholy/S1.2.3.html, accessed May 25, 2012; John Lukacs, *At the End of an Age* (New Haven, CT: Yale University Press, 2002); Irving Kirsch, *The Emperor's New Drugs: Exploding the Antidepressant Myth* (New York: Basic Books, 2010); Michel Foucault, *The Birth of the Clinic: An Archaeology of Medical Perception* (New York: Pantheon Books, 1973); Thomas Kuhn, *The Structure of Scientific Revolutions* (Chicago: University of Chicago Press, 1962); Susan Lederer, *Subjected to Science: Human Experimentation in*

America Before the Second World War (Baltimore: Johns Hopkins University Press, 1995); R. Barker Bausell, *Snake Oil Science: The Truth About Complementary and Alternative Medicine* (New York: Oxford University Press, 2007).

23. T. Kaptchuk, "Subjectivity and the Placebo Effect in Medicine: An Interview by Bonnie Horrigan," *Alternative Therapies* 7 (2001): 108.

24. L. Dossey, "How Should Alternative Therapies Be Evaluated? An Examination of Fundamentals," *Alternative Therapies in Health and Medicine* 1 (1995): 6; C. J. Schneider and W. B. Jonas, "Are Alternative Treatments Effective? Issues and Methods Involved in Measuring Effectiveness of Alternative Treatments," *Subtle Energies* 5 (1994): 69; L. A. Moye et al., "Research Methodology in Psychoneuroimmunology: Rationale and Design of the IMAGES-P Clinical Trial," *Alternative Therapies in Health and Medicine* 1 (1995): 34.

25. I. Smith, "Commissioning Complementary Medicine," *British Medical Journal* 310 (1995): 1151. See also T. A. Sheldon, "Please Bypass the PORT," *British Medical Journal* 309 (1994): 142–43.

1. EVIDENCE-BASED MEDICINE

1. Abraham Flexner, *Medical Education in the United States and Canada: A Report to the Carnegie Foundation on the Advancement of Teaching* (New York: Carnegie Foundation, 1910), 156.

2. As late as 1900, there were estimates of 8,000 to 10,000 eclectics and a comparable number of homeopaths, along with smaller numbers of other sectarians practicing their respective systems of healing among the 117,749 physicians self-identified in the US Census. See US Department of Commerce, *Historical Statistics of the United States: Colonial Times to 1970*, vol. 2: *Work and Welfare* (Washington, DC: US Department of Commerce, 1975), 541. According to a survey taken in 1894, regulars numbered 72,028; eclectics, 10,292; homeopaths, 9,648; and physios, 1,553. See "Statistics," *Eclectic Medical Journal* 54 (1894): 396; R. G. Leland, *Distribution of Physicians in the United States* (Chicago: American Medical Association, 1936), 7. Read also William G. Rothstein, *American Physicians in the Nineteenth Century: From Sects to Science* (Baltimore: Johns Hopkins University Press, 1972), 305–26; William G. Rothstein, *American Medical Schools and the Practice of Medicine: A History* (New York: Oxford University Press, 1987); W. I. Wardwell, "Alternative Medicine in the United States," *Social Science and Medicine* 31 (1994): 913–23; John S. Haller Jr., *Sectarian Reformers in American Medicine, 1800–1910* (New York: AMS Press, 2011), *The History of American Homeopathy: The Academic Years, 1820–1935* (New York: Haworth Press, 2005), and *Kindly Medicine: Physio-medicalism in America, 1836–1911* (Kent, OH: Kent State University Press, 1997).

3. J. B. McKinlay and L. D. Marceau, "The End of the Golden Age of Doctoring," *International Journal of the Health Sciences* 32 (2002): 379–416; R. L. Numbers, "The Fall and Rise of the American Medical Profession," in Nathan O. Hatch, ed., *The Professions in Ameri-*

can History (Notre Dame, IN: University of Notre Dame Press, 1985), 57–67; J. H. Warner, "Ideals of Science and Their Discontents in Late 19th Century American Medicine," *Isis* 82 (1991): 454–78. See also John Harley Warner, *The Therapeutic Perspective: Medical Practice, Knowledge, and Identity in America, 1820–1885* (Cambridge, MA: Harvard University Press, 1986); Rosemary Stevens, *American Medicine and the Public Interest: A History of Specialization* (New Haven, CT: Yale University Press, 1971); Kenneth M. Ludmerer, *Learning to Heal: The Development of American Medical Education* (New York: Basic Books, 1985); Richard H. Shryock, *Medical Licensing in America, 1650–1965* (Baltimore: Johns Hopkins University Press, 1967); Charles E. Rosenberg and Morris J. Vogel, eds., *The Therapeutic Revolution: Essays in the Social History of American Medicine* (Philadelphia: University of Pennsylvania Press, 1979); Andrew Cunningham and Perry Williams, eds., *The Laboratory Revolution in Medicine* (Cambridge: Cambridge University Press, 1992).

4. William Osler, *The Principles and Practice of Medicine* (New York: Appleton, 1892). See P. J. Edelson, "Adopting Osler's Principles: Medical Textbooks in American Medical Schools, 1891–1906," *Bulletin of the History of Medicine* 68 (1994): 67–84.

5. Some sixty-nine eclectic colleges were organized in the United States, twenty-six before 1860, thirty-two during the remainder of the century, and eleven in the early twentieth century. The last of the eclectic colleges closed its doors in 1939. The schools eschewed theories and dogmas, preferring an approach to medical therapeutics that was cumulative, drawing from all theories and practices that proved beneficial and using only those therapies that best served the needs of the patient. Over time, however, the schools settled on a more nativistic approach consisting of herbal medicines as substitutes for mineral-based drugs, a distrust of foreign influences, and a distinctly democratic approach to education. See Haller, *Sectarian Reformers in American Medicine*, 88–91.

6. Council on Medical Education, "New Policy of the American Medical Association on Medical Education," http://www.ncbi.nlm.nih.gov/pmc/articles/PMC1759914/pdf/calwestmed00405-0067b.pdf, accessed July 19, 2011.

7. T. A. Winnick, "From Quackery to 'Complementary' Medicine: The American Medical Profession Confronts Alternative Therapies," *Social Problems* 52 (2005): 40.

8. D. C. Swain, "The Rise of a Research Empire: NIH, 1930–1950," *Science* 138 (1962): 1233–37. See also Stevens, *American Medicine and the Public Interest*; Joseph D. Bronzino, Vincent H. Smith, and Maurice L. Wade, *Medical Technology and Society* (Cambridge, MA: MIT Press, 1990); Richard H. Shryock, *American Medical Research, Past and Present* (New York: Commonwealth Fund, 1947); Harry M. Marks, *The Progress of Experiment: Science and Therapeutic Reform in the United States, 1900–1990* (New York: Cambridge University Press, 1997); George W. Corner, *A History of the Rockefeller Institute, 1901–1953: Origins and Growth* (New York: Rockefeller Institute Press, 1965).

9. Read Edward Shorter, *Bedside Manners: The Troubled History of Doctors and Patients* (New York: Simon and Schuster, 1985).

10. Charles Rosenberg, *The Care of Strangers: The Rise of America's Hospital System* (New York: Basic Books, 1987), 166–89, 348; G. Laderman, "The Cult of Doctors: Harvey Cushing and

the Religious Culture of Modern Medicine," *Journal of Religion and Health* 45 (2006): 533–48. See also R. Stevens, "The Curious Career of Internal Medicine: Functional Ambivalence, Social Success," in Russell C. Maulitz and Diana E. Long, eds., *Grand Rounds: One Hundred Years of Internal Medicine* (Philadelphia: University of Pennsylvania Press, 1988), 339–64.

11. Claude Bernard, *An Introduction to the Study of the Experimental Method* (New York: Dover, 1957); William Coleman and Frederick Holmes, eds., *The Investigative Enterprise: Experimental Physiology in 19th Century Medicine* (Berkeley: University of California Press, 1988); Charles Rosenberg, *No Other Gods: On Science and American Social Thought* (1976; reprint, Baltimore: Johns Hopkins University Press, 1997); Bruno Latour, *Laboratory Life: The Social Construction of Scientific Facts* (Beverly Hills, CA: Sage, 1979); Peter Achinstein and Owen Hannaway, eds., *Observation, Experiment, and Hypothesis in Modern Physical Science* (Cambridge, MA: MIT Press, 1955); Marks, *The Progress of Experiment*, 17–41; G. L. Geison, "Divided We Stand: Physiologists and Clinicians in the American Context," in Rosenberg and Vogel, eds., *The Therapeutic Revolution*, 67–90.

12. C. Rosenberg, "The Therapeutic Revolution: Medicine, Meaning, and Social Change in 19th Century America," in Rosenberg and Vogel, eds., *The Therapeutic Revolution*, 3–25; P. Beeson, "Changes in Medical Therapy During the Past Half Century," *Medicine* 59 (1980): 79–99. See also Karin D. Knorr-Cetina and Michael Mulkay, eds., *Science Observed: Perspectives on the Social Study of Science* (London: Sage, 1983); Lewis Thomas, *The Youngest Science: Notes of a Medicine Watcher* (New York: Viking Press, 1983).

13. J. Rosser Matthews, *Quantification and the Quest for Medical Certainty* (Princeton, NJ: Princeton University Press, 1995), 10–13, 86–130.

14. J. P. Bull, "The Historical Development of Clinical Therapeutic Trials," *Journal of Chronic Diseases* 10 (1959): 218–48.

15. Ted Kaptchuk notes confusion and inaccuracy in Abraham M. Lilienfeld's article "*Ceteris paribus:* The Evolution of the Clinical Trial," *Bulletin of the History of Medicine* 56 (1982): 1–18; see T. Kaptchuk, "Intentional Ignorance: A History of Blind Assessment and Placebo Controls in Medicine," *Bulletin of the History of Medicine* 72 (1998): 389–433. See also J. P. Bull, "The Historical Development of Clinical Therapeutic Trials," *Journal of Chronic Diseases* 10 (1959): 218–48; M. D. Rawlins, "Development of a Rational Practice of Therapeutics," *British Medical Journal* 301 (1990): 729–33; Scott H. Podolsky, *Pneumonia Before Antibiotics: Therapeutic Evolution and Evaluation in Twentieth Century America* (Baltimore: Johns Hopkins University Press, 2006), 147–49; Ian Hacking, *The Taming of Chance* (Cambridge: Cambridge University Press, 1990).

16. Edward Kremers and George Urdang, *The History of Pharmacy* (Philadelphia: Lippincott, 1963), 4–5; Pierre Charles Alexandre Louis, *Researches on the Effects of Bloodletting in Some Inflammatory Diseases and on the Influence of Tartarized Antimony and Vesication in Pneumonitis* (Boston: Hilliard, Gray, 1836) (interestingly, Louis did not compare patients who underwent venesection and those who did not, but rather those bled early rather than those bled late in their treatment); Ulrich Tröhler, "Quantification in British Medicine and Surgery, 1750–1830, with Special Reference to Its Introduction Into Thera-

peutics," PhD diss., University of London, 1978; Matthews, *Quantification and the Quest for Medical Certainty*; Michael J. Cullen, *The Statistical Movement in Early Victorian Britain: The Foundations of Empirical Social Research* (New York: Barnes and Noble, 1975); Abraham Lilienfeld, ed., *Times, Places, and Persons: Aspects of the History of Epidemiology* (Baltimore: Johns Hopkins University Press, 1980); Lorenz Krüger, Gerd Gigerenzer, and Mary S. Morgan, eds., *The Probabilistic Revolution*, vol. 2: *Ideas in the Sciences* (Cambridge, MA: MIT Press, 1987); Theodore M. Porter, *The Rise of Statistical Thinking, 1820–1900* (Princeton, NJ: Princeton University Press, 1986); British Parliamentary Papers, *Reports on the Epidemics of 1854 and 1856 and Other Reports on Cholera with Appendices 1854–96. Report on the Results of the Different Methods of Treatment Pursued in Epidemic Cholera* (Shannon: Irish University Press, 1970), 657–84; Lorraine J. Daston, *Classical Probability in the Enlightenment* (Princeton, NJ: Princeton University Press, 1988); John E. Lesch, *Science and Medicine in France: The Emergence of Experimental Physiology, 1790–1855* (Cambridge, MA: Harvard University Press, 1984), 100–165.

17. I. P. Semmelweis, "The Etiology, the Concept, and the Prophylaxis of Childbed Fever," *Medical Classics* 5 (1941): 350–734.

18. P. Greenwald et al., "Vaginal Cancer After Maternal Treatment with Synthetic Estrogens," *New England Journal of Medicine* 285 (1971): 390.

19. L. E. Moses, "The Series of Consecutive Cases as a Device for Assessing Outcomes of Interventions," in John C. Bailar and Frederick Mosteller, eds., *Medical Uses of Statistics* (Waltham, MA: New England Journal of Medicine Books, 1992), 125; Kenneth W. Goodman, *Ethics and Evidence-Based Medicine: Fallibility and Responsibility in Clinical Science* (Cambridge: Cambridge University Press, 2003), 33; N. E. Breslow, "Statistics in Epidemiology: The Case–Control Study," *Journal of the American Statistical Association* 91 (1996): 14–28; Norman E. Breslow and Nicholas E. Day, *Statistical Methods in Cancer Research I: The Analysis of Case–Control Studies* (Lyon, France: International Agency for Research on Cancer, 1980).

20. J. P. Bunker, *The National Halothane Study: Report of the Subcommittee on the National Halothane Study of the Committee on Anesthesia, Division of the Medical Sciences, National Academy of Sciences—National Research Council* (Washington, DC: US Government Printing Office, 1969).

21. "Retrospective Studies," in Samuel Kotz, Norman L. Johnson, and Campbell B. Read, eds., *Encyclopedia of Statistical Science*, 16 vols. (New York: Wiley, 1982), 8:120; R. B. D'Agostino and H. Kwan, "Measuring Effectiveness: What to Expect Without a Randomized Control Group," *Medical Care* 33 (1995), 100; C. R. Weinberg and S. Wacholder, "The Design and Analysis of Case–Control Studies with Biased Sampling," *Biometrics* 46 (1990): 963; N. E. Breslow and W. Powers, "Are There Two Logistic Regressions from Retrospective Studies?" *Biometrics* 34 (1978): 100; N. Mantel and W. Haenszel, "Statistical Aspects of the Analysis of Data from Retrospective Studies of Disease," *Journal of the National Cancer Institute* 22 (1959): 719–48. See also "Link Between Hair Loss and Treatment Success?" http://altmed.creighton.edu/HIV/retrovspro.htm, accessed May 29, 2012.

22. "Historical Control," in Kotz, Johnson, and Read, eds., *Encyclopedia of Statistical Science*, 2:13; "Clinical Trials," in Kotz, Johnson, and Read, eds., *Encyclopedia of Statistical Science*, 2:640; R. Micciolo, P. Valagussa, and E. Marubini, "The Use of Historical Controls in Breast Cancer," *Controlled Clinical Trials* 6 (1985): 259; E. A. Gehan, "The Evaluation of Therapies: Historical Control Studies," *Statistics in Medicine* 3 (1984): 315–24; L. E. Moses, "Statistical Concepts Fundamental to Investigations," in Bailar and Mosteller, eds., *Medical Uses of Statistics*, 5.

23. S. M. McKinlay, "The Design and Analysis of the Observational Study: A Review," *Journal of the American Statistical Association* 70 (1975): 503; "Observational Studies," in Kotz, Johnson, and Read, eds., *Encyclopedia of Statistical Science*, 6:397; W. G. Cochran, "The Planning of Observational Studies of Human Populations," *Journal of the Royal Statistical Society: Series A* (1965): 234; R. Doll, "Proof of Causality: Deduction from Epidemiological Observation," *Perspectives in Biology and Medicine* 45 (2002): 499–515.

24. "Prospective Studies," in Kotz, Johnson, and Read, eds., *Encyclopedia of Statistical Science*, 7:315; M. Olschewski, M. Schumacher, and K. B. Davis, "Analysis of Randomized and Nonrandomized Patients in Clinical Trials Using the Comprehensive Cohort Follow-up Study Design," *Controlled Clinical Trials* 13 (1992): 226. See also Brian MacMahon, Thomas F. Pugh, and Johanes Ipsen, *Epidemiologic Methods* (Boston: Little, Brown, 1960).

25. Alison Lingo, "Empirics and Charlatans in Early Modern France: The Genesis of the Classification of 'Other' in Medical Practice," *Journal of Social History* 19 (1986): 583–604. Read also Robert C. Fuller, *Mesmerism and the American Cure of Souls* (Philadelphia: University of Pennsylvania Press, 1982); Robert Darnton, *Mesmerism and the End of the Enlightenment* (Cambridge, MA: Harvard University Press, 1968); Joseph P. F. Deleuze, *Practical Instructions in Animal Magnetism* (New York: Wells, 1843); Charles Poyen, *Progress of Animal Magnetism in New England* (Boston: Weeks, Jordan, 1837); Franz Anton Mesmer, *Mesmerism: A Translation of the Original Scientific and Medical Writings of F. A. Mesmer*, comp. and trans. George J. Bloch (Los Angeles: Kaufmann, 1980).

26. Kaptchuk, "Intentional Ignorance"; C-A. Lopez, "Franklin and Mesmer: An Encounter," *Yale Journal of Biology and Medicine* 66 (1993): 325–31. See also Vladimir A. Gheorghiu and Klaus Fiedler, eds., *Suggestion and Suggestibility: Theory and Research* (Heidelberg, Germany: Springer, 1989); Mark A. Best, Duncan Neuhauser, and Lee Slaven, eds., *Benjamin Franklin: Verification and Validation of the Scientific Process in Health Care as Demonstrated by the "Report of the Royal Commissioner on Animal Magnetism and Mesmerism"* (Victoria, Canada: Trafford, 2003).

27. R. Barker Bausell, *Snake Oil Science: The Truth About Complementary and Alternative Medicine* (New York: Oxford University Press, 2007), 33.

28. Read Alan Gaud, *A History of Hypnotism* (Cambridge: Cambridge University Press, 1992); Jan Ehrenwald, *The History of Psychotherapy: From Magic Healing to Encounter* (New York: Aronson, 1976); Donald K. Freedheim, *History of Psychotherapy: A Century of Change* (Washington, DC: American Psychological Association, 1992); John C. Norcross, Gary H. R. Vanden Bos, and Donald K. Freedheim, *History of Psychotherapy: Continuity*

and Change (Washington, DC: American Psychological Association, 2011); Philip Gushman, *Constructing the Self, Constructing America: A Cultural History of Psychotherapy* (Boston: Addison-Wesley, 1995).

29. W. Guy, "On the Value of the Numerical Method as Applied to Science, but Especially to Physiology and Medicine," *Journal of the Royal Statistical Society* 2 (1839): 26–38; J. H. Warner, "Therapeutic Explanation and the Edinburgh Bloodletting Controversy: Two Perspectives on the Medical Meaning of Science in the Mid-19th Century," *Medical History* 24 (1980): 241–58; J. S. Haller Jr., "The Decline of Bloodletting: A Study in 19th Century Ratiocinations," *Southern Medical Journal* 79 (April 1986): 469–75; J. S. Haller Jr., "The Use and Abuse of Tartar Emetic in the 19th Century Materia Medica," *Bulletin of the History of Medicine* 49 (1975): 235–57; J. S. Haller Jr., "Samson of the Materia Medica: Medical Theory and the Use and Abuse of Calomel in 19th Century America," *Pharmacy in History* 12 (1971): 27–34, 67–76. See also James H. Cassedy, *American Medicine and Statistical Thinking, 1800–1860* (Cambridge, MA: Harvard University Press, 1984), chap. 3, and *Medicine and American Growth, 1800–1860* (Madison: University of Wisconsin Press, 1986); Erwin H. Ackerknecht, *Medicine at the Paris Hospital, 1794–1848* (Baltimore: Johns Hopkins University Press, 1967); Matthews, *Quantification and the Quest for Medical Certainty*, 8–38; Stephen M. Stigler, *The History of Statistics: The Measurement of Uncertainty Before 1900* (Cambridge, MA: Harvard University Press, 1986); Charles Bartlett, *An Essay on the Philosophy of Medical Science* (Philadelphia: Lea and Blanchard, 1844).

30. "Homeopathic Organization," *American Homeopathic Review* 6 (1865–66): 394; Haller, *The History of American Homeopathy: The Academic Years*, 111–20.

31. Dr. F. W. Irvine, "M. Andral's Homeopathic Experiments at La Pitié," in William Henderson, *Homeopathy Fairly Represented: A Reply to Professor Simpson's "Homeopathy" Misrepresented* (Philadelphia: Lindsay and Blakiston, 1854), appendix, 289–91, 295–98; "Statistics of Homeopathic and Allopathic Hospitals," *North American Journal of Homeopathy* 13 (1865): 516–21; "Hospital Reports," *North American Journal of Homeopathy* 4 (1855): 293–98; J. Hooper, "Homeopathy: What Are Its Claims on Public Confidence?" *American Homeopathic Observer* 3 (1866): 87; "Homeopathic Statistics," *North American Homeopathic Journal* 3 (1853): 146; Haller, *The History of American Homeopathy: The Academic Years*, 93–120. See also Jean-Paul Tessier, *Clinical Researches Concerning the Homeopathic Treatment of Asiatic Cholera. Preceded by a Review on the Abuse of the Numerical Method in Medicine* (New York: Radde, 1855).

32. A. Trousseau, "Expériences homéopathiques tentées a l'Hôtel-Dieu de Paris," *Journal des Connaissances Médico-Chirurgicales 8 (1834): 238–41*; M. E. Dean, "A Homeopathic Origin for Placebo Controls: 'An Invaluable Gift of God,' " *Alternative Therapies in Health and Medicine* 6 (2000): 58–66. See also Jean-Paul Tessier, *Lectures on Clinical Medicine, Delivered in the Hospital Saint-Jacques, of Paris* (London: New Sydenham Society, 1872).

33. G. Rankin, "Professional Organization and the Development of Medical Knowledge: Two Interpretations of Homeopathy," in Roger Cooter, ed., *Studies in the History of Alternative Medicine* (New York: St Martin's Press, 1988), 46–62.

34. Sir John Forbes, *Homeopathy, Allopathy, and Young Physic* (New York: Radde, 1846), 17.

35. John S. Haller Jr., *Swedenborg, Mesmer, and the Mind/Body Connection: The Roots of Complementary Medicine* (West Chester, PA: Swedenborg Foundation, 2010), 152–57. Read also R. Laurence Moore, *In Search of White Crows: Spiritualism, Parapsychology, and American Culture* (New York: Oxford University Press, 1977); Janet Oppenheim, *The Other World: Spiritualism and Psychical Research in England, 1850–1914* (Cambridge: Cambridge University Press, 1985); and James McClenon, *Deviant Science: The Case of Parapsychology* (Philadelphia: University of Pennsylvania Press, 1984).

36. Matthews, *Quantification and the Quest for Medical Certainty*, 62–85. See also Bernard, *An Introduction to the Study of Experimental Medicine*; Stanley Joel Reiser, *Medicine and the Reign of Technology* (Cambridge: Cambridge University Press, 1978); Carl Auguste Wunderlich, *On the Temperature in Diseases: A Manual of Medical Thermometry* (London: New Sydenham Society, 1871); Gustav Radicke, *On the Importance and Value of Arithmetic Means* (London: New Sydenham Society, 1861).

37. A. Flint, "A Contribution Toward the Natural History of Articular Rheumatism; Consisting of a Report of Thirteen Cases Treated Solely with Palliative Measures," *American Journal of Medical Science* 46 (1862): 17–36.

38. C. E. Brown-Séquard, "Notes on the Effect Produced on Man by Subcutaneous Injections of a Liquid Obtained from the Testicles of Animals," *Lancet* 2 (1889): 105–7; Merriley Bonell, "Brown-Séquard's Organotherapy and Its Appearance in America at the End of the 19th Century," *Bulletin of the History of Medicine* 50 (1976): 309–20.

39. E. Behring, O. Boer, and H. Kossel, "Zur Behandlung Diphtheriekranker Menschen mit Diphtherieheil-Serum," *Deutsche Medizinische Wochenschrift* 19 (1893): 399–418; J. Fibiger, "Om Serumbehandling af difteri," *Hospitalstidende* 6 (1898): 309–25; A. Hróbjartsson, P. C. Gøtzsche, and C. Gluud, "The Controlled Clinical Trial Turns 100 Years: Fibiger's Trial of Serum Treatment of Diphtheria," *British Medical Journal* 317 (1998): 1243–45.

40. E. G. Boring, "The Nature and History of Experimental Control," *American Journal of Psychology* 67 (1954): 573. See also E. L. Thorndike and R. S. Woodworth, "The Influence of Improvement in One Mental Function Upon the Efficiency of Other Functions," *Psychological Review* 8 (1901): 247–61, 384–95, 553–64; E. L. Thorndike, "A Note on the Specialization of Mental Functions with Varying Content," *Journal of Philosophy, Psychology, and Scientific Methods* 6 (1909): 239–40.

41. W. H. Winch, "The Transfer of Improvement of Memory in School-Children," *British Journal of Psychology* 2 (1908): 284–93.

42. D. I. Macht, N. B. Herman, and C. S. Levy, "A Quantitative Study of the Analgesic Produced by Opium Alkaloids, Individually and in Combination with Each Other, in Normal Man," *Journal of Pharmacology and Experimental Therapeutics* 8 (1916): 1–37; D. I. Macht, "Contributions to the Phytopharmacology or the Applications of Plant Physiology to Medical Problems," *Science* 71 (1930): 302–6.

43. U. Tröhler, "Adolf Bingel's Blinded, Controlled Comparison of Different Anti-diphtheritic Sera in 1918," James Lind Library, http://www.jameslindlibrary.org/illustrating/

articles/adolf-bingels-bl, accessed September 3, 2012; Medical Research Council Therapeutic Trials Committee, "The Serum Treatment of Lobar Pneumonia," *British Medical Journal* 1 (1934): 241–45; P. P. De Deyn and R. D'Hooge, "Placebos in Clinical Practice and Research," *Journal of Medical Ethics* 22 (1996): 140–46; S. H. Podolsky and G. Davey Smith, "Park's Story and Winters' Tale: Alternate Allocation Clinical Trials in Turn of the Century America," James Lind Library, http://www.jameslindlibrary.org/illustrating/articles/parks-story-and-winters-tale-alternate-allocation-clinica, accessed May 30, 2012; Kaptchuk, "Intentional Ignorance," 420–21.

44. Medical Research Council Therapeutic Trials Committee, "The Serum Treatment of Lobar Pneumonia," 241–45; Medical Research Council Patulin Trials Committee, "Clinical Trial of Patulin in the Common Cold," *Lancet* 2 (1944): 373–74.

45. Matthews, *Quantification and the Quest for Medical Certainty*, 115–40; Podolsky, *Pneumonia Before Antibiotics*, 22–23, 35–37. See also Ronald A. Fisher, *Statistical Methods for Research Workers*, 14th ed. (Edinburgh: Oliver and Boyd, 1970), and *The Design of Experiments* (1935; reprint, London: Hafner, 1966); Austin Bradford Hill, *Principles of Medical Statistics* (1937; reprint, New York: Oxford University Press, 1971).

46. For examples of randomization, see R. A. Fisher and W. A. Mackenzie, "Studies in Crop Variation: II. The Manurial Response of Different Potato Varieties," *Journal of Agricultural Science* 13 (1923): 315; J. Burnes Amberson Jr., B. T. McMahon, and M. Pinner, "A Clinical Trial of Sanocrysin in Pulmonary Tuberculosis," *American Review of Tuberculosis* 24 (1931): 401–35.

47. J. B. Hill, "The Clinical Trial," *New England Journal of Medicine* 247 (1952): 113–19; Otho B. Ross Jr., "Use Controls in Medical Research," *JAMA* 145 (1951): 72–75; T. C. Chalmers, "Randomization of the First Patient," *Medical Clinics of North America* 59 (1975): 1035–38. See also H. Marks, "Notes from the Underground: The Social Organization of Therapeutic Research," in Maulitz and Long, eds., *Grand Rounds*, 297–336; David Sackett, R. Bryan Haynes, and Peter Tugwell, *Clinical Epidemiology: A Basic Science for Clinical Medicine* (Boston: Little, Brown, 1985).

48. Goodman, *Ethics and Evidence-Based Medicine*, 1–23.

49. Medical Research Council Whooping-Cough Immunization Committee, "The Prevention of Whooping-Cough by Vaccination," *British Medical Journal* 1 (1951): 1463–71. Read also R. A. Fisher, "The Arrangement of Field Experiments," *Journal of the Ministry of Agriculture* 33 (1926): 503–13; Hill, *Principles of Medical Statistics*.

50. Medical Research Council Streptomycin in Tuberculosis Trials Committee, "Streptomycin Treatment for Pulmonary Tuberculosis," *British Medical Journal* 2 (1948): 769–82; A. Yoshioka, "Use of Randomization in the Medical Research Council's Clinical Trial of Streptomycin in Pulmonary Tuberculosis in the 1940s," *British Medical Journal* 317 (1998): 1220–23; A. B. Hill, "Memories of the British Streptomycin Trial in Tuberculosis," *Controlled Clinical Trials* 1 (1990): 77–79.

51. I. Chalmers, "Why Transition from Alternation to Randomization in Clinical Trials Was Made," *British Medical Journal* 319 (1999): 1372.

52. J. D. Ratcliff, "New Surgery for Ailing Hearts," *Reader's Digest* 71 (1957): 70–73; L. A. Cobb et al., "An Evaluation of Internal-Mammary-Artery Ligation by a Double-Blind Technique," *New England Journal of Medicine* 260 (1959): 1115–18; E. G. Diamond, C. F. Kittle, and J. E. Crockett, "Evaluation of Internal Mammary Artery Ligation and Sham Procedure in Angina Pectoris," *Circulation* 18 (1958): 712–13.

53. H. K. Beecher, "Surgery as Placebo: A Quantitative Study of Bias," *JAMA* 1876 (1961): 1102–7; S. H. Podolsky, "Quintessential Beecher: 'Surgery as Placebo: A Quantitative Study of Bias,' *J Am Med Assoc.* 1961; 176:1102–07," *International Anesthesiology Clinics* 45 (2007): 47.

54. David L. Sackett, R. Bryan Haynes, and Gordon Guyatt, *Evidence-Based Medicine: How to Practice and Teach EBM* (New York: Churchill-Livingstone, 1997), 94.

55. S. Senn, "Are Placebo Run Ins Justified?" *British Medical Journal* 314 (1997): 1191; see also B. Freedman, "Placebo-Controlled Trials and the Logic of Clinical Purpose," *IRB: A Review of Human Subjects Research* 12 (1996): 1–6.

56. Steven S. Coughlin and Tom L. Beauchamp, *Ethics and Epidemiology* (Oxford: Oxford University Press, 1996); S. Yusuf, R. Collins, and R. Peto, "Why Do We Need Some Large, Simple Randomized Trials?" *Statistics in Medicine* 3 (1984): 971–80; Jonathan Baron, *Thinking and Deciding*, 3rd ed. (Cambridge: Cambridge University Press, 2000); David M. Eddy, *Clinical Decision Making: From Theory to Practice* (Boston: Jones and Bartlett, 1996); B. J. Cohen, "Is Expected Utility Theory Normative for Clinical Decision Making?" *Medical Decision Making* 16 (1996): 1–6; M. D. Cabana et al., "Why Don't Physicians Follow Clinical Practice Guidelines? A Framework for Improvement," *JAMA* 282 (1999): 1458–65.

57. M. Enserink, "Can the Placebo Be the Cure?" *Science* 284 (1999): 238–40. Interestingly, in the MK-869 trial, Merck included an established Prozac-generation drug that also failed to surpass the placebo.

58. H. K. Benson and D. P. McCallie Jr., "Angina Pectoris and the Placebo Effect," *New England Journal of Medicine* 300 (1979): 1424–29. See also A. H. Roberts et al., "The Power of Nonspecific Effects in Healing: Implications for Psychosocial and Biological Treatments," *Clinical Psychological Review* 13 (1993): 375–91.

59. H. Steele, "The Fortunes of Economic Reform Legislation: The Case of the Drug Amendments Act of 1962," *American Journal of Economics and Sociology* 25 (1966): 39–51. See also *Study of Administered Prices in the Drug Industry, Report of the Subcommittee on Antitrust and Monopoly of the Senate Judiciary Committee, Pursuant to Senate Resolution 52, Eighty-Seventh Congress, First Session* (Washington, DC: US Government Printing Office, 1961); *Drug Amendments of 1962: Conference Report, No. 2526, House of Representatives, Eighty-Seventh Congress, Second Session* (Washington, DC: US Government Printing Office, 1962).

60. R. E. Ferer, "The Influence of Big Pharma: Wide Ranging Report Identifies Many Areas of Influence and Distortion," *British Medical Journal* 330 (2005): 855–56; House of Commons Health Committee, *The Influence of the Pharmaceutical Industry*, http://www.parliament.the-stationary-office.co.uk/pa/cm200405, accessed September 4, 2012; B. Agnew, "Ahen Pharma Merges, R&D Is the Dowry," *Science* 287 (2000): 1952–53. Read

also Marcia Angell, *The Truth About the Drug Companies: How They Deceive Us and What to Do About It* (New York: Random House, 2004); Jerome P. Kassirer, *On the Take: How Medicine's Complicity with Big Business Can Endanger Your Health* (New York: Oxford University Press, 2005); Jerry Avorn, *Powerful Medicines: The Benefits, Risks, and Costs of Prescription Drugs* (New York: Knopf, 2004).

61. Richard L. Kradin, *The Placebo Response and the Power of Unconscious Healing* (New York: Routledge, 2008): 76; Jackie Law, *Big Pharma* (New York: Carroll and Graff, 2006), 70; Gerald N. Grob and Allan V. Horwitz, *Diagnosis, Therapy, and Evidence: Conundrums in Modern American Medicine* (New Brunswick, NJ: Rutgers University Press, 2010), 2, 11, 96

62. J. Worrall, "What Evidence in Evidence-Based Medicine?" *Philosophy of Science* 69 (2002): 319.

63. J. W. Tukey, "Some Thoughts on Clinical Trials, Especially Problems of Multiplicity," *Science* 52 (1977): 679.

64. S. M. Gore, "Assessing Clinical Trials—Why Randomize?" *British Medical Journal* 282 (1981): 1958.

65. Read Archie L. Cochrane, *Effectiveness and Efficiency: Random Reflections on Health Services* (London: Nuffield Provincial Hospitals Trust, 1972); Thomas McKeown, *The Role of Medicine: Dream, Mirage, or Nemesis?* (London: Nuffield Hospitals Trust, 1976); Ivan Illich, *Medical Nemesis: The Expropriation of Health* (Middlesex, UK: Penguin, 1976); Ann Oakley, *Women Confined: Towards a Sociology of Childbirth* (Oxford: Martin Robertson, 1980); Gena Corea, *The Mother Machine: Reproductive Technologies from Artificial Insemination to Artificial Wombs* (New York: Harper and Row, 1985).

66. Jeanne Daly, *Evidence-Based Medicine and the Search for a Science of Clinical Care* (Berkeley: University of California Press, 2005), 130–39; A. L. Cochrane, "Tuberculosis Among Prisoners of War in Germany," *British Medical Journal* 10 (1945): 656; Archie L. Cochrane, with Max Blythe, *One Man's Medicine: An Autobiography of Professor Archie Cochrane* (London: BMJ Books, 1989); A. L. Cochrane, J. G. Cox, and T. F. Jarman, "Pulmonary Tuberculosis in the Rhondda Fach: An Interim Report of a Survey of a Mining Community," *British Medical Journal* (1952): 843–53; L. K. Atuhaire et al., "Specific Causes of Death in Miners and Ex-miners in the Rhondda Fach, 1959–1980," *British Journal of Industrial Medicine* 43 (1980): 497–99.

67. Daly, *Evidence-Based Medicine and the Search for a Science of Clinical Care*, 154–81; J. Lomas, J. E. Sisk, and B. Stocking, "From Evidence to Practice in the United States, the United Kingdom, and Canada," *Milbank Quarterly* 71 (1993): 405–9. See also Matthews, *Quantification and the Quest for Medical Certainty*; Richard J. Light and David B. Pillemer, *Summing Up: The Science of Reviewing Research* (Cambridge, MA: Harvard University Press, 1984); I. Chalmers, "The Cochrane Collaboration: Preparing, Maintaining, and Disseminating Systematic Reviews of the Effects of Health Care," *Annals of the New York Academy of Science* 703 (1993): 156–63. See Cochrane, *Effectiveness and Efficiency*; Trisha Greenhalgh, *How to Read a Paper: The Basics of Evidence Based Medicine*, 2nd ed. (London: BMJ Books, 2000); Andrew Stevens, Keith R. Abrams, and John Brazier, *The Advanced Handbook of Methods in Evidence Based Healthcare* (London: Sage, 2001).

68. M. Egger, M. Schneider, and G. D. Smith, "Spurious Precision? Meta-analysis of Observational Studies," *British Medical Journal* 316 (1998): 140–45. Read also C. B. Begg and L. Pilote, "A Model for Incorporating Historical Controls Into a Meta-analysis," *Biometrics* 47 (1991): 899–906; M. Susser and E. Susser, "Choosing a Future for Epidemiology: I. Eras and Paradigms," *American Journal of Public Health* 88 (1996): 668–73; G. Taubes, "Epidemiology Faces Its Limits," *Science* 269 (1995): 164–69; I. Kristiansen and G. Mooney, "Evidence-Based Medicine: Method, Collaboration, Movement or Crusade?" in Ivar Sønbø Kristiansen and Gavin H. Mooney, eds., *Evidence-Based Medicine: In Its Place* (New York: Routledge, 2004), 10–12; A. R. Feinstein, "Meta-analysis: Statistical Alchemy for the Twenty-First Century," *Journal of Clinical Epidemiology* 48 (1995): 71–79.

69. C. Mann, "Meta-analysis in the Breach," *Science* 249 (1990): 476–80.

70. K. Linde et al., "Are the Clinical Effects of Homeopathy Placebo Effects? A Meta-analysis of Placebo-Controlled Trials," *Lancet* 350 (1997): 834–43; Gene V. Glass, "Primary, Secondary, and Meta-analysis," *Educational Researcher* 5 (1976): 3–8. See also Harris Cooper and Larry V. Hedges, eds., *The Handbook of Research Synthesis* (New York: Russell Sage Foundation, 1994).

71. P. C. Gøtzsche, "Why We Need a Broad Perspective on Meta-analysis," *British Medical Journal* 321 (2000): 586; see also D. Lewin, "Meta-analysis: A New Standard or Clinical Fool's Gold," *Journal of NIH Research* 8 (1996): 30–31.

72. Linde et al., "Are the Clinical Effects of Homeopathy Placebo Effects?"

73. M. Foley, "Providers Have Much to Gain from Homeopathy Being Accepted," *British Medical Journal* 325 (2002): 41.

74. Quoted in M. Orleans, "The Cochrane Collaboration," *Public Health Reports* 110 (1995): 634.

75. Kristiansen and Mooney, "Evidence-Based Medicine," 1–19.

76. Ibid., 3.

77. I. Chalmers, "Trying to Do More Good Than Harm in Policy and Practice: The Role of Rigorous, Transparent, Up-to-Date Evaluations," *Annals of the American Academy of Political and Social Science* 589 (2003): 25.

78. M. Clarke, "The Cochrane Collaboration: Providing and Obtaining the Best Evidence About the Effects of Health Care," *Evaluation and the Health Professions* 25 (2005): 8–11; Chalmers, "Trying to Do More Good than Harm in Policy and Practice," 33–34; J. Traub, "Does It Work?" *New York Times*, November 10, 2002; F. Godlee, "The Cochrane Collaboration," *British Medical Journal* 309 (1994): 969–70; Bausell, *Snake Oil Medicine*, 201–3. See also Robert F. Boruch, *Randomized Experiments for Planning and Evaluation: A Practical Guide* (Thousand Oaks, CA: Sage, 1997).

79. K. O'Rourke and A. S. Detsky, "Meta-analysis in Medical Research: Strong Encouragement for Higher Quality in Individual Research Efforts," *Journal of Clinical Epidemiology* 42 (1989): 1021.

80. D. Tovey and R. Dellavalle, "Cochrane in the United States of America," Cochrane Library, http://www.thecochranelibrary.com/details/editorial/847239/Cochrane, accessed September 2, 2012.

81. J. Ezzo et al., "Complementary Medicine and the Cochrane Collaboration," *JAMA* 280 (1998): 1628–30. See also L. A. Bero and J. R. Jadad, "How Consumers and Policymakers Can Use Systematic Reviews for Decision Making," *Annals of Internal Medicine* 127 (1997): 37–42; E. A. Hofmans, "Acupuncture and MEDLINE," *Lancet* 336 (1990): 57; D. J. Cook et al., "Should Unpublished Data Be Included in Meta-analyses? Current Convictions and Controversies," *JAMA* 269 (1993): 2749–53; M. L. Callaham et al., "Positive-Outcome Bias and Other Limitations in the Outcome of Research Abstracts Submitted to a Scientific Meeting," *JAMA* 280 (1998): 254–57; K. S. Khan, S. Daya, and A. Jadad, "The Importance of Quality of Primary Studies in Producing Unbiased Systematic Reviews," *Archives of Internal Medicine* 156 (1996): 363–66.

82. J. Ezzo, K. Streitberger, and A. Schneider, "Cochrane Systematic Reviews Examine P6 Acupuncture-Point Stimulation for Nausea and Vomiting," *Journal of Alternative and Complementary Medicine* 12 (2006): 489–95. See also D. O'Regan and J. Filshie, "Acupuncture and Cancer," *Autonomic Neuroscience* 157 (2010): 96–100. Other studies were carried out on music during caesarean section, Chinese herbs for angina, water gymnastics for pelvic pain in pregnancy, and dietary interventions for multiple sclerosis.

83. J. S. Levin et al., "Quantitative Methods in Research on Complementary and Alternative Medicine: A Methodological Manifesto," *Medical Care* 35 (1997): 1080.

84. D. L. Sackett, "Clinical Epidemiology: What, Who, and Whither," *Journal of Clinical Epidemiology* 52 (2002): 1161–66; R. Smith and I. Chambers, "Britain's Gift: A 'Medline' of Synthesized Evidence," *British Medical Journal* 323 (2001): 1437–38; J. Lomas, J. E. Sisk, and B. Stocking, "From Evidence to Practice in the United States, the United Kingdom, and Canada," *Milbank Quarterly* 71 (1993): 405–9; Gordon H. Guyatt and Drummond Rennie, eds., *Users' Guides to the Medical Literature: A Manual for Evidence-Based Clinical Practice* (Chicago: American Medical Association Press, 2002); J. Grimshaw and M. Eccles, "Identifying and Using Evidence-Based Guidelines in General Practice," in Andrew Haines and Anna Donald, eds., *Getting Research Findings Into Practice* (London: BMJ Books, 1998), 120–34.

85. B. G. Charlton, "Restoring the Balance: Evidence-Based Medicine Put in Its Place," *Journal of Evaluation in Clinical Practice* 3 (1997): 87–98; D. W. Light, "Effectiveness and Efficiency Under Competition: The Cochrane Test," *British Medical Journal* 303 (1991): 1253–54. See also Rudolf Klein and Janet Lewis, *The Politics of Consumer Representation: A Study of Community Health Councils* (London: Centre for Studies in Social Policy, 1976); N. Black, "Evidence-Based Policy: Proceed with Care," *British Medical Journal* 323 (2001): 275–78; R. B. Haynes, "Loose Connections Between Peer-Reviewed Clinical Journals and Clinical Practice," *Annals of Internal Medicine* 113 (1990), 724–27; Haines and Donald, eds., *Getting Research Findings Into Practice*; S. E. Straus and D. L. Sackett, "Getting Research Findings Into Practice Using Research Findings in Clinical Practice," *British Medical Journal* 317 (1998): 339–42; D. G. Covell, G. C. Uman, and P. R. Manning, "Information Needs in Office Practice: Are They Being Met?" *Annals of Internal Medicine* 103 (1985): 596–99; C. Sanders et al., "Reporting on Quality of Life in Randomized Controlled Trials: Bibliographic Study," *British Medical Journal* 317 (1998): 1191–94.

86. D. Atkins et al., "Grading Quality of Evidence and Strength of Recommendations," *British Medical Journal* 328 (2004): 1490; A. Gafni, C. Charles, and T. Whelan, "The Physician–Patient Encounter: The Physician as a Perfect Agent for the Patient Versus the Informed Treatment Decision-Making Model," *Social Science and Medicine* 47 (1998): 347–54. As an aside, the challenge of disseminating new evidence beyond the narrow confines of the political science researchers resulted in the Campbell Collaboration (based on the precedent established by the Cochrane Collaboration), designed to provide systematic reviews of evidence-based research for its application to social issues such as crime and delinquency, public money management, educational reform, drug abuse, and so on, as well as for its application to the pressures placed on politicians and administrators to implement laws and procedures. See A. Petrosino et al., "Meeting the Challenges of Evidence-Based Policy: The Campbell Collaboration," *Annals of the American Academy of Political and Social Science* 578 (2001): 14–34. See also Huw T. O. Davies, Sandra Nutley, and Peter C. Smith, eds., *What Works? Evidence-Based Policy and Practice in Public Services* (Bristol, UK: Policy Press, 2000).

87. R. Doll, "Controlled Trials: The 1948 Watershed," *British Medical Journal* 317 (1998): 1217–20. See also Shryock, *American Medical Research, Past and Present*.

88. K. J. Rothman and K. B. Michels, "The Continuing Unethical Use of Placebo Controls," *New England Journal of Medicine* 331 (1994): 394–98; A. Kessel, "On Failing to Understand Informed Consent," *British Journal of Hospital Medicine* 52 (1994): 235–38; W. Silverman, "The Myth of Informed Consent: In Daily Practice and in Clinical Trials," *Journal of Medical Ethics* 15 (1989): 6–11; J. Tobias and R. Souhami, "Fully Informed Consent Can Be Needlessly Cruel," *British Medical Journal* 307 (1993): 1199–201; D. Brahams, "Consent to Research in Presence of Incapacity," *Lancet* 341 (1993): 1143–44; C. Lavelle-Jones et al., "Factors Affecting Quality of Informed Consent," *British Medical Journal* 306 (1993): 885–90. See also Susan E. Lederer, *Subjected to Science: Human Experimentation in America Before the Second World War* (Baltimore: Johns Hopkins University Press, 1995), 1–26.

89. P. D. Wall, "The Placebo Effect, an Unpopular Topic," *Pain* 51 (1992): 1–3.

90. N. Freemantle et al., "Promoting Cost Effective Prescribing," *British Medical Journal* 310 (1993): 955–56; M. Drummond et al., "Economic Evaluation of Pharmaceuticals: A European Perspective," *Pharmacoeconomics* 4 (1993): 173–76; G. H. Brieger, "Human Experimentation: History," in Warren T. Reich, ed., *Encyclopedia of Bioethics* (New York: Macmillan, 1995), 5:684–92.

91. A. B. Hill, "Medical Ethics and Controlled Trials," *British Medical Journal* 1 (1963): 1043–49; Rothman and Michels, "The Continuing Unethical Use of Placebo Controls," 394–98; P. I. Clark and P. E. Leaverton, "Scientific and Ethical Issues in the Use of Placebo Controls in Clinical Trials," *Annual Review of Public Health* 15 (1994): 19–38; R. Temple and S. S. Ellenberg, "Placebo-Controlled Trials and Active Control Trials in the Evaluation of New Treatments: I. Ethical and Scientific Issues," *Annals of Internal Medicine* 133 (2000): 455–63; R. Simon, "Are Placebo-Controlled Clinical Trials Ethical or Needed with Alternative

Treatment Exists?" *Annals of Internal Medicine* 133 (2000): 474–75; E. J. Emanuel and P. G. Miller, "The Ethics of Placebo-Controlled Trials—a Middle Ground," *New England Journal of Medicine* 345 (2001): 915–19.

92. "Protection of Human Subjects, Part 46," http://www.access.gpo.gov/nara/cfr/waisidx_oo/45cfr46_oo.html, accessed July 20, 2011. See also P. Weindling, "The Origins of Informed Consent: The International Scientific Commission on Medical War Crimes and the Nuremberg Code," *Bulletin of the History of Medicine* 75 (2001): 37–71.

93. See George J. Annas and Michael A. Grodin, eds., *The Nazi Doctors and the Nuremberg Code: Human Rights in Human Experimentation* (New York: Oxford University Press, 1992).

94. "Declaration of Helsinki, as Revised," in Reich, ed., *Encyclopedia of Bioethics*, 5:2765–67.

95. Read R. J. Levine, "International Codes and Guidelines for Research Ethics: A Critical Appraisal," in Harold Y. Vanderpool, ed., *The Ethics of Research Involving Human Subjects: Facing the 21st Century* (Frederick, MD: University Publishing Group, 1996).

96. "WMA Declaration of Helsinki-Ethical Principles for Medical Research Involving Human Subjects," http://www.wma.net/en/30publications/10policies/b3/index.html, accessed October 30, 2013. See also Rothman and Michels, "The Continuing Unethical Use of Placebo Controls," 394–98; J. Collier, "Confusion Over Use of Placebos in Clinical Trials," *British Medical Journal* 311 (1995): 821–22; and the 1989, 1996, and 2000 editions of World Medical Association, *Declaration of Helsinki* (Ferney-Voltaire, France: World Medical Association).

97. D. Marquis, "Leaving Therapy to Chance," *Hastings Center Report* 13 (1983): 40–47.

98. Freedman, "Placebo-Controlled Trials and the Logic of Clinical Purpose," 5. See also B. Freedman, "Equipoise and the Ethics of Clinical Research," *New England Journal of Medicine* 317 (1987): 141; B. Freedman, K. C. Glass, and C. Weijer, "Placebo Orthodoxy in Clinical Research. II. Ethical, Legal and Regulatory Myths," *Journal of Law, Medicine, and Ethics* 24 (1996): 252–59.

99. Freedman, "Placebo-Controlled Trials and the Logic of Clinical Purpose," 1–6; Freedman, "Equipoise and the Ethics of Clinical Research," 141–45; Robert J. Levine, *Ethics and Regulation of Clinical Research* (New Haven, CT: Yale University Press, 1986); C. Weijer, "The Ethical Analysis of Risk," *Journal of Law, Medicine, and Ethics* 28 (2000): 344–61; C. Weijer and P. B. Miller, "Therapeutic Obligation in Clinical Research," *Hastings Center Report* 33 (2003): 3; S. Joffe and F. G. Miller, "Bench and Bedside: Mapping the Moral Terrain of Clinical Research," *Hastings Center Report* 38 (2008): 30–42; Rothman and Michels, "The Continuing Unethical Use of Placebo Controls," 394–98.

100. D. E. Snider Jr. and D. F. Stroup, "Defining Research When It Comes to Public Health," *Public Health Reports* 112 (1997): 29–32.

101. W. K. Mariner, "Counterpoint on Human Subjects Research," *Public Health Reports* 112 (1997): 36. See also Jay Katz, *Experimentation with Human Beings* (New York: Russell Sage Foundation, 1972).

102. C. Grady, "Science in the Service of Healing," *Hastings Center Report* 28 (1998): 34–38.

103. M. A. Hall, "Law, Medicine, and Trust," *Stanford Law Review* 55 (2002): 495.

104. "Side-by-Side Comparison of 1996 and 2000 Declaration of Helsinki," http://www.hhs.gov/ohrp/archive/nhrpac/mtg12-00/h2000-1996.pdf, accessed September 26, 2013. See also Freedman, "Equipoise and the Ethics of Clinical Research," 141–45; M. Angell, "The Ethics of Clinical Research in the Third World," *New England Journal of Medicine* 337 (1997): 847–49; J. Saba and A. Amman, "A Cultural Divide on AIDS Research," *New York Times*, September 20, 1977; W. Raspberry, "Shades of Tuskegee," *Washington Post*, September 22, 1997; S. Okie, "In the Researcher's Code of Conduct, Contradictions Abound," *Washington Post*, September 28, 1997; and the most recent revision of the Helsinki Declaration: World Medical Association, *Declaration of Helsinki* (Ferney-Voltaire, France: World Medical Association, 2013). This latest revision further states that "no national or international ethical, legal or regulatory requirement should reduce or eliminate any of the protections for research subjects set for in this Declaration" ("WMA Declaration of Helsinki-Ethical Principles for Medical Research Involving Human Subjects").

105. Charles Fried, *Medical Experimentation: Personal Integrity and Social Policy* (Amsterdam: North Holland, 1974); F. G. Miller and H. Brody, "A Critique of Clinical Equipoise—Therapeutic Misconception in the Ethics of Clinical Trials," *Hastings Center Report* 33 (2003): 19–28.

106. "Declaration of Helsinki Revised," *IRB: Ethics and Human Research* 22 (2000): 10.

107. World Medical Association, "Declaration of Helsinki, 5th Revision," October 2000, http://www.wma.net/e/policy/b3.htm, accessed April 21, 2011.

108. R. Temple and S. S. Ellenberg, "Placebo-Controlled Trials and Active-Control Trials in the Evaluation of New Treatments," *Annals of Internal Medicine* 133 (2000): 455–63; B. Jones et al., "Trials to Assess Equivalence: The Importance of Rigorous Methods," *British Medical Journal* 313 (1996): 36–39; I. Kirsch and J. J. Rosadino, "Do Double-Blind Studies with Informed Consent Yield Externally Valid Results?" *Psychopharmacology* 110 (1993): 347–52.

109. G. Mooney, "Evidence-Based Medicine: Objectives and Values," in Kristiansen and Mooney, eds., *Evidence-Based Medicine*, 62–72; V. Wiseman, "Caring: The Neglected Health Outcome? Or Input?" *Health Policy* 39 (1997): 43–54; M. Little, "Assignments of Meaning in Epidemiology," *Social Science and Medicine* 47 (1998): 1135–45. See also Cochrane, *Effectiveness and Efficiency*; Ian Hacking, *The Emergence of Probability* (Cambridge: Cambridge University Press, 1975); and James Le Fanu, *The Rise and Fall of Modern Medicine* (London: Little, Brown, 1999).

110. Quoted in Daly, *Evidence-Based Medicine and the Search for a Science of Clinical Care*, 104.

111. D. L. Sackett, "The Sins of Expertness and a Proposal for Redemption," *British Medical Journal* 320 (2000): 1283. See also David L. Sackett et al., *Evidence-Based Medicine: How to Practice and Teach EBM*, 2nd ed. (Edinburgh: Churchill Livingstone, 2000).

112. Daly, *Evidence-Based Medicine and the Search for a Science of Clinical Care*, 19, 239, 241.

2. POSTMODERNIST MEDICINE

1. On postmodernism, read Frederick Jameson, *Postmodernism, or, The Cultural Logic of Late Capitalism* (Durham, NC: Duke University Press, 1991); Terry Eagleton, *The Illusions of Postmodernism* (Oxford: Blackwell, 1996); Charles C. Lemert, *Postmodernism Is Not What You Think: Why Globalization Threatens Modernity* (Oxford: Blackwell, 1997); Thomas Docherty, ed., *Postmodernism: A Reader* (New York: Columbia University Press, 1993); Trisha Greenhalgh and Brian Hurwitz, eds., *Narrative-Based Medicine: Dialogue and Discourse in Clinical Practice* (London: BMJ Books, 1998); John Lukacs, *At the End of an Age* (New Haven, CT: Yale University Press, 2002).

2. Quoted in Karin Bauer, *Adorno's Nietzschean Narratives: Critiques of Ideology, Readings of Wagner* (New York: State University of New York Press, 1999), 92.

3. Read Richard Appignanesi and Chris Garratt, *Introducing Postmodernism* (New York: Totem Books, 1995); Hubert Dreyfus and Paul Rabinow, *Michel Foucault, Beyond Structuralism and Hermeneutics*, 2nd ed. (Chicago: University of Chicago Press, 1983); M. Foucault, "The Subject and Power," *Critical Inquiry* 8 (1982): 777–95; Vaclav Hubinger, ed., *Grasping the Changing World* (New York: Routledge, 1996); Bryan S. Turner, *Theories of Modernity and Postmodernity* (London: Sage, 1990).

4. D. B. Morris, "How to Speak Postmodern: Medicine, Illness, and Cultural Change," *Hastings Center Report* 30 (2000): 7–17. See also Lawrence Cahoone, *From Modernism to Post Modernism* (Oxford: Blackwell, 1996); Peter Coveney and Roger Highfield, *Frontiers of Complexity: The Search for Order in a Chaotic World* (London: Faber and Faber, 1995).

5. B. Charlton, "Medicine and Postmodernity," *Journal of the Royal Society of Medicine* 86 (1993): 497–99; M. Parker, "Postmodern Organizations or Postmodern Organization Theory?" *Organizational Studies* 13 (1992): 1–17.

6. P. Hodgkin, "Medicine, Postmodernism, and the End of Certainty: Where One Version of the Truth Is as Good as Another, Anything Goes," *British Medical Journal* 313 (1996): 1568.

7. D. P. Frost, "Complex Systems Result in a New Kind of Fundamental Uncertainty," *British Medical Journal* 314 (1997): 1045.

8. I. Morrison and R. Smith, "Hamster Health Care: Time to Stop Running Faster and Redesign Health Care," *British Medical Journal* 321 (2000): 1541–42; D. Mechanic, D. D. McAlpine, and M. Rosenthal, "Are Patients' Office Visits with Physicians Getting Shorter?" *New England Journal of Medicine* 344 (2001): 198–204; D. Mechanic, "General Practice in England and Wales: Results from a Survey of a National Sample of General Practitioners," *Medical Care* 6 (1968): 245–60.

9. Morris, "How to Speak Postmodern," 7–16. See also E. S. More, "Empathy Enters the Profession of Medicine," in Ellen S. More and Maureen A. Milligan, eds., *The Empathetic Practitioner: Empathy, Gender, and Medicine* (New Brunswick, NJ: Rutgers University Press, 1994), 19–39; David B. Morris, *Illness and Culture in the Postmodern Age* (Berkeley: University of California Press, 1998); C. E. Rosenberg, "Meanings, Policies, and Medicine: On the Bioethical Enterprise and History," *Daedalus* (1999): 27–46; Eli Ginzburg,

The Medical Triangle: Physicians, Politicians, and the Public (Cambridge, MA: Harvard University Press, 1990); Robert Aronowitz, *Making Sense out of Illness: Science, Society, and Disease* (New York: Cambridge University Press, 1998); Dianna B. Dutton, Thomas A. Preston, and Nancy E. Pfund, *Worse Than the Disease: Pitfalls of Medical Progress* (New York: Cambridge University Press, 1988); John H. Knowles, ed., *Doing Better and Feeling Worse: Health in the United States* (New York: Norton, 1977); Kenneth M. Ludmerer, *Time to Heal: American Medical Education from the Turn of the Century to the Era of Managed Care* (New York: Oxford University Press, 1999).

10. M. H. Kottow, "Classical Medicine v. Alternative Medical Practices," *Journal of Medical Ethics* 18 (1992): 20.

11. Read Thomas S. Kuhn, *The Structure of Scientific Revolutions* (Chicago: University of Chicago Press, 1962).

12. Robert Burton, *The Anatomy of Melancholy* (1621), http://ebooks.adelaide.edu.au/b/burton/robert/melancholy/S1.2.3.html, accessed May 25, 2012.

13. M. J. Martin, "Psychosomatic Medicine: A Brief History," *Psychosomatics* 19 (1978): 697–700. Also read Franz G. Alexander and Sheldon T. Selesnick, *The History of Psychiatry* (New York: Harper and Row, 1966); Gregory Zilboorg, *A History of Medical Psychology* (New York: Norton, 1941); Armand M. Nicholi, ed., *The Harvard Guide to Modern Psychiatry* (Cambridge, MA: Harvard University Press, 1978); Franz G. Alexander and Thomas Morton French, *Studies in Psychosomatic Medicine* (New York: Ronald Press, 1948).

14. "The Balance of Passions," in *Emotion and Disease*, US National Library of Medicine, National Institutes of Health, http://www.nlm.nih.gov/exhibition/emotions/balance.html, accessed May 25, 2012. See also Austin Flint, *A Treatise on the Principles and Practice of Medicine* (London: Lea's, 1881), and William Osler, *The Principles and Practice of Medicine* (New York: Appleton, 1892).

15. R. A. Cleghorn, J. M. Cleghorn, and F. H. Lowy, "Contributions of Behavioral Sciences to Health Care: An Historical Perspective," *Milbank Memorial Fund Quarterly* 49 (1971): 161. See also Wilhelm Wundt, *Grundzüge der physiologischen Psychologie* (Principles of physiological psychology) (Leipzig: Engelmann, 1874).

16. A. T. Schofield, "Mind in Medicine," *British Medical Journal* 2 (1906): 765–66.

17. Cleghorn, Cleghorn, and Lowy, "Contributions of Behavioral Sciences to Health Care," 162–63. See also Paul M. Schilder, *The Image and Appearance of the Human Body: Studies in the Constructive Energies of the Psyche* (1935; reprint, London: Routledge, 1999); Walter Bradford Cannon, *The Wisdom of the Body* (New York: Norton, 1932); Stanley Cobb, *Borderlands of Psychiatry* (N.p.: n.p., 1943) and *Foundations of Neuropsychiatry* (Baltimore: Williams and Wilkins, 1952); Hans Selye, *The Stress of Life*, rev. and exp. ed. (Chicago: McGraw-Hill, 1956).

18. Cleghorn, Cleghorn, and Lowy, "Contributions of Behavioral Sciences to Health Care," 162–63. See also Roy R. Grinker and John P. Spiegel, *War Neuroses in North Africa: The Tunisian Campaign, January to May 1943* (New York: Arno Press, 1943) and *Men Under Stress* (Philadelphia: Blakiston, 1945).

19. Cleghorn, Cleghorn, and Lowy, "Contributions of Behavioral Sciences to Health Care," 165–66; J. S. Callender, "Ethics and Aims in Psychotherapy: A Contribution from Kant," *Journal of Medical Ethics* 24 (1998): 274–78.

20. Theodore M. Brown, "The Rise and Fall of American Psychosomatic Medicine," paper read before the New York Academy of Medicine, November 29, 2000, http://human-nature.com/free-associations/riseandfall.html, accessed October 30, 2013.

21. E. D. Wittkower, "News of the Society: Twenty Years of North American Psychosomatic Medicine," *Psychosomatic Medicine* 22, no. 4 (1960): 312, http://www.psychosomaticmedi-cine.org/content/22/4/308.full.pdf, *accessed May 25, 2012. See also* L. Stevens, "The Case Against Psychotherapy," http://www.antipsychiatry.org/psychoth.htm, accessed September 10, 2012; Jeffrey Masson, *Against Therapy: Emotional Tyranny and the Myth of Psychological Healing* (New York: Atheneum, 1988); Garth Wood, *The Myth of Neurosis: Overcoming the Illness Excuse* (New York: Harper and Row, 1986); William Kirk Kilpatrick, *The Emperor's New Clothes: The Naked Truth About the New Psychology* (Westchester, IL: Crossway Books, 1985); K. Edward Renner, *What's Wrong with the Mental Health Movement* (Chicago: Nelson-Hall,1975).

22. Read Cai Song and B. E. Leonard, *Fundamentals of Psychoneuroimmunology* (New York: Wiley, 2000); Robert E. Ornstein and Charles Swencionis, *The Healing Brain: A Scientific Reader* (New York: Guilford Press, 1990); Howard S. Friedman and Roxane Cohen Silver, *Foundations of Health Psychology* (New York: Oxford University Press, 2007); G. Wilkinson, "Psychoanalysis and Analytic Psychology in NHS—a Problem for Medical Ethics," *Journal of Medical Ethics* 12 (1986): 87–90; J. D. Greenwood, "Placebo Control Treatments and the Evaluation of Psychotherapy," *Philosophy of Science* 64 (1997): 497–510; T. C. Owen, "Populist Psychotherapy," *Journal of Religion and Health* 12 (1973): 386–94; A. Christenson and N. S. Jacobson, "Who (or What) Can Do Psychotherapy: The Status and Challenge of Non-professional Therapies," *Psychological Science* 56 (1994): 8–14. See also A. Storr, "The Concept of Cure," in Charles Rycroft, ed., *Psychoanalysis Observed* (London: Constable, 1966), 52–53; A. K. Shapiro and L. A. Morris, "The Placebo Effect in Medical and Psychological Therapies," in Sol L. Garfield and Allen E. Bergen, eds., *The Handbook of Psychotherapy and Behavioral Change*, 3rd ed. (New York: Wiley, 1978), 369–410.

23. Morris, "How to Speak Postmodern," 12. See also Bill Moyers's 1993 PBS television series *Healing and the Mind.* Among the celebrities interviewed were Andrew Weil, Deepak Chopra, C. Everett Koop, Barry Sears, Julian Whitaker, Drew Pinsky, and Susan Love.

24. M. Schlesinger, "A Loss of Faith: The Sources of Reduced Political Legitimacy for the American Medical Profession," *Milbank Quarterly* 80 (2002): 185–235; G. Southon and J. Braithwaite, "The End of Professionalism?" *Social Science and Medicine* 46 (1998): 23–28; Margali S. Larson, *The Rise of Professionalism* (Berkeley: University of California Press, 1977).

25. M. Olfson and H. A. Pincus, "Outpatient Psychotherapy in the United States, I: Volume, Costs, and User Characteristics," *Journal of Consulting and Clinical Psychology* 62 (1994): 75–82.

26. M. E. P. Seligman, "The Effectiveness of Psychotherapy: The *Consumer Reports* Study," *American Psychologist* 50 (1995): 965–74. Read also Mary Lee Smith, Gene V. Glass, and Thomas I. Miller, *The Benefit of Psychotherapy* (Baltimore: Johns Hopkins University Press, 1980); D. Shapiro and D. Shapiro, "Meta-analysis of Comparative Therapy Outcome Studies: A Replication and Refinement," *Psychological Bulletin* 92 (1982): 581–604.

27. D. M. Eisenberg, "The Institute of Medicine Report on Complementary and Alternative Medicine in the United States—Personal Reflections on Its Content and Implications," *Alternative Therapies in Health and Medicine* 11 (2005): 10–11.

28. H. A. Baer, "The Work of Andrew Weil and Deepak Chopra—Two Holistic Health/New Age Gurus: A Critique of the Holistic Health/New Age Movements," *Medical Anthropology Quarterly* 17 (2003): 233–50.

29. Read the following works by Andrew Weil: *The Natural Mind: A Revolutionary Approach to the Drug Problem* (New York: Houghton Mifflin, 1972); *Health and Healing: Understanding Conventional and Alternative Medicine* (Boston: Houghton Mifflin, 1983); *Eight Weeks to Optimum Health: A Proven Program for Taking Full Advantage of Your Body's Natural Healing Power* (New York: Knopf, 1997).

30. Read Deepak Chopra, *Ageless Body, Timeless Mind: The Quantum Alternative to Growing Old* (New York: Harmony Books, 1993) and *Quantum Healing: Discovering the Power to Fulfill Your Dreams* (New York: Bantam, 1991).

31. See Deepak Chopra, *Unconditional Life—Discovering the Power to Fulfill Your Dreams* (New York: Bantam Books, 1992) and *Creating Affluence—Wealth Consciousness in the Field of All Possibilities* (San Rafael, CA: New World Library, 1993). See also John S. Haller Jr., *Swedenborg, Mesmer, and the Mind/Body Connection: The Roots of Complementary Medicine* (West Chester, PA: Swedenborg Foundation, 2010), 158–87, and *The History of New Thought: From Mind-Cure to Positive Thinking and the Prosperity Gospel* (West Chester, PA: Swedenborg Foundation, 2012).

32. J. Durlak, "Comparative Effectiveness of Paraprofessional and Professional Helpers," *Psychological Bulletin* 86 (1979): 80–92; J. A. Hattie, C. F. Sharpley, and H. J. Rogers, "Comparative Effectiveness of Professional and Paraprofessional Helpers," *Psychological Bulletin* 95 (1894): 534–41; D. M. Stern and M. J. Lambert, "On the Relationship Between Therapist Experience and Psychotherapy Outcome," *Clinical Psychology Review* 4 (1984): 127–42; D. A. Shapiro and D. Shapiro, "Meta-analysis of Comparative Therapy Outcome Studies: A Replication and Refinement," *Psychological Bulletin* 92 (1982): 581–604.

33. Edward Erwin, *Philosophy of Psychotherapy: Razing the Troubles of the Brain* (London: Sage, 1997), chap. 8; H. J. Eysenck, "The Effects of Psychotherapy: An Evaluation," *Journal of Consulting Psychology* 16 (1952): 319–24.

34. Eric Fromm, *The Crisis of Psychoanalysis* (New York: Fawcett, 1970), 12, 16, 40.

35. Herbert Benson, *The Relaxation Response* (New York: HarperTorch, 1975) and *Timeless Healing: The Power and Biology of Belief* (New York: Simon and Schuster, 1996); Rhonda Byrne, *The Secret* (New York: Atria Books, 2006) and *The Power* (New York: Atria Books, 2010).

36. F. Scogin et al., "Efficacy of Self-Administered Treatment Programs: Meta-analytic Review," *Professional Psychology: Research and Practice* 21 (1990): 42–47.

37. J. D. Frank, "The Placebo Is Psychotherapy," *Behavioral and Brain Sciences* 6 (1983): 291–92.

38. S. Starker, "Self-Help Treatment Books: The Rest of the Story," *American Psychologist* 43 (1988): 599–600.

39. D. H. Novack, "Realizing Engel's Vision: Psychosomatic Medicine and the Education of Physician-Healers," *Psychosomatic Medicine* 65 (2003): 925–30. See also G. L. Engel, "The Need for a New Medical Model: A Challenge for Biomedicine," *Science* 196 (1977): 129–36, and "The Clinical Application of the Biopsychosocial Model," *American Journal of Psychiatry* 137 (1980): 535–44; S. R. Waldstein et al., "Teaching Psychosomatic (Biopsychosocial) Medicine in United States Medical Schools: Survey Findings," *Psychosomatic Medicine* 63 (2001): 335–43; K. Kroenke, "Symptoms in Medical Patients: An Untended Field," *American Journal of Medicine* 92 (1992): 3S–6S; D. H. Novack, R. M. Epstein, and R. H. Paulsen, "Toward Creating Physician-Healers: Fostering Medical Students' Self-Awareness, Personal Growth, and Well-Being," *Academic Medicine* 74 (1999): 516–20.

40. William James, *The Varieties of Religious Experience: A Study of Human Nature* (New York: Modern Library, 1902), 77–124. See also J. S. Levin and P. L. Schiller, "Is There a Religious Factor in Health?" *Journal of Religion and Health* 26 (1987): 9–36; J. S. Levin and H. Y. Vanderpool, "Is Religion Therapeutically Significant for Hypertension?" *Social Science and Medicine* 29 (1989): 69–78; J. Levin, "God, Love, and Health: Findings from a Clinical Study," *Review of Religious Research* 42 (2001): 277–93.

41. M. Wills, "Connection, Action, and Hope: An Invitation to Reclaim the 'Spiritual' in Health Care," *Journal of Religious Health* 46 (2007): 430–31.

42. W. Roush, "Herbert Benson: Mind–Body Maverick Pushes the Envelope," *Science* 276 (1997): 357–58. See also Benson, *Timeless Healing*.

43. Wills, "Connection, Action, and Hope," 424.

44. C. Cohen et al., "Prayer as Therapy: A Challenge to Both Religious Belief and Professional Ethics," *Hastings Center Report* 30 (2000): 43. See also M. J. Hanson, "The Religious Differences in Clinical Healthcare," *Cambridge Quarterly of Healthcare Ethics* 7 (1998): 57–67; C. Wallis, "Faith and Healing," *Time*, June 24, 1996; E. G. Howe, "Influencing a Patient's Religious Beliefs: Mandate or No-Man's Land?" *Journal of Clinical Ethics* 6 (1995): 194–201; T. F. Dagi, "Prayer, Piety, and Professional Propriety: Limits on Religious Expression in Hospitals," *Journal of Clinical Ethics* 6 (1995): 274–79.

45. L. K. George, C. G. Ellison, and D. B. Larson, "Explaining the Relationships Between Religious Involvement and Health," *Psychological Inquiry* 13 (2002): 190–200.

46. R. A. Cooper and H. J. McKee, "Chiropractic in the United States: Trends and Issues," *Milbank Quarterly* 81 (2003): 107–38; K. R. Pelletier et al., "Current Trends in the Integration and Reimbursement of Complementary and Alternative Medicine by Managed Care, Insurance Carriers, and Hospital Providers," *American Journal of Health Promotion* 12 (1997): 112–22. See also Michael H. Cohen, *Complementary and Alternative Medi-*

cine: Legal Boundaries and Regulatory Perspectives (Baltimore: Johns Hopkins University Press, 1998).

47. F. M. Frohock, "Moving Lines and Variable Criteria: Differences/Connections Between Allopathic and Alternative Medicine," *Annals of the American Academy of Political and Social Science* 583 (2002): 214.

48. B. M. Hughes, "Regional Patterns of Religious Affiliation and Availability of Complementary and Alternative Medicine," *Journal of Religion and Health* 45 (2006): 549–57. See also A. D. Watkins and G. Lewith, "Mind–Body Medicine: Its Popularity and Perception," in Alan D. Watkins, ed., *Mind–Body Medicine: A Clinician's Guide to Psychoneuroimmunology* (New York: Churchill Livingston, 1997), 27–40.

49. Hughes, "Regional Patterns of Religious Affiliation and Availability of Complementary and Alternative Medicine," 550–53. See also M. Saks, "Medicine and Complementary Medicine: Challenge and Change," in Graham Scambler and Paul Higgs, eds., *Modernity, Medicine, and Health: Medical Sociology Towards 2000* (London: Routledge, 1998), 198–215.

50. E. Ernst, "Complementary Medicine: Common Misconceptions," *Journal of the Royal Society of Medicine* 88 (1995): 244–47; White House Commission on Complementary and Alternative Medicine Policy, *Final Report, March 2002* (Washington, DC: White House Commission on Complementary and Alternative Medicine Policy, 2002), 12, http://gov-info.library.unt.edu/whccamp/pdfs/fr2002_document.pdf, accessed April 23, 2011.

51. D. M. Eisenberg, T. L. Delbanco, and R. C. Kessler, "Unconventional Medicine," *New England Journal of Medicine* 329 (1993): 1203–4.

52. L. Rees and A. Weil, "Integrated Medicine Imbues Orthodox Medicine with the Values of Complementary Medicine," *British Medical Journal* 322 (2001): 119; see also A. Weil, "The Significance of Integrative Medicine for the Future of Medical Education," *American Medical Journal* 18 (2000): 441–43.

53. Tracy Deliman and John S. Smolowe, *Holistic Medicine: Harmony of Body, Mind, Spirit* (Upper Saddle River, NJ: Prentice-Hall, 1982); Barbara Montgomery Dossey, *Holistic Health Promotion: A Guide for Practice* (Rockville, MD: Aspen, 1989); Robert C. Fuller, *Alternative Medicine and American Religious Life* (New York: Oxford University Press, 1989); M. Goldstein et al., "Holistic Physicians and Family Practitioners: Similarities, Differences, and Implications for Health Policy," *Social Science and Medicine* 26 (1988): 853–61; Daniel Goldman and Joel Gurin, *Mind Body Medicine: How to Use Your Mind for Better Health* (New York: Consumer's Union, 1993).

54. For more on the journal *Evidence-Based Complementary and Alternative Medicine*, see http://www.hindawi.com/journals/ecam/osi/, accessed June 10, 2013.

55. See Michael Dixon and Kieran Sweeney, *The Human Effect in Medicine: Theory, Research, and Practice* (Abingdon, UK: Radcliffe Medical Press, 2000).

56. Health Care Financing Administration, "National Health Expenditure Projections, 2000–2010," http://www.hcfa.gov/stats, accessed April 22, 2011.

57. H. S. Merliner and J. W. Salmon, "The Holistic Alternative to Scientific Medicine: History and Analysis," *International Journal of Health Services* 10 (1980): 133–47; R. A. Deyo,

"Practice Variations, Treatment Fads, and Rising Disability," *Spine* 18 (1993): 21–54; Stefan Timmermans and Marc Berg, *The Gold Standard: The Challenge of Evidence-Based Medicine and Standardization in Health Care* (Philadelphia: Temple University Press, 2003): 166–94. See also J. C. Whorton, "The History of Complementary and Alternative Medicine," in Wayne B. Jonas, Jeffrey S. Levin, and Brian Berman, eds., *The Essentials of Complementary and Alternative Medicine* (Philadelphia: Lippincott Williams and Wilkins, 1999); June S. Lowenberg, *Caring and Responsibility: The Crossroads Between Holistic Practice and Traditional Medicine* (Philadelphia: University of Pennsylvania Press, 1989).

58. T. A. Winnick, "From Quackery to 'Complementary' Medicine: The American Medical Profession Confronts Alternative Therapies," *Social Problems* 52 (2005): 44.

59. Ibid., 45–46, 50. By 1985, chiropractors had won not only a successful antitrust suit against the American Medical Association but hospital privileges as well.

60. E. Ernst and C. H. Hentschel, "Diagnostic Methods in Complementary Medicine: Whichcraft or Witchcraft?" *International Journal of Risk and Safety Medicine* 7 (1995): 55–63; E. Ernst et al., "Complementary Medicine—a Definition," *British Journal of General Practice* 45 (1995): 506. See also Marc S. Micozzi, ed., *Fundamentals of Complementary and Alternative Medicine* (New York: Churchill Livingstone, 1996).

61. Bonnie Blair O'Connor, *Healing Traditions: Alternative Medicine and the Health Professions* (Philadelphia: University of Pennsylvania Press, 1995).

62. Read Donald W. Novey, ed., *Clinician's Complete Reference to Complementary and Alternative Medicine* (St. Louis: Mosby, 2000).

63. Ernst et al., "Complementary Medicine—a Definition," 506; Ernst and Hentschel, "Diagnostic Methods in Complementary Medicine," 55–63.

64. Winnick, "From Quackery to 'Complementary' Medicine," 38–61; M. Goldner, "Expanding Political Opportunities and Changing Collective Identities in the Complementary and Alternative Medicine Movement," *Political Opportunities, Social Movements, and Democratization* 23 (2001): 69–102; H. A. Baer et al., "The Holistic Health Movement in the San Francisco Bay Area: Some Preliminary Observations," *Social Science and Medicine* 47 (1998): 1495–501.

65. "State Laws Protecting Health Freedom," http://www.cancure.org/legislation_already_passed.htm, accessed April 22, 2011.

66. Nicola J. Newton, "The Road Taken: Women's Life Paths and Personality Development in Late Midlife," PhD diss., University of Michigan, 2011, http://deepblue.lib.umich.edu/bitstream/2027.42/86410/1/nickynew_1.pdf, accessed May 25, 2012; L. Grant and L. A. Simpson, "Marriage and Relationship Satisfaction of Physicians," *Sociological Focus* 27 (1994): 327–42; "Psychology of Women," http://www.scribd.com/doc/29167058/Psychology-of-Women, accessed May 25, 2012.

67. Department of Professional Employees, AFL-CIO, "Professional Women: Vital Statistics," http://www.pay-equity.org/PDFs/ProfWomen.pdf, accessed September 23, 2011.

68. K. S. Sibert, "Don't Quit This Day Job," *New York Times*, June 11, 2011, http://www.nytimes.com/2011/06/12/opinion/12sibert.html?pagewanted=all, accessed May 9, 2012. Through

much of postmodernist medicine, women physicians have been overrepresented in pediatrics, psychiatry, and public health while underrepresented in internal medicine, the surgical subspecialties, research, and academic medicine. Although broad shifts in the workforce have occurred, especially where women were more normative in the past, generational changes depend as much on patients' expectations as they do on a woman physician's individual choice. More recent research suggests that women physicians prefer to be engaged in careers with more of the communication behaviors valued by patients. See J. Cuca, "The Specialization and Career Preferences of Women and Men Recently Graduated from U.S. Medical Schools," *Journal of the American Medical Women's Association* 34 (1979): 1161–62; J. Braslow and M. Heins, "Women in Medical Education: A Decade of Change," *New England Journal of Medicine* 304 (1981): 1129–34; L. Grant, "Peer Expectations About Outstanding Competencies of Men and Women Medical Students," *Sociology of Health and Illness* 5 (1983): 42–61; N. J. Farber et al., "Physicians' Experiences with Patients Who Transgress Boundaries," *Journal of General Internal Medicine* 15 (2000): 770–75; J. Schmittdiel et al., "Effect of Physician and Patient Sex Concordance on Patient Satisfaction and Preventive Care Practices," *Journal of General Internal Medicine* 15 (2000): 761–69; M. C. Beach and D. L. Roter, "Interpersonal Expectations in the Patient–Physician Relationship," *Journal of General Internal Medicine* 15 (2000): 825–27.

69. For these numbers, see "U.S. Yoga Statistics" at the Namasta (North American Studio Alliance) website, http://www.namasta.com/pressresources.php, accessed September 23, 2011, and C. Sawhney, "Holistic Recipes: The Second Coming," http://www.lifepositive.com/body/homeopathy/homeopathic-treatment.asp, accessed September 28, 2011. See also D. C. Cherkin et al., "Characteristics of Licensed Acupuncturists, Chiropractors, Massage Therapists, and Naturopathic Physicians," *Journal of the American Board of Family Practice* 15 (2002): 378–90.

70. "White House Commission on Complementary and Alternative Medicine Policy— March 2002," 9, http://www.whccamp.hhs.gov/pdfs/fr2002_document.pdf, accessed September 25, 2013.

71. Ernst et al., "Complementary Medicine—a Definition," 506; see also E. Ernst, M. H. Cohen, and J. Stone, "Ethical Problems Arising in Evidence Based Complementary and Alternative Medicine," *Journal of Medical Ethics* 30 (2000): 156. This definition was adopted by the Cochrane Collaboration.

72. Read Benson, *Timeless Healing*; Beata Bishop, *A Time to Heal* (London: Arkana, 1996); Ursula Sharma, *Complementary Medicine Today: Practitioners and Patients* (London: Tavistock/Routledge, 1992).

73. D. M. Eisenberg et al., "Unconventional Medicine in the United States: Prevalence, Costs, and Patterns of Use," *New England Journal of Medicine* 328 (1993): 246–52. See also M. B. Blecher, "Alternative Medicine on Pins and Needles No More: Acupuncturists and Others Get Mainstream Nod," *Crain's Chicago Business*, January 27, 1997; D. M. Eisenberg, "Advising Patients Who Seek Alternative Medical Therapies," *Annals of Internal Medicine* 127 (1997): 61–69.

74. D. Eisenberg et al., "Trends in Alternative Medicine Use in the United States, 1990–1997," *JAMA* 280 (1998): 1569–75. The research team came from the Center for Alternative Medicine Research and Education at Beth Israel Deaconess Medical Center and the Department of Health Care Policy at Harvard Medical School.

75. Ni Hanyu, C. Simile, and A. M. Hardy, "Utilization of Complementary and Alternative Medicine by United States Adults: Results from the 1999 National Health Interview Survey," *Medical Care* 40 (2002): 353–58.

76. H. A. Tindle et al., "Trends in Use of Complementary and Alternative Medicine by U.S. Adults: 1997–2002," *Alternative Therapies in Health and Medicine* 11 (2005): 42–49.

77. N. C. Sharts-Hopko, "Spirituality and Health Care," in Joseph T. Catalano, ed., *Nursing Now: Today's Issues, Tomorrow's Trends*, 2nd ed. (Philadelphia: Davis, 2003), 347–71; S. Maimes, "Spirituality and Healing in Medicine," *Healthcare Review* 15 (2002): 7.

78. L. Clark Paramore, "Use of Alternative Therapies: Estimates from the 1994 Robert Wood Johnson Foundation National Access to Care Survey," *Journal of Pain Symptom Management* 13 (1997): 83–89; M. Kelner and B. Wellman, "Health Care and Consumer Choice: Medical and Alternative Therapies," *Social Science and Medicine* 45 (1997): 203–12.

79. J. A. Astin, "Why Patients Use Alternative Medicine," *JAMA* 279 (1998): 1548–53; Kelner and Wellman, "Health Care and Consumer Choice," 203–12; R. Parker Bausel, Wen-Lin Lee, and B. Berman, "Demographic and Health Related Correlates of Visits to Complementary and Alternative Medicine Providers," *Medical Care* 39 (2001): 190–96.

80. L. Keegan, "Use of Alternative Therapies Among Mexican Americans in the Texas Rio Grande Valley," *Journal of Holistic Nursing* 14 (1996): 277–99; A. Zaldivar and J. Smolowitz, "Perceptions of the Importance Placed on Religion and Folk Medicine by Non-Mexican-American Hispanic Adults with Diabetes," *Diabetes Education* 20 (1994): 303–6; C. Kim and V. S. Kwok, "Navajo Use of Native Healers," *Archives of Internal Medicine* 158 (1998): 2245–49.

81. Astin, "Why Patients Use Alternative Medicine," 1548–53; Eisenberg et al., "Trends in Alternative Medicine Use in the United States, 1990–1997," 1569–75; H. Eastwood, "Why Are Australian GPs Using Alternative Medicine? Postmodernism, Consumerism, and the Shift Toward Holistic Health," *Journal of Sociology* 35 (2000): 133–56; M. Siahpush, "Postmodern Values, Dissatisfaction with Conventional Medicine, and Popularity of Alternative Therapies," *Journal of Sociology* 34 (1998): 58–70.

82. Winnick, "From Quackery to 'Complementary' Medicine," 38.

83. J. Bland, "Alternative Therapies—a Moving Target," *Alternative Therapies in Health and Medicine* 11 (2005): 20.

84. D. E. King et al., "Experiences and Attitudes About Faith Healing Among Family Physicians," *Journal of Family Practice* 35 (1992): 158–62.

85. M. J. Verhoef and L. R. Sutherland, "Alternative Medicine and General Practitioners: Opinions and Behavior," *Canadian Family Physician* 41 (1995): 1005–11.

86. "Alternative and Complementary Medicine: What's a Doctor to Do?" *Hastings Center Report* 30 (2000): 47–48.

87. *American Medical Association Council on Medical Education, Encouraging Medical Student Education in Complementary Health Care Practices (Chicago: American Medical Association Press, 1997); M. S. Wetzel, D. M. Eisenberg, and T. J. Kaptchuk, Courses Involving Complementary and Alternative Medicine at U.S. Medical Schools, JAMA 280 (1998): 784–87; B. Barzansky, H. S. Jonas, and S. I. Etzel, "Educational Programs in US Medical Schools, 1999–2000," JAMA 284 (2000): 1114–20. See also M. S. Wetzel et al., "Complementary and Alternative Medical Therapies: Implications for Medical Education," Annals of Internal Medicine 138 (2003): 191–96.*

88. M. A. Burg et al., "Personal Use of Alternative Medicine Therapies by Health Science Center Faculty," *JAMA* 280 (1998): 1563.

89. J. Udani, "Integrating Alternative Medicine Into Practice," *JAMA* 280 (1998): 1620; see also Astin, "Why Patients Use Alternative Medicine," 1548–53.

90. D. Josefson, "Complementary Medicine Is Booming Worldwide," *British Medical Journal* 313 (1996): 133.

91. V. Maizes and O. Caspio, "The Principles and Challenges of Alternative Medicine: More Than a Combination of Traditional and Alternative Therapies," *Western Journal of Medicine* 171 (1999): 148–49.

92. B. Berman, "Complementary Medicine and Medical Education," *British Medical Journal* 322 (2001): 121–22; Wetzel, Eisenberg, and Kaptchuk, "Courses Involving Complementary and Alternative Medicine at U.S. Medical Schools," 784–87; R. A. Chez, W. B. Jonas, and C. Crawford, "A Survey of Medical Students' Opinions About Complementary and Alternative Medicine," *American Journal of Obstetrics and Gynecology* 185 (2001): 754–57.

93. Wetzel et al., "Complementary and Alternative Medical Therapies," *191–96.*

94. *Ibid.*

95. "Trend Watch: Complementary Growth," *AHA News,* http://www.ahastatitics.org, accessed April 23, 2011; D. Podolsky, "A New Age of Healing Hands: Cancer Centers Embrace Alternative Therapies as 'Complementary Care,'" *U.S. News & World Report,* February 5, 1996, 71–74.

96. M. E. Koch et al., "The Sedative and Analgesic Sparing Effect of Music," *Anesthesiology* 89 (1998): 300–306.

97. I. D. Coulter and R. Khorsan, "Is Health Services Research the Holy Grail of Complementary and Alternative Medicine Research?" *Alternative Therapies in Health and Medicine* 14 (2008): 40.

98. "Overview of CAM in the United States," in White House Commission on Complementary and Alternative Medicine Policy, *Final Report, March 2002,* 22.

99. V. E. Tyler, "What a Pharmacist Should Know About Herbal Remedies," *Journal of the American Pharmaceutical Association* 36 (1996): 29–37; "Herbal Roulette," *Consumer Reports,* November 1995; E. Ernst, "Risks Associated with Complementary Therapies," in M. N. G. Dukes and Jeffrey K. Aronson, eds., *Meyler's Side Effects of Drugs,* 14 ed. (Amsterdam: Elsevier Science, 2000), 1649–81.

100. See Karen Rappaport, *Directory of Schools for Alternative and Complementary Health Care*, 2nd ed. (Phoenix: Oryx, 1999); Larson, *The Rise of Professionalism*.

101. Wetzel, Eisenberg, and Kaptchuk, "Courses Involving Complementary and Alternative Medicine at U.S. Medical Schools," 784–87.

102. P. R. Wolpe, "The Dynamics of Heresy in a Profession," *Social Science and Medicine* 39 (1994): 1133–48, and "The Holistic Heresy: Strategies of Ideological Challenge in the Medical Profession," *Social Science and Medicine* 31 (1990): 913–23.

3. "THE POWERFUL PLACEBO"

1. Read J. Gold, "Cartesian Dualism and the Current Crisis in Medicine—a Plea for a Philosophical Approach: Discussion Paper," *Journal of the Royal Society of Medicine* 78 (1985): 663–66. See also Ivan Illich, *Medical Nemesis: The Expropriation of Health* (Middlesex, UK: Penguin, 1981); Ian Kennedy, *The Unmasking of Medicine* (London: Paladin/Granada, 1983).

2. Quoted in H. V. Neal, "The Basis of Individuality in Organisms: A Defense of Vitalism," *Science* 44 (1916): 82.

3. Abraham Flexner, *Medical Education in the United States and Canada: A Report to the Carnegie Foundation for the Advancement of Teaching* (New York: Carnegie Foundation, 1910), 157.

4. M. H. Kottow, "Classical Medicine v. Alternative Medical Practices," *Journal of Medical Ethics* 18 (1992): 21.

5. A. K. Shapiro, "The Placebo Effect in the History of Medical Treatment: Implications for Psychiatry," *American Journal of Psychiatry* 116 (1959): 198–304, and "A Contribution to the History of the Placebo Effect," *Behavioral Science* 5 (1960): 109–35; J. C. Whitehorn, "Psychiatric Implications of the Placebo Effect," *American Journal of Psychiatry* 114 (1958): 662–64. See also R. G. Gallimore and J. L. Turner, "Faith and Psychotherapy: Some Problems in Theories of Psychotherapy," in Murray E. Jarvik, ed., *Psychopharmacology in the Practice of Medicine* (New York: Appleton-Century-Crofts, 1977), 93–116.

6. "The Bottle of Medicine," *British Medical Journal* 1 (1952): 149. See also R. Barker Bausell, *Snake Oil Science: The Truth About Complementary and Alternative Medicine* (New York: Oxford University Press, 2007), 24.

7. A. Hróbjartsson and M. Norup, "The Uses of Placebo in Medical Practice—a National Questionnaire Survey of Danish Clinicians," *Evaluation and the Health Professions* 26 (2003): 153–65.

8. Daniel Boorstin, *The Discoverers* (New York: Random House, 1983), xv; Henry Sigerist, "The History of Medicine and the History of Disease," *Bulletin of the Institute of the History of Medicine* 4 (1936): 1–13; J. T. Patterson, "How Do We Write the History of Disease?" *Health and History* 1 (1998): 5–29. See also Michel Foucault, *The Birth of the Clinic: An Archaeology of Medical Perception* (New York: Pantheon Books, 1973); Charles Rosenberg

and Janet Golden, eds., *Framing Disease: Studies in Cultural History* (New Brunswick, NJ: Rutgers University Press, 1992).

9. H. K. Beecher, "The Powerful Placebo," *JAMA* 159 (1955): 1602–6.

10. A. Hrøbjartsson and P. C. Gøtzsche, "Is the Placebo Powerless? An Analysis of Clinical Trials Comparing Placebos with No Treatment," *New England Journal of Medicine* 344 (2001): 1599. See also T. E. Einarson, M. Hemels, and P. Stolk, "Is the Placebo Powerless?" *New England Journal of Medicine* 345 (2001): 1277; G. S. Klienle and H. Kiene, "The Powerful Placebo's Effect: Fact or Fiction?" *Journal of Clinical Epidemiology* 50 (1997): 1311–18.

11. Richard Kradin, *The Placebo Response and the Power of Unconscious Healing* (New York: Routledge, 2008), 53; B. Jacobs, "Biblical Origins of Placebo," *Journal of the Royal Society of Medicine* 93 (2000): 213–14; P. D. Wall, "The Placebo and the Placebo Response," in Patrick D. Wall and Ronald Melzak, eds., *Text Book of Pain* (Edinburgh: Churchill Livingston, 1999), 1297–308. See also Arthur K. Shapiro and Elaine Shapiro, *The Powerful Placebo: From Ancient Priest to Modern Physician* (Baltimore: Johns Hopkins University Press, 1997).

12. George Motherby, *New Medical Dictionary* (London: n.p., 1785), q.v. "placebo"; E. Ernst, "Towards a Scientific Understanding of Placebo Effects," in David Peters, ed., *Understanding the Placebo Effect in Complementary Medicine: Theory, Practice, and Research* (Edinburgh: Churchill Livingstone, 2001), 17–30.

13. D. E. Moerman, "Edible Symbols: The Effectiveness of Placebos," *Annals of the New York Academy of Sciences* 77 (1981): 256. See also J. H. Warner, "The Nature-Trusting Heresy: American Physicians and the Concept of the Healing Power of Nature in the 1850s and 1860s," *Perspectives in American History* 11 (1977–1978): 291–324.

14. Beecher, "The Powerful Placebo"; H. Brody, "The Symbolic Power of the Modern Personal Physician: The Placebo Response Under Challenge," *Journal of Drug Issues* 18 (1988): 149–61; J. S. Welch, "Ritual in Western Medicine and Its Role in Placebo Healing," *Journal of Religion and Health* 42 (2003): 21–33; M. J. Bass et al., "The Physician's Actions and the Outcome of Illness in Family Practice," *Journal of Family Practice* 23 (1986): 43–47; A. M. Kleinman, "Medicine's Symbolic Reality," *Inquiry* 16 (1985): 206–13; K. B. Thomas, "The Consultation and the Therapeutic Illusion," *British Medical Journal* 1 (1978): 1327–28; M. A. Hall et al., "Trust in Physicians and Medical Institutions: What Is It, Can It Be Measured, and Does It Matter?" *Milbank Quarterly* 79 (2001): 613–39.

15. A. K. Shapiro, "Attitudes Toward the Use of Placebos in Treatment," *Journal of Nervous Mental Disorders* 130 (1960): 200–211; Shapiro, "A Contribution to the History of the Placebo Effect," 109–35.

16. Quoted in M. Enserink, "Can the Placebo Be the Cure?" *Science* 284 (1999): 238. See also T. Kaptchuk, "Powerful Placebo: The Dark Side of the Randomized Controlled Trial," *Lancet* 354 (1998): 1722–25.

17. S. Stewart-Williams, "The Placebo Puzzle: Putting Together the Pieces," *Health Psychology* 23 (2004): 198–206. Read also Richard Totman, *The Social Causes of Illness* (London: Souvenir Press, 1987); Ernst, "Towards a Scientific Understanding of Placebo Effects."

18. Eric J. Cassell, *The Nature of Suffering* (Oxford: Oxford University Press, 2004), 113.

19. Beecher, "The Powerful Placebo," 1602–6. See also A. K. Shapiro and L. A. Morris, "The Placebo Effect in Medical and Psychological Therapies," in Sol L. Garfield and Allen E. Bergin, eds., *The Handbook of Psychotherapy and Behavioral Change* (New York: Wiley, 1978), 369–410; Howard Brody, *Placebos and the Philosophy of Medicine: Clinical, Conceptual, and Ethical Issues* (Chicago: University of Chicago Press, 1980); Bausell, *Snake Oil Science*, 24–25.

20. H. K. Beecher, "Placebos for Relief of Pain," *Science* 132 (1960): 1567–69.

21. E. J. Wayne, "Placebos," *British Medical Journal* 2 (1956): 157; S. Bok, "The Ethics of Giving Placebos," *Scientific American* 231 (1974): 17–23.

22. Read the following works by Sissela Bok: *Lying: Moral Choice in Public and Private Life* (New York: Vintage, 1978); "Secrecy and Openness in Science: Ethical Considerations," *Science, Technology, and Human Values* 7 (1982): 32–41; and "The Ethics of Giving Placebos."

23. Bok, "The Ethics of Giving Placebos," 22.

24. B. Simmons, "Problems in Deceptive Medical Procedures: An Ethical and Legal Analysis of the Administration of Placebos," *Journal of Medical Ethics* 4 (1978): 179.

25. P. Lichtenberg, U. Heresco-Levy, and U. Nitzan, "The Ethics of the Placebo in Clinical Practice," *Journal of Medical Ethics* 30 (2004): 553. See also D. E. Moerman and W. B. Jonas, "Deconstructing the Placebo Effect and Finding the Meaning Response," *Annals of Internal Medicine* 136 (2002): 471–76; G. L. Engel, "The Need for a New Medical Model: A Challenge for Biomedicine," *Science* 196 (1977): 129–36; K. B. Thomas, "The Placebo in General Practice," *Lancet* 344 (1994): 1066–67; P. P. De Deyn and R. d'Hooge, "Placebos in Clinical Practice and Research," *Journal of Medical Ethics* 12 (1965): 336–45; H. Spiro, "Clinical Reflections on the Placebo Phenomenon," in Anne Harrington, ed., *The Placebo Effect: An Interdisciplinary Exploration* (Cambridge, MA: Harvard University Press, 1997), 37–55.

26. J. C. Tilburt et al., " 'Placebo Treatments': Results of a National Survey of U.S. Internists and Rheumatologists," *British Medical Journal* 337 (2008): 1097–1100. Read also Hróbjartsson and Norup, "The Uses of Placebo Interventions in Medical Practice," 153–65; R. Sherman and J. Hicker, "Academic Physicians Use Placebos in Clinical Practice and Believe in the Mind–Body Connection," *Journal of General Internal Medicine* 23 (2008): 7–10.

27. H. Brody, "The Lie That Heals: The Ethics of Giving Placebos," *Annals of Internal Medicine* 97 (1982): 117–18. Read also Tom H. Beauchamp and James F. Childress, *Principles of Biomedical Ethics* (New York: Oxford University Press, 1979); Howard Brody, *Ethical Decisions in Medicine*, 2nd ed. (Boston: Little, Brown, 1981); P. S. Jensen, "The Doctor–Patient Relationship: Headed for Impasse or Improvement?" *Annals of Internal Medicine* 95 (1981): 769–71; L. C. Park and L. Covi, "Nonblind Placebo Trial: An Exploration of Neurotic Outpatients' Response to Placebo When Its Inert Content Is Disclosed," *Archives of General Psychiatry* 12 (1965): 105–9; A. Soble, "Deception in Social Science Research: Is Informed Consent Possible?" *Hastings Center Report* 8 (1978): 40–46.

28. Moerman and Jonas, "Deconstructing the Placebo Effect and Finding the Meaning Response," 471–76.

29. D. Christensen, "Medicinal Mimicry: Sometimes, Placebos Work—but How?" *Science News* 159 (2001): 74.

30. A. K. Shapiro, "A Historic and Heuristic Definition of the Placebo," *Psychiatry* 27 (1964): 52–58; Shapiro and Shapiro, *The Powerful Placebo*, 41 (quote). See also P. C. Gøtzsche, "Is There Logic in the Placebo?" *Lancet* 344 (1994): 925–26; M. Shepherd, "The Placebo: From Specificity to the Non-specific and Back," *Psychological Medicine* 23 (1993): 569–78; Kaptchuk, "Powerful Placebo," 1722–25.

31. An alternative view is presented in the work of Martina Amanzio and Fabrizio Benedetti, who demonstrate how through the placebo's mediating influence on endorphins the mind can have a specific effect on the body. See M. Amanzio and F. Benedetti, "Neuropharmacological Dissection of Placebo Analgesia: Expectation Activated Opioid Systems Versus Conditioning Activated Specific Subsystems," *Journal of Neuroscience* 19 (1999): 484–94.

32. Shapiro and Shapiro, *The Powerful Placebo*, 41. For an alternate definition, see A. K. Shapiro, "Factors Contributing to the Placebo Effect," *American Journal of Psychotherapy* 18 (1961): 73–88.

33. P. Lacono et al., "Placebo Effect in Cardiovascular Clinical Pharmacology," *International Journal of Clinical Pharmacology Research* 12 (1992): 53.

34. S. Stewart-Williams, "The Placebo Puzzle: Putting Together the Pieces," *Health Psychology* 23 (2004): 200.

35. Shapiro, "A Historic and Heuristic Definition of the Placebo"; K. L. Melmon, H. F. Morrelli, and H. R. Bourne, "Rational Use of Placebo," in Kenneth L. Melmon and Howard F. Morrelli, eds., *Clinical Pharmacology: Basic Principles in Therapeutics*, 2nd ed. (New York: Macmillan, 1978), 1052–62.

36. Moerman and Jonas, "Deconstructing the Placebo Effect and Finding the Meaning Response," 471–76.

37. Daniel E. Moerman, *Meaning, Medicine, and the "Placebo Effect"* (Cambridge: Cambridge University Press, 2002), 14.

38. Quoted in "The Placebo Effect: Benefiting from Belief," http://www.angelfire.com/hi/The Seer/placebo.html, accessed July 7, 2011.

39. W. P. Kennedy, "The Nocebo Reaction," *Medical World* 95 (1961): 203–5, http://priory.com/medicine/Nocebo.htm, accessed July 8, 2011.

40. M. Ross and J. Olson, "An Expectancy–Attribution Model of the Effect of Placebos," *Psychological Review* 88 (1981): 409–37; A. E. Skodol, R. Plutchick, and T. B. Karasu, "Expectations of Hospital Treatment: Conflicting Views of Patients and Staff," *Journal of Nervous and Mental Diseases* 150 (1980): 73.

41. R. J. Connelly, "Deception and the Placebo Effect in Biomedical Research," *IRB: Ethics and Human Research* 9 (1987): 5; D. Lester, "Voodoo Death: Some New Thoughts on an Old Phenomenon," *American Anthropologist* 74 (1972): 386–90; W. B. Canon, "Voodoo Death," *American Anthropologist* 44 (1942): 169–81.

42. "Informed Consent May Be Hazardous to Health," *Science* 204 (1979): 11.

43. T. D. Wager, "The Neural Bases of Placebo Effects in Pain," *Current Directions in Psychological Science* 14 (2005): 175–79.

44. J. D. Levin, N. C. Gordon, and H. L. Fields, "The Mechanism of Placebo Analgesia," *Lancet* 2 (1978): 654–57; see also R. Prince, "The Endorphins: A Review for Psychological Anthropologists," *Ethos* 10 (1982): 411.

45. Examples of the research on the latter include E. Abramson and R. A. Arky, "Treatment of the Obese Diabetic: A Comparative Study of Placebo, Sulfonylurea, and Phenformin," *Metabolism: Clinical and Experimental* 16 (1967): 204–12; F. K. Abbot, M. Mack, and S. Wolf, "The Action of Banthine on the Stomach and Duodenum of Man, with Observations on the Effects of Placebos," *Gastroenterology* 29 (1952): 249–61.

46. R. W. Wilson and B. J. Elmassian, "Endorphins," *American Journal of Nursing* 81 (1981): 724.

47. S. W. Perry and G. Heidrich, "Placebo Response: Myth and Matter," *American Journal of Nursing* 81 (1981): 721.

48. Prince, "The Endorphins," 411; J. L. Henry, "Possible Involvement of Endorphins in Altered States of Consciousness," *Ethos* 10 (1982): 405.

49. V. M. S. Oh, "The Placebo Effect: Can We Use It Better?" *British Medical Journal* 309 (1994): 69–70.

50. I. Kirsch, "Response Expectancy as a Determinant of Experience and Behavior," *American Psychologist* 40 (1985): 1189–202; R. A. Hahn and A. Kleinman, "Belief as Pathogen, Belief as Medicine: 'Voodoo Death' and the 'Placebo Phenomenon' in Anthropological Perspective," *Medical Anthropology Quarterly* 14 (1983): 16–19.

51. S. Fisher, "The Placebo Reactor: Thesis, Antithesis, Synthesis, and Hypothesis," *Diseases of the Nervous System* 28 (1967): 17–23; J. H. Conn, "Cultural and Clinical Aspects of Hypnosis, Placebos, and Suggestibility," *International Journal of Clinical and Experimental Hypnosis* 7 (1959): 175–85; F. J. Evans, "The Placebo Response in Pain Reduction," in John J. Bonica, ed., *Advances in Neurology*, 5 vols. (New York: Raven, 1974), 4:289–96.

52. Kradin, *The Placebo Response and the Power of Unconscious Healing*, 85; see also W. R. Houston, "Doctor Himself as a Therapeutic Agent," *Annals of Internal Medicine* 11 (1938): 1416–25.

53. A. K. Shapiro, "The Curative Waters and Warm Poultices of Psychotherapy," paper delivered at the American Psychiatric Association Divisional Meeting, November 21, 1964, Philadelphia; Welch, "Ritual in Western Medicine and Its Role in Placebo Healing," 21–33; P. Lowinger and S. Dobie, "What Makes the Placebo Work," *Archives of General Psychiatry* 26 (1969): 84–88; Shapiro, "A Contribution to the History of the Placebo Effect," 109–35; J. Z. Smith, "The Bare Facts on Ritual," *History of Religions* 20 (1980): 112–27.

54. Michael Balint, *The Doctor, His Patient, and the Illness* (London: International Universities Press, 1972). See also H. Brody, "The Doctor as Therapeutic Agent: A Placebo Effect Research Agenda," in Harrington, ed., *The Placebo Effect*, 77–92; I. Wickramasekera, "A Conditioned Response Model of the Placebo Effect: Predictions From the Model," in

Leonard White, Bernard Tursky, and Gary E. Schwartz, eds., *Placebo: Theory, Research, and Mechanisms* (New York: Guilford Press, 1985), 255–87.

55. "Placebos," *British Medical Journal* 1 (1961): 43–44.

56. "Power of the Placebo," *Science News* 108 (1975): 20.

57. K. W. Berblinger, "The Influence of Personalities on Drug Therapy," *American Journal of Nursing* 59 (1959): 1130; see also B. Roueche, "Placebo," *New Yorker* 15 (1960): 85–103.

58. C. E. Goshen, "The Placebo Effect: For Whom?" *American Journal of Nursing* 66 (1966): 293–94.

59. R. Squires, "Confidence Tricks," *Philosophy* 69 (1994): 371–72.

60. See A. K. Shapiro, "Iatroplacebogenics," *International Pharmacopsychiatry* 2 (1969): 215–48.

61. Jerome D. Frank, *Persuasion and Healing: A Comparative Study of Psychotherapy* (Baltimore: Johns Hopkins University Press, 1961), 144. See also Charles G. Sorer, *Healing: Biblical, Medical, and Pastoral* (London: Christian Medical Fellowship, 1979); Louis Rose, *Faith Healing* (London: Gollanz, 1968); William A. Nolen, *Healing: A Doctor in Search of a Miracle* (New York: Fawcett, 1974).

62. Hall et al., "Trust in Physicians and Medical Institutions," 630. See also Jay Katz, *The Silent World of Doctor and Patient* (New York: Free Press, 1984); D. E. Moerman, "Cultural Variations in the Placebo Effect: Ulcers, Anxiety, and Blood Pressure," *Medical Anthropology Quarterly* 14 (2000): 25–26. See also D. D. Price, S. W. Harkins, and C. Baker, "Sensory-Affective Relationships Among Different Types of Clinical and Experimental Pain," *Pain* 28 (1987): 297–307; A. M. Kleinman, "Medicine's Symbolic Reality," *Inquiry* 16 (1985): 206–13.

63. See Bok, "The Ethics of Giving Placebos"; Beauchamp and Childress, *Principles of Biomedical Ethics*; S. J. Reiser, "Words as Scalpels: Transmitting Evidence in the Clinical Dialogue," *Annals of Internal Medicine* 92 (1980): 837–42; B. Simmons, "Problems in Deceptive Medical Procedures: An Ethical and Legal Analysis of the Administration of Placebos," *Journal of Medical Ethics* 4 (1978): 172–81; Robert M. Veatch, *A Theory of Medical Ethics* (New York: Basic Books, 1981).

64. See, for example, Talcott Parsons, *The Social System* (Glencoe, IL: Free Press, 1951); F. W. Peabody, "The Care of the Patient," *JAMA* 88 (1927): 877–82; D. Mechanic, "Changing Medical Organization and the Erosion of Trust," *Milbank Quarterly* 74 (1996): 171–89 ; Edmund D. Pellegrino, Robert M. Veatch, and John P. Langan, *Ethics, Trust, and the Professions: Philosophical and Cultural Aspects* (Washington, DC: Georgetown University Press, 1991).

65. M. A. Hall, "Law, Medicine, and Trust," *Stanford Law Review* 55 (2002): 470–71, 481–82. See also Hall et al., "Trust in Physicians and Medical Institutions," 613–39; Bass et al., "The Physician's Actions and the Outcome of Illness in Family Practice," 43–47; Brody, "The Symbolic Power of the Modern Personal Physician," 149–61; A. M. Kleinman, "Medicine's Symbolic Reality," *Inquiry* 16 (1985): 206–13. See also Tom F. Driver, *The Magic of Ritual: Our Need for Liberating Rites That Transform Our Lives and Our Communities* (San Francisco: HarperCollins, 1991).

66. Z. Di Blasi et al., "The Influence of Context Effects on Health Outcomes: A Systematic Review," *Lancet* 357 (2001): 757–62; J. Z. Smith, "The Bare Facts on Ritual," *History of Religions* 20 (1980): 112–27, http://www.doloreskrieger.com/, accessed July 7, 2011.

67. I. D. Coulter et al., "Patients Using Chiropractors in North America: Who Are They and Why Are They in Chiropractic Care?" *Spine* 27 (2002): 291–97; I. D. Coulter, R. D. Hayes, and C. D. Danielson, "The Chiropractic Satisfaction Questionnaire," *Topics in Clinical Chiropractic* 1 (1994): 40–43; C. Goertz et al., "The Chiropractic Report Card: Patient Satisfaction Study," *Journal of the American Chiropractic Association* 34 (1997): 40–47.

68. T. Kaptchuk, "The Placebo Effect in Alternative Medicine: Can the Performance of a Healing Ritual Have Clinical Significance?" *Annals of Internal Medicine* 136 (2002): 817–25; W. Brown, "The Placebo Effect," *Scientific American* 278 (1998): 90–95.

69. R. A. Cooper and H. J. McKee, "Chiropractic in the United States: Trends and Issues," *Milbank Quarterly* 81 (2003): 114. See also J. A. Astin, "Why Patients Use Alternative Medicine: Results of a National Study," *JAMA* 279 (1998): 1548–53; P. G. Shekelle, M. Markovich, and R. Louie, "An Epidemiologic Study of Episodes of Back Pain Care," *Spine* 20 (1995): 1668–73; P. G. Shekelle, M. Markovich, and R. Louie, "Factors Associated with Choosing a Chiropractor for Episodes of Back Pain Care," *Medical Care* 33 (1995): 842–50.

70. Shapiro, "A Historic and Heuristic Definition of the Placebo"; Melmon, Morrelli, and Bourne, "Rational Use of Placebo," 1052–62; Beecher, "The Powerful Placebo," 1602–6.

71. M. J. DiNubile, "Skepticism: A Lost Clinical Art," *Clinical Infectious Diseases* 32 (2000): 514.

72. H. Walach and W. B. Jonas, "Placebo Research: The Evidence Base for Harnessing Self-Healing Capacities," *Journal of Alternative and Complementary Medicine* 10 (2004): S108.

73. T. Kaptchuk, "Subjectivity and the Placebo Effect in Medicine: An Interview by Bonnie Horrigan," *Alternative Therapies* 7 (2001): 102; see also Ted J. Kaptchuk, *The Web That Has No Weaver: Understanding Chinese Medicine* (Chicago: Contemporary Press, 2000).

74. Frank, *Persuasion and Healing*, 24–35.

75. Hrøbjartsson and Gøtzsche, "Is the Placebo Powerless?" 1594–602.

76. E. Ernst and K. L. Resch, "Concept of True and Perceived Placebo Effects," *British Medical Journal* 311 (1995): 551–53; see also Bausell, *Snake Oil Science*, 95–97.

77. P. C. Gøtzsche, "Concept of Placebo Should Be Discarded," *British Medical Journal* 311 (1995): 1640.

78. R. M. Coe, "The Magic of Science and the Science of Magic: An Essay on the Process of Healing," *Journal of Health and Social Behavior* 38 (1997): 1–8.

79. D. E. Moerman, "General Medical Effectiveness and Human Biology: Placebo Effects in the Treatment of Ulcer Disease," *Medical Anthropology Quarterly* 14 (1983): 3, 13. See also Hahn and Kleinman, "Belief as Pathogen, Belief as Medicine," 3, 16–19; H. Brody, "Does Disease Have a Natural History?" *Medical Anthropology Quarterly* 14 (1983): 20; Beecher, "The Powerful Placebo," 1102–7.

80. Brody, "Does Disease Have a Natural History?" 20; Beecher, "The Powerful Placebo," 1102–7.

81. H. Brody, "On Placebos," *Hastings Center Report* 5 (1975): 17–18.

82. Brody, "The Doctor as Therapeutic Agent," 78.

83. Shapiro, "A Historic and Heuristic Definition of the Placebo"; Beecher, "The Powerful Placebo," 1602–6; Andrew Weil, *The Natural Mind: A Revolutionary Approach to the Drug Problem* (Boston: Houghton, Mifflin, 1972).

84. M. Meldrum, "Review," *Isis* 90 (1999): 353.

85. Oh, "The Placebo Effect," 69–70.

86. H. Benson and R. Friedman, "Harnessing the Power of the Placebo Effect and Renaming It 'Remembered Wellness,'" *Annual Review of Medicine* 47 (1996): 193–99; H. Benson and D. P. McCallie Jr., "Angina Pectoris and the Placebo Effect," *New England Journal of Medicine* 300 (1979): 1424–29; UK Gabapentin Study Group, "Gabapentin in Partial Epilepsy," *Lancet* 335 (1990): 1114–17; S. M. Downer et al., "Pursuit and Practice of Complementary Therapies by Cancer Patients Receiving Conventional Treatment," *British Medical Journal* 309 (1994): 86–89.

87. P. Bennett, "Placebo and Healing," in Joseph E. Pizzorno and Michael T. Murray, eds., *Textbook of Natural Medicine*, 2 vols. (New York: Churchill Livingstone, 1999), 1:51–71.

88. A. Harrington, "Introduction," in Harrington, ed., *The Placebo Effect*, 1–2.

89. A. Harrington, "The Placebo Effect and Alternative Medicine: Reimagining the Relationship," in Michael I. Weintraub and Marc S. Micozzi, eds., *Alternative and Complementary Treatment in Neurologic Illness* (New York: Churchill Livingstone, 2001), 152–54. See also Moerman, "General Medical Effectiveness and Human Biology," 14–16; R. Bennett, "The Power of Placebos: Shaking Off Their Image as 'Inert Substances,' Placebos Are Finding New Respect," http://oregonlive.com/news/99/07/st072820.html, accessed April 22, 2011.

90. Harrington, "The Placebo Effect and Alternative Medicine," 154.

91. Kaptchuk, "Subjectivity and the Placebo Effect in Medicine," 106.

92. Howard Spiro, *The Power of Hope: A Doctor's Perspective* (New Haven, CT: Yale University Press, 1998), 18; Moerman, "Cultural Variations in the Placebo Effect," 51–72.

4. POLITICS OF HEALING

1. "OAM Legislative History," in *Seventh Meeting of the Alternative Medicine Program Advisory Council, Office of Alternative Medicine, National Institutes of Health* (Bethesda, MD: Office of Alternative Medicine, 1996), 41. See also J. Warren Salmon, ed., *Alternative Medicine: Popular and Policy Perspectives* (New York: Tavistock, 1984).

2. G. Kolata, "In Quests Outside Mainstream, Medical Projects Rewrite Policy," *New York Times*, June 18, 1996.

3. D. Brown, "A New Look at Alternative Therapies," *Washington Post*, June 23, 1992; E. Marshall, "The Politics of Alternative Medicine," *Science* 265 (1994): 2000–2002; S. Budiansky, "Cures or Quackery?" *U.S. News & World Report*, July 17, 1995, 48–51; F. Wiewel, "Alternative Medicine Warrants Study," *Des Moines Register*, December 21, 1994.

4. Quoted in Marshall, "The Politics of Alternative Medicine," 2000.

5. J. H. Young, "The Development of the Office of Alternative Medicine in the National Institutes of Health, 1991–1996," *Bulletin of the History of Medicine* 72 (1998): 279–98.

6. Quoted in Budiansky, "Cures or Quackery?" 50. See also Workshop on Alternative Medicine, *Alternative Medicine: Expanding Medical Horizons—a Report to the National Institutes of Health on Alternative Medical Systems and Practices in the United States* (Bethesda, MD: National Institutes of Health, 1995).

7. D. McLellan, "Medicine Man," *Washingtonian*, May 1993: 46–47, 124–25; C. Wallis, J. M. Horowitz, and E. Lafferty, "Why New Age Medicine Is Catching On," *Time*, November 4, 1991, 46–57.

8. J. Price, "Alternative-Medicine Unit Told to Get Busy," *Washington Times*, June 25, 1993.

9. Quoted in Marshall, "The Politics of Alternative Medicine," 2000–2001.

10. Ibid., 2002.

11. J. E. Pizzorno, "Naturopathic Medicine—a Ten-Year Perspective (from a 35-Year View)," *Alternative Therapies in Health and Medicine* 11 (2005): 24–26.

12. H. A. Baer, "The Sociopolitical Status of U.S. Naturopathy at the Dawn of the 21st Century," *Medical Anthropology Quarterly* 15 (2001): 330–31, 339. See also Andrew Weil, *Health and Healing: Understanding Conventional and Alternative Medicine* (Boston: Houghton Mifflin, 1983), 138; J. Jagtenberg et al., "Evidence-Based Medicine and Naturopathy," *Journal of Alternative and Complementary Medicine* 12 (2006): 323–28; P. McKnight, "Naturopathy's Main Article of Faith Cannot Be Validated," http://vancouversun.com/story_print.html, accessed September 9, 2011.

13. N. Angier, "U.S. Head of Alternative Medicine Quits," *New York Times*, August 1, 1994.

14. K. A. Gazella and S. Snyder, "Wayne B. Jonas, M.D.: Supporting the Scientific Foundation of Integrative Medicine," *Alternative Therapies in Health and Medicine* 11 (2005): 69–74.

15. Wayne Jonas and Jennifer Jacobs, *Healing with Homeopathy: The Complete Guide* (New York: Warner, 1996) and *Healing with Homeopathy: The Doctor's Guide* (New York: Warner, 1998).

16. Young, "The Development of the Office of Alternative Medicine in the National Institutes of Health,," 291–92.

17. W. B. Jonas, "Policy, the Public, and Priorities in Alternative Medicine Research," *Annals of the American Academy of Political and Social Science* 583 (2002): 37–38; see also Daniel Callahan, ed., *The Role of Complementary and Alternative Medicine: Accommodating Pluralism* (Washington, DC: Georgetown University Press, 2002).

18. Jonas, "Policy, the Public, and Priorities in Alternative Medicine Research," 33.

19. Gazella and Snyder, "Wayne B. Jonas, M.D.," 69–74.

20. See Harris L. Coulter, *The Controlled Clinical Trial: An Analysis* (Washington, DC: Center for Empirical Medicine, 1991).

21. W. B. Jonas, "Alternative Medicine—Learning from the Past, Examining the Present, Advancing to the Future," *JAMA* 280 (1998): 1617. See also Hastings Center, *The Goals of Medicine: Setting New Priorities* (New York: Hastings Center, 1996).

22. J. S. Levin et al., "Quantitative Methods in Research on Complementary and Alternative Medicine: A Methodological Manifesto," *Medical Care* 35 (1997): 1079–81. Larry Dossey, the editor of *Alternative Therapies in Health and Medicine*, used the journal's inaugural issue to encourage a reexamination of how alternative therapies should and ought to be studied. See L. Dossey, "How Should Alternative Therapies Be Evaluated? An Examination of Fundamentals," *Alternative Therapies in Health and Medicine* 1 (1995): 13–14.

23. Levin et al., "Quantitative Methods in Research on Complementary and Alternative Medicine," 1083–84.

24. Read George T. Lewith and David Aldridge, eds., *Clinical Research Methodology for Complementary Therapies* (London: Hodder and Stoughton, 1993).

25. D. M. Eisenberg et al., "Unconventional Medicine in the United States: Prevalence, Costs, and Patterns of Use," *New England Journal of Medicine* 328 (1993): 246–52.

26. Levin et al., "Quantitative Methods in Research on Complementary and Alternative Medicine," 1082–84.

27. Practice and Policy Guidelines Panel, NIH Office of Alternative Medicine, "Clinical Practice Guidelines in Complementary and Alternative Medicine: An Analysis of Opportunities and Obstacles," *Archives of Family Medicine* 6 (1997): 149–54.

28. Levin et al., "Quantitative Methods in Research on Complementary and Alternative Medicine," 1086–92.

29. Ibid., 1079.

30. Ibid., 1089.

31. Ibid., 1090.

32. Ibid., 1092.

33. F. M. Frohock, "Moving Lines and Variable Criteria: Differences/Connections Between Allopathic and Alternative Medicine," *Annals of the American Academy of Political and Social Science* 583 (2002): 227.

34. P. B. Fontanarosa and G. D. Lundberg, "Alternative Medicine Meets Science," *JAMA* 280 (1998): 1619.

35. M. Angell and J. P. Kassirer, "Alternative Medicine—the Risks of Untested and Unregulated Remedies," *New England Journal of Medicine* 339 (1998): 839.

36. Quoted in M. Crane, "Let's Stop Giving Alternative Medicine a Free Ride," *Medical Economic*, February 21, 2000, http://medicaleconomics.modernmedicine.com/memag/Alternative+Medicine/Lets-stop-giving-alternative-medicine-a-free-ride/ArticleStandard/Article/detail/121128, accessed September 9, 2012.

37. NCCAM, "Five Year Strategic Plan," http://nccam.nih.gov/about/plans/fiveyear/, accessed April 28, 2011. See also W. R. Harlan, "New Opportunities and Proven Approaches in Complementary and Alternative Medicine Research at the National Institutes of Health," *Journal of Alternative and Complementary Medicine* 7 (2001): 53–59; S. E. Straus, "Complementary and Alternative Medicine: Challenges and Opportunities for American Medicine," *Academic Medicine* 75 (2000): 572–73.

38. Jonas, "Policy, the Public, and Priorities in Alternative Medicine Research," 34–35.

39. Quoted in J. Couzin, "Beefed-Up NIH Center Probes Unconventional Therapies," *Science* 282 (1998): 2175–76.

40. H. Varmus, "Proliferation of National Institutes of Health," *Science* 291 (2001): 1903–4.

41. E. Stokstad, "Stephen Straus's Impossible Job," *Science* 288 (2000): 1568. See also K. C. Atwood, "The Ongoing Problem with the National Center for Complementary and Alternative Medicine," *Skeptical Inquirer* 27 (2003): 3–11.

42. Stokstad, "Stephen Straus's Impossible Job," 1568.

43. S. Maimes, "Spirituality and Healing in Medicine," *Healthcare Review* 15 (2002): 7; D. Bessinger and T. Kuhne, "Medical Spirituality: Defining Domains and Boundaries," *Southern Medical Journal* 95 (2002): 1385–426; T. Daaleman, A. K. Cobb, and B. Frey, "Spirituality and Well Being: An Exploratory Study of the Patient Perspective," *Social Science and Medicine* 53 (2001): 1503–11; D. B. Larson and S. B. Larson, "Spirituality's Potential Relevance to Physical and Emotional Health: A Brief Review of Quantitative Research," *Journal of Psychology and Theology* 31 (2003): 37–52. The Gonzalez Protocol, named after Nicholas James Gonzalez of New York City, was based on the assumption that cancer and other degenerative diseases are caused by toxins and physiological imbalances. Gonzalez offered individualized nutritional/enzyme protocols as treatment.

44. Stokstad, "Stephen Straus's Impossible Job," 1570.

45. Ibid., 1569; "Two Dietary Supplements Supported by Study," *New York Times*, March 15, 2000.

46. Couzin, "Beefed-Up NIH Center Probes Unconventional Therapies," 2175–76; J. Raloff, "A Fishy Therapy," *Science News* 167 (2005): 154–56; P. Falardeau et al., "Neovastat, a Naturally Occurring Multifunctional Antiangiogenic Drug, in Phase III Clinical Trials," *Seminars in Oncology* 28 (2001): 620–25; D. J. Newman and G. M. Cragg, "Advanced Preclinical and Clinical Trials of Natural Products and Related Compounds from Marine Sources," *Current Medicinal Chemistry* 11 (2004): 1693–713; C. L. Loprinzi et al., "Evaluation of Shark Cartilage in Patients with Advanced Cancer: A North Central Cancer Treatment Group Trial," *Cancer* 104 (2005): 176–82; National Cancer Institute, NIH, "Cartilage (Bovine and Shark)," http://www.cancer.gov/cancertopics/pdq/cam/cartilage/Healthprofes, accessed September 13, 2012.

47. E. Ernst, "Chelation Therapy for Coronary Heart Disease," *American Heart Journal* 140 (2000): 139–41; M. L. Knudtson et al., "Chelation Therapy for Ischemic Heart Disease," *JAMA* 287 (2002): 481–86, http://clinicaltrials.gov, accessed June 17, 2011; for links to sites on questionable cancer treatments, go to http://www.quackwatch.org/01Quackery Related Topics/Cancer/kg.html, accessed June 17, 2011.

48. J. S. Markowitz et al., "Effect of St. John's Wort on Drug Metabolism by Induction of Cytochrome P450 3A4 Enzyme," *JAMA* 290 (2003): 1500–1504; R. B. Turner et al., "An Evaluation of *Echinacea anguistifolia* in Experimental Rhinovirus Infections," *New England Journal of Medicine* 353 (2005): 341–48; S. Bent et al., "Saw Palmetto for Benign Prostatic Hyperplasia," *New England Journal of Medicine* 354 (2006): 1950–51.

49. Quoted in D. A. Taylor, "Botanical Supplements: Weeding Out the Health Risks," *Environmental Health Perspectives* 112 (2004): 753.

50. G. Kolata, "Study Says Echinacea Has No Effect on Colds," *New York Times*, July 28, 2005.

51. V. Adams, "Randomized Controlled Crime: Postcolonial Sciences in Alternative Medicine Research," *Social Studies of Science* 32 (2002): 670.

52. Ibid., 671–76.

53. "Coordination of Research," in White House Commission on Complementary and Alternative Medicine Policy, *Final Report, March 2002* (Washington, DC: White House Commission on Complementary and Alternative Medicine Policy, 2002), 31, http://govinfo .library.unt.edu/whccamp/pdfs/fr2002_document.pdf, accessed April 23, 2011.

54. D. M. Marcus and A. P. Grollman, "Response," *Science* 314 (2006): 1084.

55. J. S. Gordon, "The Chairman's Vision," in White House Commission on Complementary and Alternative Medicine Policy, *Final Report, March 2002*, x.

56. Ibid., x.

57. "Introduction," in White House Commission on Complementary and Alternative Medicine Policy, *Final Report, March 2002*, 5–6. See also M. Angell and J. P. Kassirer, "Alternative Medicine—the Risks of Untested and Unregulated Remedies," *New England Journal of Medicine* 339 (1998): 839–41.

58. "Executive Summary," in White House Commission on Complementary and Alternative Medicine Policy, *Final Report, March 2002*, xvi, http://www.whccamp.hhs.gov/es.html, accessed April 5, 2011.

59. Tracy Deliman and John H. Smolowe, *Holistic Medicine: Harmony of Body, Mind, Spirit* (Upper Saddle River, NJ: Prentice-Hall, 1982); Barbara Montgomery Dossey, *Holistic Health Promotion: A Guide for Practice* (Rockville, MD: Aspen, 1989); Robert Fuller, *Alternative Medicine and American Religious Life* (New York: Oxford University Press, 1989); M. Goldstein et al., "Holistic Physicians and Family Practitioners: Similarities, Differences, and Implications for Health Policy," *Social Science and Medicine* 26 (1988): 853–61; Daniel Goldman and Joel Gurin, *Mind Body Medicine: How to Use Your Mind for Better Health* (New York: Consumer's Union, 1993).

60. "Executive Summary," xvi.

61. A. Williams, "Therapeutic Landscapes in Holistic Medicine," *Social Science and Medicine* 46 (1998): 1193–203.

62. Gordon, "The Chairman's Vision," xiii.

63. "Executive Summary."

64. N. R. Slifman et al., "Contamination of Dietary Supplements by Digitalis Ianata," *New England Journal of Medicine* 339 (1998): 806–11; R. J. Ko, "Adulterants in Asian Patent Medicines," *New England Journal of Medicine* 339 (1998): 847.

65. "Executive Summary," xxiv.

66. Ibid.

67. "Coordination of Research," 47.

68. "Education and Training of Health Care Practitioners," in White House Commission on Complementary and Alternative Medicine Policy, *Final Report, March 2002*, 52. See also

D. M. Marcus, "How Should Alternative Medicine Be Taught to Medical Students and Physicians?" *Academic Medicine* 76 (2001): 224–29; W. Sampson, "The Need for Educational Reform in Teaching About Alternative Therapies," *Academic Medicine* 76 (2001): 248–50; T. W. Gaudet, "Integrative Medicine: The Evolution of a New Approach to Medicine and Medical Education," *Integrative Medicine* 1 (1998): 30–33.

69. L. A. Moyé et al., "Research Methodology in Psychoneuroimmunology: Rationale and Design of the IMAGES-P Clinical Trial," *Alternative Therapies in Health and Medicine* 1 (1995): 34; C. Marwick, "Complementary, Alternative Therapies Should Face Rigorous Testing, IOM Concludes," *Journal of the National Cancer Institute* 97 (2005): 255–56; D. Riley and B. Berman, "Complementary and Alternative Medicine in Outcomes Research," *Alternative Therapies in Health and Medicine* 8 (2002): 36–37; N. Vuckovic, "Integrating Qualitative Methods in Randomized Controlled Trials: The Experience of the Oregon Center for Complementary and Alternative Medicine," *Journal of Alternative and Complementary Medicine* 8 (2002): 225–27; E. Ernst, "Intangible Principles of Good Research in Complementary and Alternative Medicine," *Alternative Therapies in Health and Medicine* 8 (2002): 22; C. J. Schneider and W. B. Jonas, "Are Alternative Treatments Effective? Issues and Methods Involved in Measuring Effectiveness of Alternative Treatments," *Subtle Energies* 5 (1994): 69; E. Marshall, "The Politics of Alternative Medicine," *Science* 265 (1994): 2000; J. Steinberg, "Alternative-Medicine Office: A Time to Heal," *Journal of NIH Research* 7 (1995): 34.

70. Quoted in Dónal P. O'Manthúna, *Alternative Medicine: A Response to the White House Commission on Complementary and Alternative Medicine Policy* (Washington, DC: Christian Medical Association, 2002), 8.

71. Ibid., 4, quoting the report.

72. K. F. Schaffner, "Assessments on Efficacy in Biomedicine: The Turn Toward Methodological Pluralism," in Callahan, ed., *The Role of Complementary and Alternative Medicine*, 1–14.

73. F. M. Frohock, "Moving Lines and Variable Criteria: Differences/Connections Between Allopathic and Alternative Medicine," *Annals of the American Academy of Political and Social Science* 583 (2002): 221–23.

74. Callahan, ed., *The Role of Complementary and Alternative Medicine.*

75. Marc S. Micozzi, *Fundamentals of Complementary and Alternative Medicine* (New York: Churchill Livingstone, 1996).

76. The committee members included Stuart Bondurant, Joyce Anastasi, Brian Berman, Margaret Buhrmaster, Gerard Burrow, Michele Chang, Larry Churchill, Florence Comite, Jeanne Drisko, David Eisenberg, Alfred Fishman, Susan Folkman, Albert Mulley, David Nerenz, Mark Nichter, Bernard Rosof, Harold Sox, Ellen Gritz, and Michael Cohen.

77. Institute of Medicine (IOM), *Complementary and Alternative Medicine in the United States* (Washington, DC: National Academies Press, 2005), 31.

78. D. M. Eisenberg, "The Institute of Medicine Report on Complementary and Alternative Medicine in the United States—Personal Reflections on Its Content and Implications," *Alternative Therapies in Health and Medicine* 11 (2005): 11.

79. IOM, *Complementary and Alternative Medicine in the United States*, 66–67, as summarized in ibid., 12.

80. Eisenberg, "The Institute of Medicine Report on Complementary and Alternative Medicine in the United States," 12; IOM, *Complementary and Alternative Medicine in the United States*, 62, 221.

81. J. P. Briggs, "Message from the Director: Listening to Different Voices," April 19, 2010, http://nccam.nih.gov/about/offices/od/2010-04.htm, accessed August 8, 2011.

82. W. Sampson, "Why the National Center for Complementary and Alternative Medicine (NCCAM) Should Be Defunded," http://www.quackwatch.org/01QuackeryRelatedTopics/nccam.html, accessed September 27, 2013; E. C. Halperin, "Let's Abolish the Office of Alternative Medicine of the National Institutes of Health," *North Carolina Medical Journal* 59 (1998): 21–23.

83. G. Weissmann, "Homeopathy: Holmes, Hogwarts, and the Prince of Wales," *Journal of the Federation of American Societies for Experimental Biology* 20 (2006): 1757.

84. D. M. Marcus and A. P. Grollman, "Review for NCCAM Is Overdue," *Science* 313 (2006): 301–2.

85. Steven Novella, "Our Visit with NCCAM," *Science-Based Medicine*, http://www.sciencebasedmedicine.org/our-visit-with-nccam/, accessed October 30, 2013.

86. T. Winnick, "From Quackery to 'Complementary' Medicine: The American Medical Profession Confronts Alternative Therapies," *Social Problems* 52 (2005): 44.

5. COMPLEMENTARY AND ALTERNATIVE MEDICINE'S CHALLENGE: A CASE STUDY

1. See Paul A. Komesaroff, *Troubled Bodies: Critical Perspectives on Postmodernism, Medical Ethics, and the Body* (Durham, NC: Duke University Press, 1995); Ronald A. Carson and Chester R. Burns, eds., *Philosophy of Medicine and Bioethics: A Twenty-Year Retrospective and Critical Appraisal* (Dordrecht, Netherlands: Kluwer, 1997); Nicholas J. Fox, *Postmodernism, Sociology, and Health* (Buckingham, UK: Open University Press, 1993); Graham Scambler and Paul Higgs, eds., *Modernity, Medicine, and Health: Medical Sociology Towards 2000* (London: Routledge, 1998).

2. S. Goldbeck-Wood et al., "Complementary Medicine Is Booming Worldwide," *British Medical Journal* 313 (1996): 131–33; N. K. Rasmussen and J. M. Morgall, "The Use of Alternative Treatments in the Danish Adult Population," *Complementary Medical Research* 4 (1990): 16–22; T. Vaskilampi et al., "The Use of Alternative Treatments in the Finnish Adult Population," in George T. Lewith and David Aldridge, eds., *Clinical Research Methodology for Complementary Therapies* (London: Hodder and Stoughton, 1993), 204–29; A. H. MacLennan, D. H. Wilson, and A. W. Taylor, "Prevalence and Cost of Alternative Medicine in Australia," *Lancet* 347 (1996): 569–73; W. J. Millar, "Use of Alternative Health Care Practitioners by Canadians," *Canadian Journal of Public Health* 88 (1997): 154–58; P.

Fisher and A. Ward, "Complementary Medicine in Europe," *British Medical Journal* 309 (1996): 107–11.

3. Ursula Sharma, *Complementary Medicine Today: Practitioners and Patients* (London: Tavistock/Routledge, 1992), 16–17.

4. Fisher and Ward, "Complementary Medicine in Europe," 107–11. See also P. Pietroni, "Beyond the Boundaries: Relationship Between General Practice and Complementary Medicine," *British Medical Journal* 305 (1992): 564–66; George T. Lewith and David Aldridge, eds., *Complementary Medicine and the European Community* (Saffron Walden, UK: Daniel, 1991).

5. Sharma, *Complementary Medicine Today*, 16–17

6. Goldbeck-Wood et al., "Complementary Medicine Is Booming Worldwide," 131.

7. Read Kate Thomas, *National Survey of Access to Complementary Health Care Via General Practice* (Sheffield, UK: Medical Care Research Unit, Sheffield University, 1995), 5.

8. C. Zollman and A. Vickers, "ABC of Complementary Medicine: Complementary Medicine in Conventional Practice," *British Medical Journal* 319 (1999): 901–4.

9. "Alternative and Complementary Medicine: What's a Doctor to Do?" *Hastings Center Report* 30 (2000): 47–48.

10. A. Vickers and C. Zollman, "ABC of Complementary Medicine: Homeopathy," *British Medical Journal* 319 (1999): 1115–18.

11. S. Hahnemann, "Essay on a New Principle for Ascertaining the Curative Powers of Drugs, with a Few Glances at Those Hitherto Employed," in *The Lesser Writings of Samuel Hahnemann*, trans. Robert E. Dudgeon (New York: Radde, 1852), 259–61. See also Samuel Hahnemann, *Organon of Homeopathic Medicine* (Allentown, PA: Academical Bookstore, 1836), and *The Chronic Diseases: Their Specific Nature and Homeopathic Treatment*, 5 vols. (New York: Radde, 1845–1846); Thomas Lindsay Bradford, *The Life and Letters of Dr. Samuel Hahnemann* (Philadelphia: Boericke and Tafel, 1895); Benjamin F. Joslin, *Principles of Homeopathy. In a Series of Lectures* (New York: Radde, 1850); John S. Haller Jr., *The History of American Homeopathy: The Academic Years, 1820–1835* (New York: Haworth Press, 2005).

12. J. S. Haller Jr., "Decline of Bloodletting: A Study in Nineteenth Century Ratiocinations," *Southern Medical Journal* 79 (1986): 469–75; J. S. Haller Jr., "Samson of the Materia Medica: Medical Theory and the Use and Abuse of Calomel in 19th Century America," *Pharmacy in History* 13 (1971): 27–34, 67–76; J. S. Haller Jr., "The Use and Abuse of Tartar Emetic in the 19th Century Materia Medica," *Bulletin of the History of Medicine* 49 (1975): 235–57.

13. H. M. Smith, "Present Position of Medical Science," *American Homeopathic Review* 1 (1858): 2–4.

14. N. Rogers, "American Homeopathy Confronts Scientific Medicine," in Robert Jütte, Guenter B. Risse, and John Woodward, eds., *Culture, Knowledge, and Healing: Historical Perspectives of Homeopathic Medicine in Europe and North America* (Sheffield, UK: European Association for the History of Medicine and Health Publications, 1998), 31.

15. Haller, *The History of American Homeopathy: The Academic Years*, 70–89.

16. W. A. Dewey, "Propagantism of Homeopathy in Universities," *Transactions of the American Institute of Homeopathy* 1905:118–26; J. B. Nichols, "Medical Sectarianism," *JAMA* 60 (1913): 331–37.

17. John S. Haller Jr., *The History of American Homeopathy: From Rational Medicine to Holistic Health Care* (New Brunswick, NJ: Rutgers University Press, 2009), 63–85; D. M. Eisenberg et al., "Trends in Alternative Medicine Use in the United States, 1990–1997: Results of a Follow-up National Survey," *JAMA* 280 (1998): 1569–75.

18. Haller, *The History of American Homeopathy: From Rational Medicine to Holistic Health Care*, 141–51.

19. Read Eliot Freidson, *Professional Powers: A Study of the Institutionalization of Formal Knowledge* (Chicago: University of Chicago Press, 1986); Gerald Larkin, *Occupational Monopoly and Modern Medicine* (London: Tavistock, 1983); Phillip Nicholls, *Homeopathy and the Medical Profession* (London: Croom Helm, 1988).

20. The new American College of Homeopathy opened in Phoenix, Arizona, in February 2011, the first homeopathic college to be established in the United States since 1920. Its success remains to be seen.

21. D. Ullman, "Homeopathy and Managed Care: Manageable or Unmanageable?" *Journal of Alternative and Complementary Medicine* 5 (1999): 63–73; R. Frank, "Integrating Homeopathy and Biomedicine: Medical Practice and Knowledge Production Among German Homeopathic Physicians," *Sociology of Health and Illness* 24 (2002): 815.

22. J. Ruusuvuori, "Empathy and Sympathy in Action: Attending to Patients' Troubles in Finish Homeopathic and General Practice Consultation," *Social Psychology Quarterly* 68 (2005): 204–22; W. A. Beach and C. N. Dixson, "Revealing Moments: Formulating Understandings of Adverse Experiences in a Health Appraisal Interview," *Social Science and Medicine* 52 (2001): 25–44; W. T. Branch and T. K. Malik, "Using 'Windows of Opportunities' in Brief Interviews to Understand Patients' Concerns," *JAMA* 269 (1993): 1667–68; J. Coulter, "Discourse and Mind," *Human Studies* 22 (1999): 163–81; J. Halpern, "Empathy: Using Resonance Emotions in the Service of Curiosity," in Howard M. Spiro et al., eds., *Empathy and the Practice of Medicine: Beyond Pills and the Scalpel* (New Haven, CT: Yale University Press, 1996), 160–73.

23. M. Van Wassenhoven and G. Ives, "An Observational Study of Patients Receiving Homeopathic Treatment," *Homeopathy* 93 (2004): 3–11; T. D. Thompson and M. Weiss, "Homeopathy—What Are the Active Ingredients? An Exploratory Study Using the UK Medical Research Council's Framework for the Evaluation of Complex Interventions," *BMC Complementary and Alternative Medicine* 6 (2006): 37.

24. "How to Use High Potencies," *Homeopathic Physician* 2 (1882): 73; W. B. Jonas and E. Ernst, "The Safety of Homeopathy," in Wayne B. Jonas, Jeffrey S. Levin, and Brian Berman, eds., *The Essentials of Complementary and Alternative Medicine* (Philadelphia: Lippincott Williams and Wilkins, 1999), 167–71.

25. In addition to homeopathy, there is also what Dr. Roy Martina of Holland calls "resonance homeopathy," whose medicines are "amplified" by ingredients known to have "energetic

signatures." See the ad for Apex Energetics and Resonance Homeopathy at http://www.ritecare.com/members/apexenergetics.asp, accessed August 1, 2011. Generally speaking, the term *"low" potencies* refers to remedies lower than Avogadro's number (as explained later in this chapter), whereas *"high" potencies* refers to those higher than it.

26. See K. C. Elliott, "A Novel Account of Scientific Anomaly: Help for the Dispute Over Low-Dose Biochemical Effects," *Philosophy of Science* 73 (2006): 790–802.

27. S. Hahnemann, "Remarks on the Extreme Attenuation of Homeopathic Medicines," in *The Lesser Writings of Samuel Hahnemann*, 765.

28. James Y. Simpson, *Homeopathy: Its Tenets and Tendencies, Theoretical, Theological, and Therapeutical* (Philadelphia: Lindsay and Blakiston, 1854), 68–69.

29. "Single Remedy Guide: Dilutions," http://www.hmedicine.com/homeopathy/information/remedy_guide/dilutions, accessed August 21, 2011.

30. Hahnemann, *Organon of Homeopathic Medicine*, 210–11; M. Dinges, "Men's Bodies 'Explained' on a Daily Basis in Letters from Patients to Samuel Hahnemann (1830–35)," in *Patients in the History of Homeopathy* (Sheffield, UK: European Association for the History of Medicine and Health, 2002), 85–118. This theory was eventually replaced with that of *comminution*, which was built on a less spiritual basis, arguing that grinding or mixing a grain of medicine increased its surface with every fracture and thus increased its distribution through the organism.

31. James Garth Wilkinson, *Swedenborg Among the Doctors: A Letter to Robert T. Cooper, M.D.* (London: Speirs, 1895), 3, 5, 9–10, 18–19, and *Epidemic Man and His Visitations* (London: Speirs, 1893), 32–33, 48, 53, 120–21.

32. See James Tyler Kent, *Lectures on Homeopathic Philosophy* (Chicago: Ehrhart and Karl, 1919), and *Kent's Minor Writings on Homeopathy* (Heidelberg, Germany: Haug, 1987).

33. James Tyler Kent, *The Art and Science of Homeopathic Medicine* (1900; reprint, New York: Dover, 2002), 133, 127; F. Treuherz, "The Origins of Kent's Philosophy," *Journal of the American Institute of Homeopathy* 77 (1983): 130–49.

34. J. S. Haller Jr., "Oliver Wendell Holmes's 1842 Lectures on 'Homeopathy and Its Kindred Delusions': A Retrospective Look," in Scott H. Podolsky and Charles S. Bryan, eds., *Oliver Wendell Holmes: Physician and Man of Letters* (Sagamore Beach, MA: Science History, 2009), 23–38. See also I. G. Rosenstein, *Theory and Practice of Homeopathy First Part, Containing a Theory of Homeopathy, with Dietetic Rules, etc.* (Louisville, KY: Henkle and Logan, 1840); B. F. Joslin, "Evidences of the Power of Small Doses of Attenuated Medicines, Including a Theory of Potentization," *American Journal of Homeopathy* 1 (1846–1847): 263–78; "Polemis Among German Homeopathists," *North American Journal of Homeopathy* 7 (1858): 250–52.

35. Dr. Kirn, "Homeopathy and the 'OD' Theory," *Homeopathic Recorder* 42 (1927): 529–41. See also Robert Rohland, *Od, or Odo-Magnetic Force: An Explanation of Its Influence on Homeopathic Medicines, from the Odic Point of View* (New York: n.p., 1916).

36. G. B. Stearns, "Physics of High Dilutions," *Homeopathic Recorder* 46 (1931): 400; Albert Abrams, *New Concepts in Diagnosis and Treatment* (San Francisco: Philopolis Press, 1916).

37. Henry C. Allen, *Materia Medica of the Nosodes and Provings of the X-Ray* (Philadelphia: Boericke and Tafel, 1910); F. K. Bellokossy, "X-Ray Potencies," *Journal of the American Institute of Homeopathy* 40 (1947): 160–62; F. Anaya-Reyes, "X-Ray and Its Application According to Homeopathy and the Law of Arndt-Schulz," *Journal of the American Institute of Homeopathy* 58 (1965): 24–25.

38. J. K. Kaplowe, "Science and Homeopathy," *Homeopathic Recorder* 50 (1935): 129–31. See also Herbert A. Roberts, *The Principles and Art of Cure by Homeopathy* (Halsworthy, UK: Health Science Press, 1942).

39. "Homeopathy and the Atomic Bomb," *Journal of the American Institute of Homeopathy* 39 (1946): 19–20; W. P. Mowry, "The Atomic Energy Principles in the Treatment of the Patient," *Journal of the American Institute of Homeopathy* 39 (1946): 346–48; K. C. Hiteshi, "Atomic Bomb and Homeopathy," *Journal of the American Institute of Homeopathy* 39 (1946): 21–22.

40. E. Davenas et al., "Human Basophil Degranulation Triggered by Very Dilute Antiserum Against 1gE," *Nature* 333 (1988): 816–18.

41. J. Maddox, J. Randi, and W. W. Stewart, "High Dilution Experiments a Delusion," *Nature* 334 (1988): 287–91.

42. R. Pool, "More Squabbling Over Unbelievable Result," *Science* 241 (1988): 658.

43. P. Fisher et al., "Effect of Homeopathic Treatment on Fibrositis (Primary Fibromyalgia)," *British Medical Journal* 299 (1989): 365–66; see also P. D. Wall, "Complementary Medicine," *British Medical Journal* 299 (1989): 1401.

44. T. A. Hoover, "Homeopathy: Setting the Record Straight," *Alternative Therapies* 16 (2010): 9.

45. Fritjof Capra, *The Tao of Physics* (New York: Bantam, 1977), 211.

46. George Vithoulkas, *The Science of Homeopathy* (New York: Grove Press, 1980), 68–69. See also Stanley Krippner and Daniel Rubin, *The Kirlian Aura* (New York: Doubleday, 1974).

47. Vithoulkas, *The Science of Homeopathy*, 81, 85, 90–91.

48. Harold Saxton Burr, *The Fields of Life: Our Links with the Universe* (New York: Ballantine, 1972).

49. D. Feinstein and D. Eden, "Six Pillars of Energy Medicine: Clinical Strengths of a Complementary Paradigm," *Alternative Therapies in Health and Medicine* 14 (2008): 44–54.

50. Frank, "Integrating Homeopathy and Biomedicine," 810.

51. H. Wallach, "Does a Highly Diluted Homeopathic Drug Act as a Placebo in Healthy Volunteers? Experimental Study of Belladonna 30C in a Double Blind Crossover Design—a Pilot Study," *Journal of Psychosomatic Research* 37 (1993): 851–60. Avogadro's number corresponds in dilution to a 24X, which is roughly equivalent to a 12C or between a 5M or 6M.

52. R. Buckman and G. Lewith, "What Does Homeopathy Do—and How?" *British Medical Journal* 309 (1994): 103.

53. Ibid., 103.

54. Ibid., 106. See also B. Brigo and G. Serpelloni, "Homeopathic Treatment of Migraines: A Randomized Double-Blind Controlled Study of Sixty Cases," *Berlin Journal of Research*

in Homeopathy 1 (1991): 98–106; D. T. Reilly et al., "Is Homeopathy a Placebo Response? Controlled Trial of Homeopathic Potency with Pollen and Hayfever as a Model," *Lancet* 2 (1986): 881–86; Fisher et al., "Effect of Homeopathic Treatment on Fibrositis," 365–66.

55. Buckman and Lewith, "What Does Homeopathy Do—and How?" 104.

56. Ibid., 104–5. As for the three randomized studies, two remained unrepeated, and one was repeated but did not confirm the initial results.

57. Ibid., 105.

58. See, for example, K. Linde et al., "Impact of Study Quality on Outcome in Placebo-Controlled Trials of Homeopathy," *Journal of Clinical Epidemiology* 52 (1999): 631–36; E. Ernst and J. Barnes, "Meta-analysis of Homeopathy Trials," *Lancet* 351 (1998): 366–68; K. Linde et al., "Are the Clinical Effects of Homeopathy Placebo Effects? A Meta-analysis of Placebo-Controlled Trials," *Lancet* 350 (1997): 834–43; E. Ernst, "Homeopathic Prophylaxis of Headaches and Migraine? A Systematic Review," *Journal of Pain and Symptom Management* 18 (1999): 353–57; J. Jacobs et al., "Homeopathy for Childhood Diarrhea: Combined Results and Meta-analysis from Three Randomized, Controlled Clinical Trials," *Pediatric Infectious Disease Journal* 22 (2003): 229–34.

59. J. Kleijnen, P. Knipschild, and G. ter Reit, "Clinical Trials of Homeopathy," *British Medical Journal* 302 (1991): 321.

60. Homeopathic Medicine Research Group, *Report to the European Commission Director General XII: Science, Research, and Development*, vol. 1 (Brussels: European Commission, 1996), 16–17.

61. J. P. Vandenbrouchke, "Homeopathy Trials: Going Nowhere," *Lancet* 350 (1997): 824.

62. Linde et al., "Are the Clinical Effects of Homeopathy Placebo Effects?" 834–43.

63. See M. A. Taylor et al., "Randomized Controlled Trial of Homeopathy Versus Placebo in Perennial Allergic Rhinitis with Overview of Four Trial Series," *British Medical Journal* 321 (2000): 471–76. Three earlier trials came to a similar conclusion. See also D. T. Reilly and M. A. Taylor, "Potent Placebo or Potency? A Proposed Study Model with Initial Findings Using Homeopathically Prepared Pollens in Hay Fever," *British Medical Journal* 74 (1985): 66–75; D. T. Reilly et al., "Is Homeopathy a Placebo Response? Controlled Trial of Homeopathic Potency, with Pollen in Hayfever as Model," *Lancet* 2 (1986): 881–86; D. T. Reilly et al., "Is Evidence for Homeopathy Reproducible?" *Lancet* 344 (1994): 1601–6.

64. T. Lancaster and A. Vickers, "Commentary: Larger Trials Are Needed," *British Medical Journal* 321 (2000): 476.

65. G. Feder and T. Katz, "Randomized Controlled Trials for Homeopathy: Who Wants to Know the Results?" *British Medical Journal* 324 (2002): 499.

66. G. T. Lewith et al., "Use of Ultramolecular Potencies of Allergen to Treat Asthmatic People Allergic to House Dust Mite: Double Blind Randomized Controlled Clinical Trial," *British Medical Journal* 324 (2002): 520–23.

67. M. Dorey, "Study Is in Effect Trying to Compare Apples and Oranges," *British Medical Journal* 325 (2002): 42; see also G. T. Lewith, M. E. Hyland, and S. Holgate, "Authors' Reply," *British Medical Journal* 325 (2002): 42–43.

68. W. B. Jonas, T. J. Kaptchuk, and K. Linde, "A Critical Overview of Homeopathy," *Annals of Internal Medicine* 138 (2003): 393.

69. A. Hróbjartsson and P. C. Gøtzsche, "Is the Placebo Powerless? An Analysis of Clinical Trials Comparing Placebo with No Treatment," *New England Journal of Medicine* 344 (2001): 1594 (quote); A. Hróbjartsson and P. C. Gøtzsche, "Is the Placebo Powerless? Update of a Systematic Review with 52 New Randomized Trials Comparing Placebo with No Treatment," *Journal of Internal Medicine* 256 (2004): 91–100.

70. Quoted in S. Boseley, "As a Fourth Study Says It's No Better Than a Placebo, Is This the End for Homeopathy?" *Guardian*, August 26, 2005. See also "The End of Homeopathy," *Lancet* 366 (2005): 690.

71. "The End of Homeopathy," 690.

72. D. Ramey, "Evidence for Homeopathy Is Lacking," *British Medical Journal* 320 (2000): 1341–42. See also Linde et al., "Impact of Study Quality on Outcome in Placebo-Controlled Trials in Homeopathy," 631–36; Ernst and Barnes, "Meta-analysis of Homeopathy Trials," 366–68.

73. "Homeopathy and the *Lancet*," http://www.ncbi.nlm.nih.gov/pmc/articles/PMC1375230/, accessed July 10, 2011; "Open Letter in Response to the Article in the *Lancet*," http://www.ncbi.nlm.nih.gov/pubmed/16781599, accessed July 10, 2011; "Prominent Doctors and Scientists Reject *Lancet* Report on Homeopathy," http://www.ncbi.nlm.nih.gov/pubmed/16670783, accessed July 10, 2011.

74. P. Fisher, "Homeopathy and the *Lancet*," *eCAM* 3 (2006): 145.

75. P. Fisher et al., "Evaluation of Specific and Non-specific Effects in Homeopathy: Feasibility Study for a Randomized Trial," *Homeopathy* 95 (2006): 215–22.

76. T. J. Kaptchuk et al., "Components of Placebo Effect: Randomized Controlled Trial in Patients with Irritable Bowel Syndrome," *British Medical Journal* 336 (2008): 998.

77. R. Lüdtke and A. L. Rutten, "The Conclusions of the Effectiveness of Homeopathy Highly Depend on the Set of Analyzed Trials," *Journal of Clinical Epidemiology* 61 (2008): 1197–204; A. Shang et al., "Are the Clinical Effects of Homeopathy Placebo Effects? Comparative Study of Placebo-Controlled Trials of Homeopathy and Allopathy," *Lancet* 366 (2005): 726–32.

78. J. Weiner, "Studies Comparing Homeopathy and Placebo Are Useful," *British Medical Journal* 325 (2002): 41; Lewith et al., "Use of Ultramolecular Potencies of Allergen to Treat Asthmatic People Allergic to House Dust Mite," 520–23; P. Fisher and D. L. Scott, "A Randomized Controlled Trial of Homeopathy in Rheumatoid Arthritis," *Rheumatology* 40 (2001): 1052–55.

79. M. Foley, "Providers Have Much to Gain from Homeopathy Being Accepted," *British Medical Journal* 325 (2002): 41.

80. Vandenbrouchke, "Homeopathy Trials," 824; A. Vickers, "Clinical Trials of Homeopathy and Placebo: Analysis of a Scientific Debate," *Journal of Alternative and Complementary Medicine* 6 (2000): 49–56.

81. C. A. Vincent and P. H. Richardson, "Placebo Controls for Acupuncture Studies," *Journal of the Royal Society of Medicine* 88 (1995): 199–202; C. Vincent, "Credibility Assessments in Trials of Acupuncture," *Complementary Medical Research* 4 (1990): 8–11.

82. T. J. Kaptchuk et al., "Sham Device Versus Inert Pill: Randomized Controlled Trial of Two Placebo Treatments," *British Medical Journal* 332 (2006): 391.

83. D. C. Cherkin et al., "Randomized Trial Comparing Traditional Chinese Medical Acupuncture, Therapeutic Massage, and Self-Care Education for Chronic Low Back Pain," *Archives of Internal Medicine* 161 (2001): 1081–88; T. M. Cummings, "Teasing Apart the Quality and Validity in Systematic Reviews of Acupuncture," *Acupuncture Medicine* 18 (2000): 104–7; A. D. Woolf and K. Akesson, "Understanding the Burden of Musculoskeletal Conditions," *British Medical Journal* 322 (2001): 1079–80; D. Eskinazi and D. Muchsam, "Factors That Shape Alternative Medicine: The Role of the Alternative Medicine Research Community," *Alternative Therapies in Health and Medicine* 6 (2000): 49–53; C. Vincent and G. Lewith, "Placebo Controls for Acupuncture Studies," *Journal of the Royal Society of Medicine* 88 (1995): 199–202; R. Hammerschlag, "Methodological and Ethical Issues in Clinical Trials of Acupuncture," *Journal of Alternative and Complementary Medicine* 4 (1998): 159–71.

84. L. Dossey, "How Should Alternative Therapies Be Evaluated? An Examination of Fundamentals," *Alternative Therapies in Health and Medicine* 1 (1995): 6; C. J. Schneider and W. B. Jonas, "Are Alternative Treatments Effective? Issues and Methods Involved in Measuring Effectiveness of Alternative Treatments," *Subtle Energies* 5 (1994): 69; L. A. Moye et al., "Research Methodology in Psychoneuroimmunology: Rationale and Design of the IMAGES-P Clinical Trial," *Alternative Therapies in Health and Medicine* 1 (1995): 34.

85. I. Smith, "Commissioning Complementary Medicine," *British Medical Journal* 310 (1995): 1151. See also T. A. Sheldon, "Please Bypass the PORT," *British Medical Journal* 309 (1994): 142–43.

86. J. Bland, "Alternative Therapies—a Moving Target," *Alternative Therapies in Health and Medicine* 11 (2005): 21.

87. Frank, "Integrating Homeopathy and Biomedicine," 810.

88. Feder and Katz, "Randomized Controlled Trials for Homeopathy," 498–99.

89. F. J. Master, "Research in Homeopathy," *Homeopathic Heritage International* 4 (2010): 10–13; Luc De Schepper, *Hahnemann Revisited* (Santa Fe: Full of Life, 1999).

90. N. Degele, "On the Margins of Everything: Doing, Performing, and Staging Science in Homeopathy," *Science, Technology, and Human Values* 30 (2005): 116; D. Eskinazi, "Homeopathy Re-visited: Is Homeopathy Compatible with Biomedical Observations?" *Archives of Internal Medicine* 159 (1991): 1981–87.

91. E. Ernst, "Harmless Herbs?" *American Journal of Medicine* 104 (1998): 170–78.

92. David Taylor, "Herbal Medicine at a Crossroads," *Environmental Health Perspectives* 104 (1966): 925.

93. E. Ernst, "The Role of Complementary and Alternative Medicine," *British Medical Journal* 321 (2000): 1134–35.

94. "Report of the Board of Science Working Party on Alternative Therapy," *British Medical Journal* 292 (1986): 1407.

6. REASSESSMENT

1. A. Shang et al., "Are the Clinical Trials of Homeopathy Placebo Effects? Comparative Study of Placebo-Controlled Trials of Homeopathy and Allopathy," *Lancet* 366 (2005): 726–32; J. Ezzo et al., "Is Acupuncture Effective for the Treatment of Chronic Pain? A Systematic Review," *Pain* 86 (2000): 217–25; E. Ernst, "Chiropractic Spinal Manipulation for Neck Pain: A Systematic Review," *Journal of Pain* 4 (2003): 417–21.

2. H. Holman, "Chronic Disease—the Need for a New Clinical Education," *JAMA* 292 (2004): 1057–59.

3. Nina Degele, "On the Margins of Everything: Doing, Performing, and Staging Science in Homeopathy," *Science, Technology, and Human Values* 30 (2005): 116–17.

4. R. L. Nahin and S. E. Straus, "Research Into Complementary and Alternative Medicine: Problems and Potential," *British Medical Journal* 322 (2001): 161–64.

5. D. Bessinger and T. Huhne, "Medical Spirituality: Defining Domains and Boundaries," *Southern Medical Journal* 95 (2002): 1385–426.

6. M. Wills, "Connection, Action, and Hope: An Invitation to Reclaim the 'Spiritual' in Health Care," *Journal of Religion and Health* 46 (2007): 433.

7. S. R. Sehon and D. E. Stanley, "A Philosophical Analysis of the Evidence-Based Medicine Debate," *BMC Health Services Research* 3 (2003): 1–10.

8. P. Vineis, "Evidence-Based Medicine and Ethics: A Practical Approach," *Journal of Medical Ethics* 30 (2004): 126–30; R. E. Ashcroft, "Current Epistemological Problems in Evidence Based Medicine," *Journal of Medical Ethics* 30 (2004): 131–35.

9. T. Kaptchuk, "Subjectivity and the Placebo Effect in Medicine: An Interview by Bonnie Horrigan," *Alternative Therapies* 7 (2001): 104.

10. F. G. Miller and T. J. Kaptchuk, "The Power of Context: Reconceptualizing the Placebo Effect," *Journal of the Royal Society of Medicine* 101 (2008): 223.

11. See R. K. Merton, "Behavior Patterns of Scientists," *Leonardo* 3 (1970): 215–16. See also R. K. Merton, "Science and Technology in a Democratic Order," *Journal of Legal and Political Sociology* 1 (1942): 115–26.

12. Friedrich Nietzsche, *The Birth of Tragedy* (New York: Modern Library, 2000), 97.

BIBLIOGRAPHY

Abadie, Marie-Jeanne. *Healing Mind, Body, Spirit*. Holbrook, MA: Adams Media, 1997.

Abbott, Andrew D. *The System of Professions: An Essay on the Division of Expert Labor*. Chicago: University of Chicago Press, 1988.

Abgrall, Jean-Marie. *Healing or Stealing? Medical Charlatans in the New Age*. New York: Algora, 2000.

Abrams, Albert. *New Concepts in Diagnosis and Treatment*. San Francisco: Philopolis Press, 1916.

Achinstein, Peter, and Owen Hannaway, eds. *Observation, Experiment, and Hypothesis in Modern Physical Science*. Cambridge, MA: MIT Press, 1955.

Ackerknecht, Erwin H. *Medicine at the Paris Hospital, 1794–1848*. Baltimore: Johns Hopkins University Press, 1967.

Adams, Jon. *Researching Complementary and Alternative Medicine*. London: Routledge, 2007.

Adams, Robert. *Foundations of Complementary Therapies and Alternative Medicine*. New York: Palgrave Macmillan, 2010.

Albanese, Catherine L. *Nature Religion in America: From the Algonkian Indians to the New Age*. Chicago: University of Chicago Press, 1990.

——. *A Republic of Mind and Spirit: A Cultural History of American Metaphysical Religion*. New Haven, CT: Yale University Press, 2007.

Aldridge, David. *Health, the Individual, and Integrated Medicine: Revisiting an Aesthetic of Health Care*. New York: Kingsley, 2004.

Alexander, Franz G., and Thomas Morton French. *Studies in Psychosomatic Medicine*. New York: Ronald Press, 1948.

Alexander, Franz G., and Sheldon T. Selesnick. *The History of Psychiatry*. New York: Harper and Row, 1966.

Alexander, Jane. *The Holistic Therapy File: A Complete Guide to Over 80 Effective Treatments to Heal the Mind, Body, and Spirit*. London: Carlton Books, 2003.

Allen, Henry C. *Materia Medica of the Nosodes and Provings of the X-Ray*. Philadelphia: Boericke and Tafel, 1910.

Allison, Kathleen Cahill, and Harvard Medical School. *Alternative Medicine: A Selection of Articles on Complementary and Integrative Therapies.* Boston: Harvard Health Publications, 2001.

Allison, Nancy. *The Complete Body, Mind, and Spirit.* Chicago: Keats, 2001.

Alster, Kristine B. *The Holistic Health Movement.* Tuscaloosa: University of Alabama Press, 1989.

Altenberg, Henry Edward. *Holistic Medicine: A Meeting of East and West.* New York: Japan, 1992.

Altshuler, Larry. *Balanced Healing: Combining Modern Medicine with Safe and Effective Alternative Therapies.* Gig Harbor, WA: Harbor Press, 2004.

American Association of Naturopathic Physicians. *Nature's Pharmacy: Your Guide to Healing Foods, Herbs, Supplements, and Homeopathic Remedies.* Lincolnwood, IL: Publications International, 2001.

American Medical Association Council on Medical Education. *Encouraging Medical Student Education in Complementary Health Care Practices.* Chicago: American Medical Association Press, 1997.

American Psychiatric Association. *Diagnostic and Statistical Manual of Mental Disorders.* 4th ed. Washington, DC: American Psychiatric Association, 1994.

Amos, Paul. *Miracle Medicine: Urgent Natural Alternatives to the Prescription Drug Crisis.* Baltimore: Healthier News, 2008.

Anderson, C. Alan, and Deborah G. Whitehouse. *New Thought: A Practical American Spirituality.* Bloomington, IN: self-published, 2002.

Angell, Marcia. *The Truth About the Drug Companies: How They Deceive Us and What to Do About It.* New York: Random House, 2004.

Ankerberg, John, and John Weldon. *Can You Trust Your Doctor? The Complete Guide to New Age Medicine and Its Threat to Your Family.* Brentwood, TN: Wolgemuth and Hyatt, 1991.

Annas, George J., and Michael A. Grodin, eds. *The Nazi Doctors and the Nuremberg Code: Human Rights in Human Experimentation.* New York: Oxford University Press, 1992.

Appelbaum, Stephen A. *The Mystery of Healing: Journeys Through Alternative Medicine.* Cambridge, MA: Lumen Editions, 1999.

Appignanesi, Richard, and Chris Garratt. *Introducing Postmodernism.* New York: Totem Books, 1995.

Aronowitz, Robert. *Making Sense out of Illness: Science, Society, and Disease.* New York: Cambridge University Press, 1998.

Atkinson, William Walker. *Self Healing by Thought Force.* Kila, MT: Kessinger, 1996.

Avedon, John. *The Buddha's Art of Healing.* New York: Rizzoli, 1998.

Avorn, Jerry. *Powerful Medicines: The Benefits, Risks, and Costs of Prescription Drugs.* New York: Knopf, 2004.

Bach, Edward. *The Essential Writings of Dr. Edward Bach: The Twelve Healers and Other Remedies and Heal Thyself.* London: Vermillion, 2005.

Badaracco, Claire. *Prescribing Faith: Medicine, Media, and Religion in American Culture.* Waco, TX: Baylor University Press, 2007.

Baer, Hans A. *Biomedicine and Alternative Healing Systems in America: Issues of Class, Race, Ethnicity, and Gender*. Madison: University of Wisconsin Press, 2001.

Baer, Hans A., Merrill Singer, and Ida Susser. *Medical Anthropology and the World System: A Critical Perspective*. Westport, CN: Bergin and Garvey, 1997.

Bailar, John C., and Frederick Mosteller, eds. *Medical Uses of Statistics*. Waltham, MA: New England Journal of Medicine Books, 1992.

Bakal, Donald A. *Minding the Body: Clinical Uses of Somatic Awareness*. New York: Guilford Press, 1999.

Baker, Sharon. *Healing with Hands: Miracles, Inspiration, and Science. Reiki and Other Related Therapies: A Holistic Approach to Healing*. Imlay City, MI: Sharon Baker, 2005.

Balint, Michael. *The Doctor, His Patient, and the Illness*. New York: International Universities Press, 1972.

Bandura, Albert. *Self-Efficacy: The Exercise of Control*. Cambridge: Cambridge University Press, 1997.

Barasch, Marc. *The Healing Path: A Soul Approach to Illness*. New York: Putnam, 1993.

Barber, Joseph, and Cheri Adrian. *Psychological Approaches to the Management of Pain*. New York: Brunner/Mazel, 1982.

Barker, Alexandra. *Relief Beyond Belief: Exploring the World of Natural Healing*. Belleville, Canada: Seraphine, 2002.

Barnes, Patricia M., Barbara Bloom, Richard L. Nahin, and the National Center for Health Statistics. *Complementary and Alternative Medicine Use Among Adults and Children: United States, 2007*. Hyattsville, MD: National Center for Health Statistics, 2008.

Barnum, Barbara Stevens. *The New Healers: Minds and Hands in Complementary Medicine*. Long Branch, NJ: Vista, 2002.

Baron, Jonathan. *Thinking and Deciding*. 3rd ed. Cambridge: Cambridge University Press, 2000.

Bartlett, Charles. *An Essay on the Philosophy of Medical Sciences*. Philadelphia: Lea and Blanchard, 1844.

Bauer, Karin. *Adorno's Nietzschean Narratives: Critiques of Ideology, Readings of Wagner*. New York: State University of New York Press, 1999.

Bausell, R. Barker. *Snake Oil Science: The Truth About Complementary and Alternative Medicine*. New York: Oxford University Press, 2007.

Beauchamp, Tom H., and James F. Childress. *Principles of Biomedical Ethics*. New York: Oxford University Press, 1979.

Becker, Carl B. *Time for Healing: Integrating Traditional Therapies with Scientific Medical Practice*. St. Paul, MN: Paragon House, 2002.

Beckman, Howard. *Mantras, Yantras, and Fabulous Gems: The Healing Secrets of the Ancient Vedas*. Faridabad, India: Balaji, 1997.

Beecher, Henry K. *Measurement of Subjective Responses: Quantitative Effects of Drugs*. New York: Oxford University Press, 1959.

Bell, Iris R. *Getting Whole, Getting Well: Healing Holistically from Chronic Illness*. New York: Morgan James, 2008.

Bellamy, David J., and Andrea Pfister. *World Medicine: Plants, Patients, and People.* Cambridge, MA: Blackwell, 1992.

Bellamy, Isabel. *Radiant Healing: The Many Paths to Personal Harmony and Planetary Wholeness.* Wentworth Falls, Australia: Donald MacLean, 2001.

Benedetti, Fabrizio. *Placebo Effects: Understanding the Mechanisms in Health and Disease.* New York: Oxford University Press, 2009.

Benson, Herbert. *The Mind/Body Effect.* New York: Berkley, 1979.

——. *The Relaxation Response.* New York: HarperTorch, 1975.

——. *Timeless Healing: The Power and Biology of Belief.* New York: Simon and Schuster, 1996.

Berkholtz, Herbert. *The FDA Follies.* New York: Basic Books, 1994.

Berloiz, L. V. J. *Memoires sur les maladies chroniques, les evacuationes sanguine et l'acupuncture.* Paris: Chez Croullebois, 1816.

Bernard, Claude. *Introduction to the Study of Experimental Medicine.* New York: Dover, 1957.

Best, Mark A., Duncan Neuhauser, and Lee Slaven, eds. *Benjamin Franklin: Verification and Validation of the Scientific Progress in Health Care as Demonstrated by the "Report of the Royal Commissioner on Animal Magnetism and Mesmerism."* Victoria, Canada: Trafford, 2003.

Billitteri, Thomas J. *Alternative Medicine.* Brookfield, CT: Twenty-First Century Books, 2001.

Bion, Wilfred R. *Elements of Psycho-analysis.* London: Heinemann, 1963.

Bishop, Beata. *A Time to Heal.* London: Arkana, 1996.

Bivins, Roberta E. *Alternative Medicine: A History.* New York: Oxford University Press, 2007.

Black, Dean. *Health at the Crossroads: Exploring the Conflict Between Natural Healing and Conventional Medicine.* Springville, UT: Tapestry Press, 1988.

Blavatsky, Helena P., William Quan Judge, and Robert Crosbie. *The Laws of Healing: Physical and Metaphysical.* Los Angeles: Theosophy, 1937.

Bloom, Harold. *The American Religion: The Emergence of the Post-Christian Nation.* New York: Simon and Schuster, 1992.

Bloom, William. *The Endorphin Effect.* London: Piatkus, 2009.

Bloom, William, Judy Hall, and David Peters. *The Complete Encyclopedia of Mind, Body, and Spirit: The Complete Guide to Healing Therapies, Esoteric Wisdom, and Spiritual Traditions.* London: Godsfield, 2009.

Bobrow, Robert S. *The Witch in the Waiting Room.* New York: Thunder's Mouth Press, 2006.

Bodhi, Bhikkhu. *Discourses of the Buddha.* Sommerville, MA: Wisdom Press, 2000.

Bodine, Echo L. *Hands That Heal.* 2nd ed. San Diego: ACS, 1997.

Bok, Sissela. *Lying: Moral Choice in Public and Private Life.* New York: Vintage, 1978.

Bonica, John J., ed. *Advances in Neurology.* 5 vols. New York: Raven, 1974.

——, ed. *Advances in Pain Research and Therapy.* New York: Raven Press, 1979.

Bonnett, O. T., MD. *What I Learned After Medical School.* Huntsville, AR: Ozark Mountain, 2006.

Boorstin, Daniel. *The Discovers.* New York: Random House, 1983.

Booth, Emmons R. *History of Osteopathy and Twentieth-Century Medical Practice.* Cincinnati: Caxton, 1924.

Boruch, Robert F. *Randomized Experiments for Planning and Evaluation: A Practical Guide.* Thousand Oaks, CA: Sage, 1997.

Boulderstone, John. *Living with Vitality: The Role of Life Force in Health and Disease.* Findhorn, Scotland: Findhorn Press, 2006.

Bowditch, Henry I. *The Past, Present, and Future Treatment of Homeopathy, Eclecticism, and Kindred Delusions Which May Hereafter Arise in the Medical Profession as Viewed from the Standpoints of the History of Medicine and of Personal Experience.* Boston: Upham, 1887.

Boyd, Hilary. *Boosting Your Energy Through Conventional and Complementary Methods.* London: Mitchell Beazley, 2004.

Bradford, Nikki. *Healing Yourself with Flowers and Other Essences.* London: Quadrille, 2005.

Bradford, Thomas Lindsay. *The Life and Letters of Dr. Samuel Hahnemann.* Philadelphia: Boericke and Tafel, 1895.

Breslow, Norman E., and Nicholas E. Day. *Statistical Methods in Cancer Research I: The Analysis of Case–Control Studies.* Lyon, France: International Agency for Research on Cancer, 1980.

British Medical Association. *Complementary Medicine: New Approaches to Good Practice.* Oxford: Oxford University Press, 1993.

British Parliamentary Papers. *Reports on the Epidemics of 1854 and 1856 and Other Reports on Cholera with Appendices 1854–96. Report on the Results of the Different Methods of Treatment Pursued in Epidemic Cholera.* Shannon: Irish University Press, 1970.

Brody, Howard. *Ethical Decisions in Medicine.* 2nd ed. Boston: Little, Brown, 1981.

——. *The Healer's Power.* New Haven, CT: Yale University Press, 1992.

——. *Placebos and the Philosophy of Medicine: Clinical, Conceptual, and Ethical Issues.* Chicago: University of Chicago Press, 1980.

Brody, Howard, and Daralyn Brody. *The Placebo Response: How You Can Release the Body's Inner Pharmacy for Better Health.* New York: Cliff Street Books, 2000.

Bromberg, Walter. *Man Above Humanity: A History of Psychotherapy.* Philadelphia: Lippincott, 1954.

Bronzino, Joseph D., Vincent H. Smith, and Maurice L. Wade. *Medical Technology and Society.* Cambridge, MA: MIT Press, 1990.

Brooksby, Robert C. *Healing from Within: Be Still and Know.* San Jose, CA: Writers Club Press, 1999.

Brown, David Jay. *Mavericks of Medicine: Conversations on the Frontiers of Medical Research.* Petaluma, CA: Smart, 2006.

Brown, Denise W., and Sandra White. *Alternative Health Therapies: The Complete Guide to Aromatherapy, Massage, and Reflexology.* New York: Todtri, 2001.

Brown, Michael F. *The Channeling Zone: American Spirituality in an Anxious Age.* Cambridge, MA: Harvard University Press, 1997.

Bruce, Debra F., and Dolores Krieger. *Miracle Touch: A Complete Guide to Hands-on Therapies That Have the Amazing Ability to Heal.* New York: Three Rivers Press, 2003.

Bruce, H. Addington. *Scientific Mental Healing.* Boston: Little, Brown, 1912.

Bruner, Jerome. *Actual Minds, Possible Worlds.* Cambridge, MA: Harvard University Press, 1986.

Bulpitt, Christopher J. *Randomised Controlled Clinical Trials*. Boston: Kluwer, 1996.

Bunker, John P. *The National Halothane Study: Report of the Subcommittee on the National Halothane Study of the Committee on Anesthesia, Division of the Medical Sciences, National Academy of Sciences—National Research Council*. Washington, DC: US Government Printing Office, 1969.

Burkholder, Lester K. *A Closer Look! A Scriptural View of Alternative Health Practices*. Ephrata, PA: Weaverland, 1996.

Burr, Harold Saxton. *The Fields of Life: Our Links with the Universe*. New York: Ballantine, 1972.

Burroughs, Hugh, and Mark Kastner. *Alternative Healing: The Complete A–Z Guide to Over 160 Different Alternative Therapies*. La Mesa, CA: Halcyon, 1993.

Byrd, Cary R. *Current Concepts in Complementary Alternative Medicine*. Baltimore: Publish America, 2005.

Byrne, Rhonda. *The Power*. New York: Atria Books, 2010.

——. *The Secret*. New York: Atria Books, 2006.

Cahoone, Lawrence, ed. *From Modernism to Post Modernism*. Oxford: Blackwell, 1996.

Callahan, Daniel, ed. *The Role of Complementary and Alternative Medicine: Accommodating Pluralism*. Washington, DC: Georgetown University Press, 2002.

Calvin, William H. *The Cerebral Code*. Cambridge, MA: MIT Press, 2000.

Cannon, Walter Bradford. *The Wisdom of the Body*. New York: Norton, 1932.

Cant, Sarah, and Ursla Sharma. *A New Medical Pluralism? Alternative Medicine, Doctors, Patients, and the State*. London: University College London Press, 1999.

Capra, Fritjof. *The Tao of Physics*. New York: Bantam, 1977.

Cargill, Marie. *Acupuncture: A Viable Medical Alternative*. Westport, CT: Praeger, 1994.

Carson, Ronald A., and Chester R. Burns, eds. *Philosophy of Medicine and Bioethics: A Twenty-Year Retrospective and Critical Appraisal*. Dordrecht, Netherlands: Kluwer, 1997.

Carver, Charles S., and Michael F. Scheir. *Self Regulation of Behavior*. Cambridge: Cambridge University Press, 1998.

Cassedy, James H. *American Medicine and Statistical Thinking, 1800–1860*. Cambridge, MA: Harvard University Press, 1984.

——. *Medicine and American Growth, 1800–1860*. Madison: University of Wisconsin Press, 1986.

Cassell, Eric J. *The Nature of Suffering*. Oxford: Oxford University Press, 2004.

Cassileth, Barrie R. *The Alternative Medicine Handbook: The Complete Reference Guide of Alternative and Complementary Therapies*. New York: Norton, 1998.

Castleman, Michael. *Blended Medicine: Combining Mainstream and Alternative Therapies*. Emmaus, PA: Rodale Press, 2000.

Catalano, Joseph T., ed. *Nursing Now: Today's Issues, Tomorrow's Trends*. 2nd ed. Philadelphia: Davis, 2003.

Cerney, J. V. *Handbook of Unusual and Unorthodox Healing Methods*. New York: Parker, 1977.

Chapman, Joseph B., and Wilhelm Heinrich Schussler. *Biochemistry: A Domestic Treatise on the Application of Schuessler's Twelve Tissue Remedies*. 3rd ed. St. Louis: Luyties, 1900.

Chin, Jacqueline M. *The Light Within: A Reiki Handbook*. Bloomington, IN: AuthorHouse, 2004.

Chopra, Deepak. *Ageless Body, Timeless Mind: The Quantum Alternative to Growing Old*. New York: Harmony Books, 1993.

——. *Creating Affluence—Wealth Consciousness in the Field of All Possibilities*. San Rafael, CA: New World Library, 1993.

——. *The Higher Self: The Magic of Inner and Outer Fulfillment*. Chicago: Nightingale-Conant, 1992.

——. *Perfect Health: The Complete Mind–Body Guide*. New York: Crown, 1990.

——. *Quantum Healing: Discovering the Power to Fulfill Your Dreams*. New York: Bantam, 1991.

——. *Unconditional Life—Discovering the Power to Fulfill Your Dreams*. New York: Bantam Books, 1992.

Clark, Carolyn C. *Integrating Complementary Health Procedures Into Practice*. New York: Springer, 2000.

Clymer, Emerson M. *The Gifts of the Spirit: The Doctor Within*. Quakertown, PA: Humanitarian Society, 1976.

Cobb, Stanley. *Borderlands of Psychiatry*. N.p.: n.p., 1943.

——. *Foundations of Neuropsychiatry*. Baltimore: Williams and Wilkins, 1952.

Cochrane, Archie L. *Effectiveness and Efficiency: Random Reflections on Health Services*. London: Nuffield Provincial Hospitals Trust, 1972.

——, with Max Blythe. *One Man's Medicine: An Autobiography of Professor Archie Cochrane*. London: BMJ Books, 1989.

Cohen, Mark Nathan. *Health and the Rise of Civilization*. New Haven, CT: Yale University Press, 1989.

Cohen, Michael H. *Beyond Complementary Medicine: Legal and Ethical Perspectives on Health Care and Human Evolution*. Ann Arbor: University of Michigan Press, 2000.

——. *Complementary and Alternative Medicine: Legal Boundaries and Regulatory Perspectives*. Baltimore: Johns Hopkins University Press, 1998.

——. *Healing at the Borderland of Medicine and Religion*. Chapel Hill: University of North Carolina Press, 2006.

Coleman, William, and Frederick Holmes, eds. *The Investigative Enterprise: Experimental Physiology in 19th Century Medicine*. Berkeley: University of California Press, 1988.

Cooper, Edwin L., and Nobuo Yamaguchi, eds. *Complementary and Alternative Approaches to Biomedicine*. New York: Kluwer Academic, 2002.

Cooper, Harris, and Larry V. Hedges, eds. *The Handbook of Research Synthesis*. New York: Russell Sage Foundation, 1994.

Cooter, Roger, ed. *Studies in the History of Alternative Medicine*. New York: St. Martin's Press, 1988.

Corea, Gena. *The Mother Machine: Reproductive Technologies from Artificial Insemination to Artificial Wombs*. New York: Harper and Row, 1985.

Corner, George W. *A History of the Rockefeller Institute, 1901–1953: Origins and Growth*. New York: Rockefeller Institute Press, 1965.

Coughlin, Steven S., and Tom L. Beauchamp. *Ethics and Epidemiology*. Oxford: Oxford University Press, 1996.

Coulter, Harris L. *The Controlled Clinical Trial: An Analysis*. Washington, DC: Center for Empirical Medicine, 1991.

——. *Divided Legacy: A History of the Schism in Medical Thought*. 4 vols. Washington, DC: Wehawken, 1973.

Coulter, Ian D. *Chiropractic: A Philosophy for Alternative Health Care*. Boston: Butterworth-Heinemann, 1999.

Council on Graduate Medical Education. *Third Report. Improving Access to Health Care Through Physician Workforce Reform: Directions for the 21st Century*. Washington, DC: US Department of Health and Human Services, 1992.

Cousins, Norman. *Anatomy of an Illness*. New York: Norton, 1995.

——. *Head First: The Biology of Hope*. New York: Dutton, 1989.

Coveney, Peter, and Roger Highfield. *Frontiers of Complexity: The Search for Order in a Chaotic World*. London: Faber and Faber, 1995.

Crellin, John K., and Fernando Ania. *Professionalism and Ethics in Complementary and Alternative Medicine*. New York: Haworth Press, 2002.

Crosley, Reginald. *Alternative Medicine and Miracles: A Grand Unified Theory*. Lanham, MD: University Press of America, 2004.

Cullen, Michael J. *The Statistical Movement in Early Victorian Britain: The Foundations of Empirical Social Research*. New York: Barnes and Noble, 1975.

Cunningham, Andrew, and Perry Williams, eds. *The Laboratory Revolution in Medicine*. Cambridge: Cambridge University Press, 1992.

Daly, Jeanne. *Evidence-Based Medicine and the Search for a Science of Clinical Care*. Berkeley: University of California Press, 2005.

Damasio, Antonio R. *Descartes' Error: Emotion, Reason, and the Human Brain*. New York: Putnam, 1994.

D'Arcy, Patrick D., James C. McElnay, and Peter G. Welling, eds. *Mechanisms of Drug Interactions*. New York: Springer, 1996.

Darnton, Robert. *Mesmerism and the End of the Enlightenment*. Cambridge, MA: Harvard University Press, 1968.

Daston, Lorraine J. *Classical Probability in the Enlightenment*. Princeton, NJ: Princeton University Press, 1988.

Davidson, John. *Subtle Energy*. 4th ed. Saffron Waldon, UK: Daniel, 1997.

Davies, Huw T. O., Sandra Nutley, and Peter C. Smith, eds. *What Works? Evidence-Based Policy and Practice in Public Services*. Bristol, UK: Policy Press, 2000.

Davis-Floyd, Robbie, and Gloria St. John. *From Doctor to Healer: The Transformative Journey*. New Brunswick, NJ: Rutgers University Press, 1998.

Dawkins, Richard. *The Selfish Gene*. Oxford: Oxford University Press, 1990.

Deleuze, Joseph P. F. *Practical Instructions in Animal Magnetism*. New York: Wells, 1843.

Deliman, Tracy, and John S. Smolowe, *Holistic Medicine: Harmony of Body, Mind, Spirit*. Upper Saddle River, NJ: Prentice-Hall, 1982.

De Schepper, Luc. *Hahnemann Revisited*. Santa Fe: Full of Life, 1999.

De Vries, Jan. *Treating Body, Mind, and Soul*. Edinburgh: Mainstream, 2003.

Diamond, John. *Holism and Beyond: The Essence of Holistic Medicine: Two Perspectives*. Bloomingdale, IL: Enhancement Books, 2001.

———. *Snake Oil and Other Preoccupations*. London: Vintage, 2001.

Diamond, W. John. *The Clinical Practice of Complementary, Alternative, and Western Medicine*. Boca Raton, FL: CRC Press, 2001.

DiGiovanna, Eileen L., Stanley Schiowitz, and Dennis J. Dowling. *An Osteopathic Approach to Diagnosis and Treatment*. Plymouth, MA: Lippincott Raven, 1996.

Dinges, Martin. *Patients in the History of Homeopathy*. Sheffield, UK: European Association for the History of Medicine and Health, 2002.

Dixon, Michael, and Kieran Sweeney. *The Human Effect in Medicine: Theory, Research, and Practice*. Abingdon Oxon, UK: Radcliffe Medical Press, 2000.

Dobbs, Horace E. *Dolphin Healing: The Extraordinary Power and Magic of Dolphins to Heal and Transform Our Lives*. London: Piatkus, 2000.

Docherty, Thomas, ed. *Postmodernism: A Reader*. New York: Columbia University Press, 1993.

Dossey, Barbara Montgomery. *Holistic Health Promotion: A Guide for Practice*. Rockville, MD: Aspen, 1989.

Dossey, Larry. *Beyond Illness*. Boston: New Science Library, 1984.

———. *The Extraordinary Healing Power of Ordinary Things*. New York: Three Rivers Press, 2006.

———. *Healing Words: The Power of Prayer in the Practice of Medicine*. San Francisco: Harper, 1993.

———. *Meaning and Medicine: A Doctor's Tales of Breakthrough and Healing*. New York: Bantam Books, 1991.

———. *The Power of Premonitions: How Knowing the Future Can Shape Our Lives*. New York: Dutton, 2009.

Dresser, Horatio W. *The Spirit of the New Thought*. London: Harrap, 1917.

Dreyfus, Hubert, and Paul Rabinow. *Michel Foucault, Beyond Structuralism and Hermeneutics*. 2nd ed. Chicago: University of Chicago Press, 1983.

Driver, Tom F. *The Magic of Ritual: Our Need for Liberating Rites That Transform Our Lives and Our Communities*. San Francisco: HarperCollins, 1991.

Drug Amendments of 1962: Conference Report, No. 2526, House of Representatives, Eighty-Seventh Congress, Second Session. Washington, DC: US Government Printing Office, 1962.

Duffy, John. *The Healers: A History of American Medicine*. Urbana: University of Illinois Press, 1976.

Dukes, M. N. G., and Jeffrey K. Aronson, eds. *Meyler's Side Effects of Drugs*. 14th ed. Amsterdam: Elsevier Science, 2000.

Duncan, Grant. "The Medical Imagination: A Study in Health Belief Systems and the Doctor–Patient Relationship." PhD diss., University of Auckland, 1989.

Dutton, Dianna B., Thomas A. Preston, and Nancy E. Pfund. *Worse Than the Disease: Pitfalls of Medical Progress*. New York: Cambridge University Press, 1988.

Eagleton, Terry. *The Illusions of Postmodernism*. Oxford: Blackwell, 1996.

Ebertin, Reinhold. *Astrological Healing: The History and Practice of Astromedicine*. Wellingborough, UK: Aquarian, 1990.

Eddy, David M. *Clinical Decision Making: From Theory to Practice*. Boston: Jones and Bartlett, 1996.

Edelman, Gerald M., and Giulio Tononi. *A Universe of Consciousness*. New York: Basic Books, 2000.

Eden, James. *Energetic Healing: The Merging of Ancient and Modern Medical Practices*. New York: Insight Books, 1993.

Ehrenwald, Jan. *The History of Psychotherapy: From Magic Healing to Encounter*. New York: Aronson, 1976.

Ellenberger, Henri F. *The Discovery of the Unconscious*. New York: Basic Books, 1970.

English-Lueck, Jan A. *Health in the New Age: A Study in California Holistic Practices*. Albuquerque: University of New Mexico Press, 1990.

Epstein, William M. *The Illusion of Psychotherapy*. Piscataway, NJ: Transaction, 1995.

Erdmann, Erika. *Beyond a World Divided: Human Values in the Brain–Mind Science of Roger Sperry*. New York: Authors Choice Press, 2000.

Ernst, Edzard. *Complementary Medicine: An Objective Appraisal*. Boston: Butterworth-Heinemann, 1996.

Ernst, Edzard, David Eisenberg, and Max H. Pittler. *The Desktop Guide to Complementary and Alternative Medicine*. London: Mosby, 2001.

Erwin, Edward. *Philosophy of Psychotherapy: Razing the Troubles of the Brain*. London: Sage, 1997.

Eskinazi, Daniel, ed. *Botanicals: A Role in U.S. Health Care*. Larchmont, NY: Liebert, 1998.

——. *What Will Influence the Future of Alternative Medicine? A World Perspective*. Hackensack, NJ: World Scientific, 2001.

Evans, Dylan. *Placebo: The Belief Effect*. London: HarperCollins, 2003.

——. *Placebo: Mind Over Matter in Modern Medicine*. New York: Oxford University Press, 2004.

Evans, Mark. *Mind, Body, Spirit: A Practical Guide to Natural Therapies for Health and Well-Being*. London: Hermes House, 2007.

——. *Natural Healing: Remedies and Therapies*. London: Hermes House, 2005.

Evans, Michael, and Iain Rodger. *Healing for Body, Soul, and Spirit: An Introduction to Anthroposophical Medicine*. Edinburgh: Floris, 2000.

Facklam, Howard. *Alternative Medicine: Cures or Myths?* New York: Twenty-First Century Books, 1996.

Featonby, Gwyn. *Aromatherapy for All: Empowering the Clinical Team*. London: Hospice Information, 2002.

Federation of the State Medical Boards of the United States. *Report on Health Care Fraud from the Special Committee on Health Care Fraud*. Austin, TX: Federation of the State Medical Boards of the United States, 1997.

Feinstein, Alvan R. *Clinical Epidemiology: The Architecture of Clinical Research*. Philadelphia: Saunders, 1985.

Ferguson, Elaine R. *Healing, Health, and Transformation: New Frontiers in Medicine.* Chicago: Lavonne Press, 1990.

Feuerman, Francine, and Marsha J. Handel. *Alternative Medicine Resource Guide.* Lanham, MD: MLA and Scarecrow Press, 1997.

Fishbein, Morris. *Medical Follies.* New York: Boni and Liveright, 1925.

——. *Quacks and Quackeries of the Healing Cults.* Girard, KS: Haldemann-Julius, 1927.

Fisher, Ronald A. *The Design of Experiments.* 1935. Reprint. London: Hafner, 1966.

——. *Statistical Methods for Research Workers.* Edinburgh: Oliver and Boyd, 1926.

Fisher, Seymour, and Roger P. Greenberg, eds. *The Limits of Biological Treatments for Psychological Distress: Comparisons with Psychotherapy and Placebo.* Hillsdale, NJ: Erlbaum Associates, 1989.

Flexner, Abraham. *Medical Education in the United States and Canada: A Report to the Carnegie Foundation on the Advancement of Teaching.* New York: Carnegie Foundation, 1910.

Flint, Austin. *A Treatise on the Principles and Practice of Medicine.* London: Lea's, 1881.

Fontaine, Karen Lee. *Healing Practices: Alternative Therapies for Nursing.* Upper Saddle River, NJ: Prentice-Hall, 2000.

Fontanarosa, Phil B. *Alternative Medicine: An Objective Assessment.* Chicago: American Medical Association, 2000.

Forbes, Sir John. *Homeopathy, Allopathy, and Young Physic.* New York: Radde, 1846.

Foucault, Michel. *The Birth of the Clinic: An Archaeology of Medical Perception.* New York: Pantheon Books, 1973.

Fox, Nicholas J. *Postmodernism, Sociology, and Health.* Buckingham, UK: Open University Press, 1993.

Frank, Jerome D. *Persuasion and Healing: A Comparative Study of Psychotherapy.* Baltimore: Johns Hopkins University Press, 1961.

Freedheim, Donald K. *History of Psychotherapy: A Century of Change.* Washington, DC: American Psychological Association, 1992.

Freeman, Lynn, and Frank Lawlis. *Mosby's Complementary Medicine and Alternative Therapies: A Research Based Approach.* St. Louis: Mosby, 2000.

Freidson, Eliot. *Professional Powers: A Study of the Institutionalization of Formal Knowledge.* Chicago: University of Chicago Press, 1986.

Fried, Charles. *Medical Experimentation: Personal Integrity and Social Policy.* Amsterdam: North Holland, 1974.

Friedman, Howard S., and Roxane C. Silver. *Foundations of Health Psychology.* New York: Oxford University Press, 2007.

Frohock, Fred M. *Healing Powers.* Chicago: University of Chicago Press, 1992.

——. *Lives of the Psychics.* Chicago: University of Chicago Press, 2000.

Fromm, Erich. *The Crisis of Psychoanalysis.* New York: Fawcett, 1970.

Fugh-Berman, Adraine. *Alternative Medicine: What Works.* Baltimore: Williams and Wilkins, 1997.

Fuller, Ray, Patricia Noonan Walsh, and Patrick McGinley, eds. *A Century of Psychology: Progress, Paradigms, and Prospects for the New Millennium.* London: Routledge, 1997.

Fuller, Robert C. *Alternative Medicine and American Religious Life*. New York: Oxford University Press, 1989.

——. *Mesmerism and the American Cure of Souls*. Philadelphia: University of Pennsylvania Press, 1982.

Garfield, Sol L., and Allen E. Bergin, eds. *The Handbook of Psychotherapy and Behavioral Change*. New York: Wiley, 1978.

Gaud, Alan. *A History of Hypnotism*. Cambridge: Cambridge University Press, 1992.

Gerber, Richard. *Vibrational Medicine: New Choices for Healing Ourselves*. Santa Fe: Bear, 2001.

Gevitz, Norman. *The Dos: Osteopathic Medicine in America*. 2nd ed. Baltimore: Johns Hopkins University Press, 2004.

——, ed. *Other Healers: Unorthodox in America*. Baltimore: Johns Hopkins University Press, 1988.

Gheorghiu, Vladimir A., and Klaus Fiedler, eds. *Suggestion and Suggestibility: Theory and Research*. Heidelberg, Germany: Springer, 1989.

Gilkeson, Jim, and Beth Budesheim. *Energy Healing: A Pathway to Inner Growth*. New York: Marlowe, 2000.

Ginzburg, Eli. *The Medical Triangle: Physicians, Politicians, and the Public*. Cambridge, MA: Harvard University Press, 1990.

Gleich, James. *Chaos*. New York: Penguin, 1988.

Godlee, Fiona, and Tom Jefferson. *Peer Review in Health Sciences*. London: BMJ Books, 2003.

Goldacre, Ben. *Bad Science*. London: Harper Perennial, 2009.

Goldman, Daniel, and Joel Gurin. *Mind Body Medicine: How to Use Your Mind for Better Health*. New York: Consumer's Union, 1993.

Goldstein, Michael S. *Alternative Health Care: Medicine, Miracle, or Mirage?* Philadelphia: Temple University Press, 1999.

Goodman, Kenneth W. *Ethics and Evidence-Based Medicine: Fallibility and Responsibility in Clinical Science*. Cambridge: Cambridge University Press, 2003.

Gordon, Benjamin Lee. *Medicine Throughout Antiquity*. Philadelphia: Davis, 1949.

Gordon, James S. *Holistic Medicine*. New York: Chelsea House, 1988.

Graham, Helen. *Time, Energy, and the Psychology of Healing*. London: J. Kingsley, 1990.

Greenhalgh, Trisha. *How to Read a Paper: The Basics of Evidence Based Medicine*. 2nd ed. London: BMJ Books, 2000.

Greenhalgh, Trisha, and Brian Hurwitz, eds. *Narrative-Based Medicine: Dialogue and Discourse in Clinical Practice*. London: BMJ Books, 1998.

Grinker, Roy R., and John P. Spiegel. *Men Under Stress*. Philadelphia: Blakiston, 1945.

——. *War Neuroses in North Africa: The Tunisian Campaign, January to May 1943*. New York: Arno Press, 1943.

Grob, Gerald N., and Alan V. Horwitz. *Diagnosis, Therapy, and Evidence: Conundrums in Modern American Medicine*. New Brunswick, NJ: Rutgers University Press, 2010.

Gross, Stan. *The Physician Within: A Practical Guide to the Natural Healing Power Within All of Us*. Needham Heights, MA: Pearson Custom, 1999.

Grossinger, Richard. *Planet Medicine: From Stone Age Shamanism to Post-industrial Healing.* Berkeley, CA: North Atlantic Books, 1990.

Guess, Harry A., Arthur Kleinman, John W. Kusek, and Linda W. Engel, eds. *The Science of the Placebo: Toward an Interdisciplinary Research Agenda.* London: BMJ Books, 2002.

Gushman, Philip. *Constructing the Self, Constructing America: A Cultural History of Psychotherapy.* Boston: Addison-Wesley, 1995.

Guyatt, Gordon H., and Drummond Rennie, eds. *Users' Guides to the Medical Literature: A Manual for Evidence-Based Clinical Practice.* Chicago: American Medical Association Press, 2002.

Hacking, Ian. *The Emergence of Probability.* Cambridge: Cambridge University Press, 1975.

——. *The Taming of Chance.* Cambridge: Cambridge University Press, 1990.

Hadler, Nortin M. *Worried Sick: A Prescription for Health in an Overtreated America.* Chapel Hill: University of North Carolina Press, 2008.

Haggard, Howard W. *Mystery, Magic, and Medicine.* New York: Doubleday Doran, 1933.

Hahn, Robert A. *Sickness and Healing: An Anthropological Perspective.* New Haven, CT: Yale University Press, 1995.

Hahnemann, Samuel. *The Chronic Diseases: Their Specific Nature and Homeopathic Treatment.* 5 vols. New York: Radde, 1845–1846.

——. *The Lesser Writings of Samuel Hahnemann.* Translated by Robert E. Dudgeon. New York: Radde, 1852.

——. *Organon of Homeopathic Medicine.* Allentown, PA: Academical Bookstore, 1836.

Haines, Andrew, and Anna Donald, eds. *Getting Research Findings Into Practice.* London: BMJ Books, 1998.

Haldeman, Scott, David Chapman-Smith, and David M. Peterson. *Guidelines for Chiropractic Quality Assurance and Practice Parameters, Proceedings of the Mercer Center Consensus Conference.* Gaithersburg, MD: Aspen, 1993.

Hall, Thomas S. *Ideas of Life and Matter: Studies in the History of General Physiology, 600 B.C.–1900 A.D.* 2 vols. Chicago: University of Chicago Press, 1969.

Haller, John S., Jr. *American Medicine in Transition, 1840–1910.* Urbana: University of Illinois Press, 1981.

——. *The History of American Homeopathy: The Academic Years, 1820–1935.* New York: Haworth Press, 2005.

——. *The History of American Homeopathy: From Rational Medicine to Holistic Health Care.* New Brunswick, NJ: Rutgers University Press, 2009.

——. *The History of New Thought: From Mind-Cure to Positive Thinking and the Prosperity Gospel.* West Chester, PA: Swedenborg Foundation, 2012.

——. *Kindly Medicine: Physio-medicalism in America, 1836–1999.* Kent, OH: Kent State University Press, 1997.

——. *Medical Protestants: The Eclectics in American Medicine, 1825–1939.* Carbondale: Southern Illinois University Press, 1994.

——. *The People's Doctors: Samuel Thomson and the American Botanical Movement, 1790–1860.* Carbondale: Southern Illinois University Press, 2000.

——. *Sectarian Reformers in American Medicine, 1800–1910.* New York: AMS Press, 2011.

——. *Swedenborg, Mesmer, and the Mind/Body Connection: The Roots of Complementary Medicine.* West Chester, PA: Swedenborg Foundation, 2010.

Harrington, Anne. *The Cure Within: A History of Mind–Body Medicine.* New York: Norton, 2008.

——, ed. *The Placebo Effect: An Interdisciplinary Exploration.* Cambridge, MA: Harvard University Press, 1997.

Hastings Center. *The Goals of Medicine: Setting New Priorities.* New York: Hastings Center, 1996.

Hatch, Nathan O., ed. *The Professions in American History.* Notre Dame, IN: University of Notre Dame Press, 1985.

Hawkey, Sue, and Robin Hayfield. *Natural Healing: Homeopathy, Herbalism, Relaxation, and Stress Relief.* London: Lorenz, 2002.

Health Policy Tracking Service. Washington, DC: National Conference of State Legislatures, 2001.

Henderson, William. *Homeopathy Fairly Represented: A Reply to Professor Simpson's "Homeopathy" Misrepresented.* Philadelphia: Lindsay and Blakiston, 1854.

Hess, David J. *Science in the New Age: The Paranormal, Its Defenders and Debunkers, and American Culture.* Madison: University of Wisconsin Press, 1993.

Hildreth, Arthur. *The Lengthening Shadow of Dr. Andrew Taylor Still.* Kirksville, MO: Journal Printing, 1942.

Hill, Austin Bradford. *Principles of Medical Statistics.* 1937. Reprint. New York: Oxford University Press, 1971.

Hodgkinson, Neville. *Will to Be Well: The Real Alternative Medicine.* London: Hutchinson, 1984.

Holmes, Oliver Wendell. *Homeopathy and Its Kindred Delusions.* Boston: Ticknor, 1842.

Holzer, Hans. *Healing Beyond Medicine: Alternative Paths to Wellness.* Stamford, CT: Longmeadow Press, 1994.

Homeopathic Medicine Research Group. *Report to the European Commission Director General XII: Science, Research, and Development.* Vol. 1. Brussels: European Commission, 1996.

Homola, Samuel. *Bonesetting, Chiropractic, and Cultism.* Panama City, FL: Critique Books, 1963.

Hover-Kramer, Dorothea. *Healing Touch: A Resource for Health Care Professionals.* Albany, NY: Delmar, 1996.

Hubinger, Vaclav, ed. *Grasping the Changing World.* New York: Routledge, 1996.

Humber, James M., and Robert F. Almeder, eds. *Alternative Medicine and Ethics.* New York: Humana Press, 1998.

Illich, Ivan. *Medical Nemesis: The Expropriation of Health.* Middlesex, UK: Penguin, 1976.

Inglis, Brian. *Fringe Medicine.* London: Faber and Faber, 1965.

——. *Natural Medicine.* London: Fontana, 1980.

Institute of Medicine. *Complementary and Alternative Medicine in the United States.* Washington, DC: National Academies Press, 2005.

Jadad, Alejandro R. *Randomized Controlled Trials*. London: BMJ Books, 1998.

James, William. *The Varieties of Religious Experience: A Study in Human Nature*. New York: Modern Library, 1902.

Jameson, Frederick. *Postmodernism, or, The Cultural Logic of Late Capitalism*. Durham, NC: Duke University Press, 1991.

Janiger, Oscar, and Philip Goldberg. *A Different Kind of Healing: Doctors Speak Candidly About Their Successes with Alternative Medicine*. New York: Putnam, 1993.

Janssen, Thierry. *The Solution Lies Within: Towards a New Medicine of Body and Mind*. London: Free Association Books, 2010.

Jarvik, Murray E., ed. *Psychopharmacology in the Practice of Medicine*. New York: Appleton-Century-Crofts, 1977.

Jesson, Lucinda E., and Stacey A. Tovino. *Complementary and Alternative Medicine and the Law*. Durham, NC: Carolina Academic Press, 2010.

Johnston, Robert D. *Politics of Healing: Histories of Alternative Medicine in Twentieth-Century North America*. New York: Routledge, 2004.

Jonas, Wayne B. *Mosby's Dictionary of Complementary and Alternative Medicine*. St. Louis: Elsevier Mosby, 2005.

Jonas, Wayne B., and Jennifer Jacobs. *Healing with Homeopathy: The Complete Guide*. New York: Warner, 1996.

——. *Healing with Homeopathy: The Doctor's Guide*. New York: Warner, 1998.

Jonas, Wayne B., Jeffrey S. Levin, and Brian Berman, eds. *The Essentials of Complementary and Alternative Medicine*. Philadelphia: Lippincott Williams and Wilkins, 1999.

Jones, James Howard. *Bad Blood: The Tuskegee Syphilis Experiment*. New York: Free Press, 1981.

Jones, R. Kenneth. *Sickness and Sectarianism: Exploratory Studies in Medical and Religious Sectarianism*. Aldershot, UK: Gower, 1985.

Jopling, David A. *Taking Cures and Placebo Effects*. New York: Oxford University Press, 2008.

Joslin, Benjamin F. *Principles of Homeopathy. In a Series of Lectures*. New York: Radde, 1850.

Jospe, Michael. *The Placebo Effect in Healing*. Lexington, MA: Lexington Books, 1978.

Judd, Sandra J. *Complementary and Alternative Medicine Sourcebook*. Detroit: Omnigraphics, 2006.

Jütte, Robert, Guenter B. Risse, and John Woodward, eds. *Culture, Knowledge, and Healing: Historical Perspectives of Homeopathic Medicine in Europe and North America*. Sheffield, UK: European Association for the History of Medicine and Health Publications, 1998.

Kane, Mark. *Research Made Easy in Complementary and Alternative Medicine*. New York: Churchill Livingstone, 2004.

Kaptchuk, Ted J. *The Web That Has No Weaver: Understanding Chinese Medicine*. Chicago: Contemporary Press, 2000.

Kaptchuk, Ted J., and Michael Croucher, *The Healing Arts: Exploring the Medical Ways of the World*. New York: Summit Books, 1987.

——. *The Healing Arts: A Journey Through the Faces of Medicine*. London: Guild, 1986.

Kassirer, Jerome P. *On the Take: How Medicine's Complicity with Big Business Can Endanger Your Health*. New York: Oxford University Press, 2005.

Katz, Jay. *Experimentation with Human Beings.* New York: Russell Sage Foundation, 1972.

——. *The Silent World of Doctor and Patient.* New York: Free Press, 1984.

Katz, Michael. *Gemstone Energy Medicine: Healing Body, Mind, and Spirit.* Portland, OR: Natural Healing Press, 2005.

Keeney, Bradford P. *Shaking Medicine: The Healing Power of Ecstatic Movement.* Rochester, VT: Destiny Books, 2007.

Kelner, Merrijoy, Beverly Wellman, Bernice Pescosolido, and Mike Saks, eds. *Complementary and Alternative Medicine: Challenge and Change.* Amsterdam: Harwood Academic, 2000.

Kennedy, Ian. *The Unmasking of Medicine.* London: Paladin/Granada, 1983.

Kent, James Tyler. *The Art and Science of Homeopathic Medicine.* 1900. Reprint. New York: Dover, 2002.

——. *Kent's Minor Writings on Homeopathy.* Heidelberg, Germany: Haug, 1987.

——. *Lectures on Homeopathic Philosophy.* Chicago: Ehrhart and Karl, 1919.

Kilpatrick, William Kirk. *The Emperor's New Clothes: The Naked Truth About the New Psychology.* Westchester, IL: Crossway Books, 1985.

King, Lester. *Medical Thinking.* Princeton, NJ: Princeton University Press, 1982.

Kirchfield, Friedhelm, and Wade Boyle. *Nature Doctors: Pioneers in Naturopathic Medicine.* Portland, OR: Medicina Biologica, 1994.

Kirsch, Irving. *The Emperor's New Drugs: Exploding the Antidepressant Myth.* New York: Basic Books, 2010.

Klein, Rudolf, and Janet Lewis. *The Politics of Consumer Representation: A Study of Community Health Councils.* London: Center for Studies in Social Policy, 1976.

Kleinman, Arthur. *Patients and Healers in the Context of Culture: An Exploration of the Borderland Between Anthropology, Medicine, and Psychiatry.* Berkeley: University of California Press, 1980.

——. *Rethinking Psychiatry.* New York: Free Press, 1988.

Knishinsky, Ran, and Gil E. Gilly. *Integrative Homeopathy.* Prescott, AZ: Hohm Press, 1996.

Knorr-Cetina, Karin D., and Michael Mulkay, eds. *Science Observed: Perspectives on the Social Study of Science.* London: Sage, 1983.

Knowles, John H., ed. *Doing Better and Feeling Worse: Health in the United States.* New York: Norton, 1977.

Knoor-Cetina, Karin D., and Michael Mulkay, eds. *Science Observed: Perspectives on the Social Study of Science.* London: Sage, 1983.

Kohlstedt, Sally G., and Margaret Rossiter, eds. *Historical Writing on American Science.* Baltimore: Johns Hopkins University Press, 1985.

Komesaroff, Paul A. *Troubled Bodies: Critical Perspectives on Postmodernism, Medical Ethics, and the Body.* Durham, NC: Duke University Press, 1995.

Kosslyn, Stephen M., and Oliver Koenig. *Wet Minds: The New Cognitive Neuroscience.* New York: Free Press, 1992.

Kotz, Samuel, Norman L. Johnson, and Campbell B. Read, eds. *Encyclopedia of Statistical Science.* 16 vols. New York: Wiley, 1982.

——, eds. *Encyclopedia of Statistical Science, Supplement Volume.* New York: Wiley, 1989.

Kradin, Richard L. *The Placebo Response and the Power of Unconscious Healing*. New York: Routledge, 2008.

Kratky, Karl W. *Complementary Medicine Systems: Comparison and Integration*. New York: Nova Science, 2008.

Krause, Elliot A. *Power and Illness: The Political Sociology of Health and Medical Care*. New York: Elsevier, 1977.

Kremers, Edward, and George Urdang. *The History of Pharmacy*. Philadelphia: Lippincott, 1963.

Krieger, Dolores. *Living the Therapeutic Touch: Healing as Lifestyle*. Wheaton, IL: Quest, 1988.

Krippner, Stanley, and Daniel Rubin. *The Kirlian Aura*. New York: Doubleday, 1974.

Kristiansen, Ivar Sønbø, and Gavin H. Mooney. *Evidence-Based Medicine: In Its Place*. New York: Routledge, 2004.

Krüger, Lorenz, Gerd Gigerenzer, and Mary S. Morgan, eds. *The Probabilistic Revolution*. Vol. 2: *Ideas in the Sciences*. Cambridge, MA: MIT Press, 1987.

Kuhn, Thomas S. *The Structure of Scientific Revolutions*. Chicago: University of Chicago Press, 1962.

Kyle, Richard. *The New Age Movement in American Culture*. Lanham, MD: University Press of America, 1995.

Landy, David. *Culture, Disease, and Healing: Studies in Medical Anthropology*. New York: Macmillan, 1977.

Larkin, Gerald. *Occupational Monopoly and Modern Medicine*. London: Tavistock, 1983.

Larson, Margali S. *The Rise of Professionalism*. Berkeley: University of California Press, 1977.

Latour, Bruno. *Laboratory Life: The Social Construction of Scientific Facts*. Beverly Hills, CA: Sage, 1979.

Law, Jacky. *Big Pharma*. New York: Carroll and Graff, 2006.

Lederer, Susan. *Subjected to Science: Human Experimentation in America Before the Second World War*. Baltimore: Johns Hopkins University Press, 1995.

Le Fanu, James. *The Rise and Fall of Modern Medicine*. London: Little, Brown, 1999.

Leland, R. G. *Distribution of Physicians in the United States*. Chicago: American Medical Association, 1936.

Lemert, Charles C. *Postmodernism Is Not What You Think: Why Globalization Threatens Modernity*. Oxford: Blackwell, 1997.

Lesch, John E. *Science and Medicine in France: The Emergence of Experimental Physiology, 1790–1855*. Cambridge, MA: Harvard University Press, 1984.

Leuret, Francois. *Modern Miraculous Cures*. New York: Farrar, Straus, and Cudahay, 1957.

Levine, Robert J. *Ethics and Regulation of Clinical Research*. New Haven, CT: Yale University Press, 1986.

Lewis, Clive S. *The Problem of Pain*. New York: Macmillan, 1947.

Lewis, I. M. *Ecstatic Religion*. London: Penguin, 1971.

Lewith, George T., and David Aldridge, eds. *Clinical Research Methodology for Complementary Therapies*. London: Hodder and Stoughton, 1993.

——, eds. *Complementary Medicine and the European Community*. Saffron Walden, UK: Daniel, 1991.

Lewith, George T., Wayne B. Jonas, and Harald Walach. *Clinical Research in Complementary Therapy: Principles, Problems, and Solutions.* Edinburgh: Churchill Livingstone, 2001.

Lewith, George T., J. N. Kenyon, and Peter J. Lewis. *Complementary Medicine: An Integrated Approach.* New York: Oxford University Press, 1996.

Light, Richard J., and David B. Pillemer. *Summing Up: The Science of Reviewing Research.* Cambridge, MA: Harvard University Press, 1984.

Lilienfeld, Abraham, ed. *Times, Places, and Persons: Aspects of the History of Epidemiology.* Baltimore: Johns Hopkins University Press, 1980.

Lindberg, David C., and Ronald L. Numbers. *God and Nature: Historical Essays on the Encounter Between Christianity and Science.* Berkeley: University of California Press, 1986.

Louis, Pierre Charles Alexandre. *Researches on the Effects of Bloodletting in Some Inflammatory Diseases and on the Influence of Tartarized Antimony and Vesication in Pneumonitis.* Boston: Hilliard, Gray, 1836.

Lowenberg, June S. *Caring and Responsibility: The Crossroads Between Holistic Practice and Traditional Medicine.* Philadelphia: University of Pennsylvania Press, 1989.

Ludmerer, Kenneth M. *Learning to Heal: The Development of American Medical Education.* New York: Basic Books, 1985.

——. *Time to Heal: American Medical Education from the Turn of the Century to the Era of Managed Care.* New York: Oxford University Press, 1999.

Lukacs, John. *At the End of an Age.* New Haven, CT: Yale University Press, 2002.

Lytle, C. D. *An Overview of Acupuncture.* Rockville, MD: Public Health Service, 1993.

Lytle, Larry. *Healing Light: Energy Medicine of the Future.* Bloomington, IN: AuthorHouse, 2004.

Maciocia, Giovanni. *The Foundations of Chinese Medicine.* Edinburg: Churchill Livingston, 1989.

MacMahon, Brian, Thomas F. Pugh, and Johanes Ipsen. *Epidemiologic Methods.* Boston: Little, Brown, 1960.

Macrae, Janet. *Therapeutic Touch: A Practical Guide.* New York: Knopf, 1994.

Majno, Guido. *The Healing Hand.* Cambridge, MA: Harvard University Press, 1975.

Mantle, Fiona. *Complementary Therapies: Is There an Evidence Base?* London: NT Books, 1999.

Marks, Harry M. *The Progress of Experiment: Science and Therapeutic Reform in the United States, 1900–1990.* New York: Cambridge University Press, 1997.

Marti, James. *The Alternative Health and Medicine Encyclopedia.* 2nd ed. Detroit: Visible Ink, 1997.

Masson, Jeffrey. *Against Therapy: Emotional Tyranny and the Myth of Psychological Healing.* New York: Atheneum, 1988.

Matthews, J. Rosser. *Quantification and the Quest for Medical Certainty.* Princeton, NJ: Princeton University Press, 1995.

Mattson, Phyllis H. *Holistic Health in Perspective.* Palo Alto, CA: Mayfield, 1982.

Maulitz, Russell C., and Diana E. Long, eds. *Grand Rounds: One Hundred Years of Internal Medicine.* Philadelphia: University of Pennsylvania Press, 1988.

Mayo Clinic. *Mayo Clinic Book of Alternative Medicine.* 2nd ed. New York: Little Brown, 2010.

McCartney, Francesca. *Intuition Medicine: The Science of Energy.* Mill Valley, CA: Intuition Library, 2000.

McClenon, James. *Deviant Science: The Case of Parapsychology.* Philadelphia: University of Pennsylvania Press, 1984.

McCullough, Michael. *Faith, Hope, and Healing.* Lincolnwood, IL: Publications International, 1998.

McGarey, Gladys, and Jess Stearn. *The Physician Within You: Medicine for the Millennium.* Scottsdale, AZ: Inkwell, 2000.

McGuire, Meredith B., and Debra Kantor. *Ritual Healing in Suburban America.* New Brunswick, NJ: Rutgers University Press, 1988.

McKeown, Thomas. *The Role of Medicine: Dream, Mirage, or Nemesis?* London: Nuffield Hospitals Trust, 1976.

McLaughlin, Chris, and Nicola Hall. *Secrets of Reflexology.* London: Dorling Kindersley, 2001.

McTaggart, Lynn. *The Field: The Quest for the Secret Force of the Universe.* New York: Harper, 2008.

Mehlman, Maxwell J. *The Price of Perfection: Individualism and Society in the Era of Biomedical Enhancement.* Baltimore: Johns Hopkins University Press, 2009.

Meissner, William W. *The Therapeutic Alliance.* New Haven, CT: Yale University Press, 1996.

Melmon, Kenneth L., and Howard F. Morrelli, eds. *Clinical Pharmacology: Basic Principles in Therapeutics.* 2nd ed. New York: Macmillan, 1978.

Melville, Arabella, and Colin Johnson. *Health Without Drugs.* New York: Simon and Schuster, 1990.

Merleau-Ponty, Maurice. *The Phenomenology of Perception.* New York: Humanities Press, 1962.

Mesmer, Franz Anton. *Mesmerism: A Translation of the Original Scientific and Medical Writings of F. A. Mesmer.* Compiled and translated by George J. Bloch. Los Angeles: Kaufmann, 1980.

Mhatre, Prabhakar R., and Geeta Desai. *Principles of Integrated Medicine: Stepping Beyond Alternative Medicine.* New Delhi: Tata McGraw-Hill, 2003.

Micozzi, Marc S. *Fundamentals of Complementary and Alternative Medicine.* New York: Churchill Livingstone, 1996.

Middleton, Carl L. *Integrative Health Care: An Emerging Approach to the Art of Healing.* Denver: Catholic Health Initiatives, 2001.

Midgley, Mary. *The Myths We Live By.* London: Routledge, 2004.

Milbank Memorial Fund. *Enhancing the Accountability of Alternative Medicine.* New York: Milbank Memorial Fund, 1998.

Miller, Jenifer. *Healing Centers and Retreats; Healthy Getaways for Every Body and Budget.* Santa Fe: Muir, 1998.

Mills, Juliet. *Mind, Body, and Soul in Balance.* Los Angeles: Mills, 1993.

Milner, Kathleen Ann. *Reiki and Other Rays of Touch Healing.* 5th ed. Scottsdale, AZ: self-published, 2003.

Minnesota Health Economics Program. *Complementary Medicine: Final Report to the Legislature.* St. Paul: Health Economics Program, 1998.

Mischoulon, David, and J. F. Rosenbaum. *Natural Medications and the Treatment of Psychiatric Disorders: Considering the Alternatives.* Philadelphia: Lippincott Williams and Wilkins, 2002.

Moerman, Daniel E. *Meaning, Medicine, and the "Placebo Effect."* Cambridge: Cambridge University Press, 2002.

Monte, Tom. *World Medicine: The East West Guide to Healing Your Body.* New York: Putnam, 1993.

Montgomery, Kathryn. *How Doctors Think: Clinical Judgment and the Practice of Medicine.* Oxford: Oxford University Press, 2006.

Moore, J. Stuart. *Chiropractic in America: The History of a Medical Alternative.* Baltimore: Johns Hopkins University Press, 1977.

Moore, R. Laurence. *In Search of White Crows: Spiritualism, Parapsychology, and American Culture.* New York: Oxford University Press, 1977.

Morand, M. *Memoir on Acupuncturation: Embracing a Series of Cases Drawn Up Under the Inspection of M. Julius Cloquet.* Philadelphia: Desiluer, 1825.

More, Ellen S., and Maureen A. Milligan, eds. *The Empathetic Practitioner: Empathy, Gender, and Medicine.* New Brunswick, NJ: Rutgers University Press, 1994.

Morris, David B. *Illness and Culture in the Postmodern Age.* Berkeley: University of California Press, 1998.

Motherby, George. *New Medical Dictionary.* London: n.p., 1785.

Moyers, Bill. *Healing and the Mind.* New York: Doubleday, 1993.

Moynihan, Ray, and Alan Cassels. *Selling Sickness: How the World's Biggest Pharmaceutical Companies Are Turning Us All Into Patients.* New York: Nation Books, 2005.

Mullen, José Miguel. *Understanding Homeopathy and Integrative Medicine.* 5th ed. Bloomington, IN: 1st Books, 2002.

Muskin, Philip R. *Complementary and Alternative Medicine and Psychiatry.* Washington, DC: American Psychiatric Press, 2000.

National Center for Complementary and Alternative Medicine (NCCAM). *Are You Considering Using Complementary and Alternative Medicine?* Gaithersburg, MD: NCCAM, 2002.

——. *CAM at the NIH: Focus on Complementary and Alternative Medicine.* Bethesda, MD: National Institutes of Health, 2005.

——. *Energy Medicine: An Overview.* Bethesda, MD: NCCAM, 2007.

——. *Expanding Horizons of Health Care: Strategic Plan 2005–2009.* Bethesda, MD: NCCAM, 2004.

——. *NCCAM National Center for Complementary and Alternative Medicine.* Bethesda, MD: NCCAM, 2008.

——. *Time to Talk: Tell Your Doctor About Your Use of Complementary and Alternative Medicine.* Bethesda, MD: NCCAM, 2007.

——. *Tips for Talking with Your Health Care Providers about CAM.* Bethesda, MD: NCCAM, 2008.

——. *The Use of CAM in the United States.* Bethesda, MD: NCCAM, 2007.

National Institute for the Clinical Application of Behavioral Medicine. *Practical Resources: A Collaboration of Experts on Mind/Body Medicine.* Mansfields Center, CT: National Institute for the Clinical Application of Behavioral Medicine, 1991.

National Institutes of Health (NIH). *Alternative Medicine: Expanding Medical Horizons. A Report to the National Institutes of Health on Alternative Medical Systems and Practices in the United States.* Bethesda, MD: NIH, 1992.

National Library of Medicine and National Center for Complementary and Alternative Medicine (NCCAM). *CAM on Pubmed.* Bethesda, MD: National Library of Medicine and NCCAM, 2006.

Needes, Robin. *Naturopathy for Self-Healing: Nutrition, Life-Style, Herbs, Homeopathy.* Delhi: Health Harmony, 1995.

Newman, Robert Bruce, and Ruth L. Miller. *Calm Healing: Methods for a New Era of Medicine.* Berkeley, CA: North Atlantic Books, 2006.

Newton, Nicola J. "The Road Taken: Women's Life Paths and Personality Development in Late Midlife." PhD diss., University of Michigan, 2011.

Nicholi, Armand M., ed. *The Harvard Guide to Modern Psychiatry.* Cambridge, MA: Harvard University Press, 1978.

Nicholls, Phillip A. *Homeopathy and the Medical Profession.* London: Croom Helm, 1988.

Nolen, William A. *Healing: A Doctor in Search of a Miracle.* New York: Fawcett, 1974.

Norcross, John C., Gary H. R. Vanden Bos, and Donald K. Freedheim. *History of Psychotherapy: Continuity and Change.* Washington, DC: American Psychological Association, 2011.

Norris, Catie, and Marjorie Rothstein. *Magnetic Miracles: Your Guide to the Use of Magnetics for Radiant Health.* Malibu, CA: Energy Essentials, 1999.

Novey, Donald W., ed. *Clinician's Complete Reference to Complementary and Alternative Medicine.* St. Louis: Mosby, 2000.

Numbers, Ronald L. *Prophetess of Health: Ellen G. White and the Origins of Seventh-Day Adventist Health Reform.* Knoxville: University of Tennessee Press, 1992.

Oakley, Ann. *Women Confined: Towards a Sociology of Childbirth.* Oxford: Martin Robertson, 1980.

O'Connor, Bonnie Blair. *Healing Traditions: Alternative Medicine and the Health Professions.* Philadelphia: University of Pennsylvania Press, 1995.

Office of Alternative Medicine. *Alternative Medicine: Expanding Medical Horizons.* Bethesda, MD: Office of Alternative Medicine, 1992.

O'Manthúna, Dónal P. *Alternative Medicine: A Response to the White House Commission on Complementary and Alternative Medicine Policy.* Washington, DC: Christian Medical Association, 2002.

Oppenheim, Janet. *The Other World: Spiritualism and Psychical Research in England, 1850–1914.* Cambridge: Cambridge University Press, 1985.

Ornstein, Robert, and Charles Swencionis, eds. *The Healing Brain: A Scientific Reader.* New York: Guilford, 1990.

Osler, William. *The Evolution of Modern Medicine.* New Haven, CT: Yale University Press, 1921.

——. *The Principles and Practice of Medicine.* New York: Appleton, 1892.

Otto, Herbert Arthur, and James W. Knight. *Dimensions in Wholistic Healing: New Frontiers in the Treatment of the Whole Person.* Chicago: Nelson-Hall, 1979.

Palmer, B. J. *The Hour Has Struck.* N.p.: n.p., 1924.

Paris, Joel. *The Fall of an Icon: Psychoanalysis and Academic Psychiatry.* Toronto: University of Toronto Press, 2005.

Parsons, Talcott. *The Social System.* Glencoe, IL: Free Press, 1951.

Paton, Scott. *Health Beyond Medicine: A Chiropractic Miracle.* Ramsey, NJ: Healthcare Unity Press, 2009.

Payer, Lynn. *Medicine and Culture: Varieties of Treatment in the United States, England, West Germany, and France.* New York: Henry Holt, 1996.

Peel, Robert. *Health and Medicine in the Christian Science Tradition.* New York: Crossroad, 1988.

Pellegrino, Edmund D., Robert M. Veatch, and John P. Langan. *Ethics, Trust, and the Professions: Philosophical and Cultural Aspects.* Washington, DC: Georgetown University Press, 1991.

Pelletier, Kenneth R. *The Best Alternative Medicine: What Works? What Does Not?* New York: Simon and Schuster, 2000.

Pennell, Maryland, and Shirlene Showel. *Women in Health Care: Chartbook for the International Conference on Women in Health.* Washington, DC: American Public Health Association, 1975.

Perl, Sheri. *Healing from the Inside Out.* New York: New American Library, 1989.

Peters, David, ed. *Understanding the Placebo Effect in Complementary Medicine: Theory, Practice, and Research.* Edinburgh: Churchill Livingstone, 2001.

Peters, David, Leon Chaitow, Gerry Harris, and Sue Morrison. *Integrating Complementary Therapies in Primary Care: A Practical Guide for Health Professionals.* Edinburgh: Churchill Livingstone, 2002.

Pizzorno, Joseph E., and Michael T. Murray, eds. *Textbook of Natural Medicine.* 2 vols. New York: Churchill Livingstone, 1999.

Podmore, Frank. *From Mesmer to Christian Science.* New York: University Books, 1963.

Podolsky, Scott H. *Pneumonia Before Antibiotics: Therapeutic Evolution and Evaluation in Twentieth Century America.* Baltimore: Johns Hopkins University Press, 2006.

Podolsky, Scott H., and Charles S. Bryan, eds. *Oliver Wendell Holmes: Physician and Man of Letters.* Sagamore Beach, MA: Science History, 2009.

Porter, Theodore M. *The Rise of Statistical Thinking, 1820–1900.* Princeton, NJ: Princeton University Press, 1986.

Poyen, Charles. *Progress of Animal Magnetism in New England.* Boston: Weeks, Jordan, 1837.

Price, Donald D. *Psychological and Neural Mechanisms of Pain.* New York: Raven Press, 1988.

Radicke, Gustav. *On the Importance and Value of Arithmetic Means.* London: New Sydenham Society, 1861.

Radin, Dean I. *The Conscious Universe: The Scientific Truth of Psychic Phenomena.* San Francisco: Harper Edge, 1997.

Rappaport, Karen. *Directory of Schools for Alternative and Complementary Health Care.* 2nd ed. Phoenix: Oryx Press, 1999.

Reed, Louis. *The Healing Cults.* Chicago: University of Chicago Press, 1932.

Reich, Warren T., ed. *Encyclopedia of Bioethics.* Vol. 5. New York: MacMillan, 1995.

Reiser, Stanley Joel. *Medicine and the Reign of Technology.* Cambridge: Cambridge University Press, 1978.

Renner, K. Edward. *What's Wrong with the Mental Health Movement.* Chicago: Nelson-Hall,1975.

Rieff, Philip. *The Triumph of the Therapeutic: Uses of Faith After Freud.* New York: Harper and Row, 1966.

Rinkel, Max. *Specific and Non-specific Factors in Psychopharmacology.* New York: Philosophic Library, 1963.

Roberts, Herbert A. *The Principles and Art of Cure by Homeopathy.* Halsworthy, UK: Health Science Press, 1942.

Robins, Natalie S. *Copeland's Cure: Homeopathy and the War Between Conventional and Alternative Medicine.* New York: Knopf, 2005.

Robinson, Daniel N. *An Intellectual History of Psychology.* Madison: University of Wisconsin Press, 1995.

Rohland, Robert. *Od, or Odo-Magnetic Force: An Explanation of Its Influence on Homeopathic Medicines, from the Odic Point of View.* New York: n.p., 1916.

Rose, Louis. *Faith Healing.* London: Gollanz, 1968.

Rosenberg, Charles E. *The Care of Strangers: The Rise of America's Hospital System.* New York: Basic Books, 1987.

——. *No Other Gods: On Science and American Social Thought.* 1976. Reprint. Baltimore: Johns Hopkins University Press, 1997.

Rosenberg, Charles E., and Janet Golden, eds. *Framing Disease: Studies in Cultural History.* New Brunswick, NJ: Rutgers University Press, 1992.

Rosenberg, Charles E., and Morris J. Vogel, eds. *The Therapeutic Revolution: Essays in the Social History of American Medicine.* Philadelphia: University of Pennsylvania Press, 1979.

Rosenstein, I. G. *Theory and Practice of Homeopathy First Part, Containing a Theory of Homeopathy, with Dietetic Rules, etc.* Louisville, KY: Henkle and Logan, 1840.

Rosenthal, Robert, and Ralph L. Rosnow. *The Volunteer Subject.* New York: Wiley, 1975.

Rossi, Ernest. *Mind Body Therapy: Methods of Ideodynamic Healing in Hypnotherapy.* New York: Norton, 1992.

Rothman, David J. *Strangers at the Bedside.* New York: Basic Books, 1991.

Rothstein, William G. *American Medical Schools and the Practice of Medicine: A History.* New York: Oxford University Press, 1987.

——. *American Physicians in the Nineteenth Century: From Sects to Science.* Baltimore: Johns Hopkins University Press, 1972.

Roy, Ranjan. *The Social Context of the Chronic Pain Sufferer.* Toronto: University of Toronto Press, 1992.

Ruggie, Mary. *Alternative Medicine in America: From Quackery to Commonplace*. New York: Cambridge University Press, 2004.

Ruzek, Sheryl. *The Women's Health Movement: Feminist Alternatives to Medical Control*. New York: Praeger, 1978.

Rycroft, Charles, ed. *Psychoanalysis Observed*. London: Constable, 1966.

Sackett, David, R. Bryan Haynes, and Gordon Guyatt. *Evidence-Based Medicine: How to Practice and Teach EBM*. New York: Churchill-Livingstone, 1997.

Sackett, David, R. Bryan Haynes, and Peter Tugwell. *Clinical Epidemiology: A Basic Science for Clinical Medicine*. Boston: Little, Brown, 1985.

Sackett, David L., Sharon E. Straus, W. Scott Richardson, William Rosenberg, and R. Brian Haynes. *Evidence-Based Medicine: How to Practice and Teach EBM*. 2nd ed. Edinburgh: Churchill Livingstone, 2000.

Saks, Mike, ed. *Alternative Medicine in Britain*. Oxford: Clarendon Press, 1992.

——. *Orthodox and Alternative Medicine: Politics, Professionalization, and Health Care*. New York: Continuum, 2003.

Salmon, J. Warren, ed. *Alternative Medicine: Popular and Policy Perspectives*. New York: Tavistock, 1984.

Scambler, Graham, and Paul Higgs, eds. *Modernity, Medicine, and Health: Medical Sociology Towards 2000*. London: Routledge, 1998.

Scarry, Elaine. *The Body in Pain*. New York: Oxford University Press, 1985.

Schenck, David, and Larry R. Churchill. *Healers: Extraordinary Clinicians at Work*. New York: Oxford University Press, 2011.

Schilder, Paul M. *The Image and Appearance of the Human Body: Studies in the Constructive Energies of the Psyche*. 1935. Reprint. London: Routledge, 1999.

Selye, Hans. *The Stress of Life*. Rev. and exp. ed. Chicago: McGraw-Hill, 1956.

Seventh Meeting of the Alternative Medicine Program Advisory Council, Office of Alternative Medicine, National Institutes of Health. Bethesda, MD: Office of Alternative Medicine, 1996.

Shapiro, Arthur K., and Elaine Shapiro. *Ethical Controversies About the Use of Placebos, the Double-Blind, and Controlled Clinical Trials*. Cambridge, MA: Harvard University Press, 1997.

——. *The Powerful Placebo: From Ancient Priest to Modern Physician*. Baltimore: Johns Hopkins University Press, 1997.

Sharma, Ursula. *Complementary Medicine Today: Practitioners and Patients*. London: Tavistock and Routledge, 1992.

Shaw, George B. *The Doctor's Dilemma*. New York: Penguin Books, 1911.

Shealy, C. Norman. *Miracles Do Happen: A Physician's Experience with Alternative Medicine*. London: Vega, 2002.

Shorter, Edward. *Bedside Manners: The Troubled History of Doctors and Patients*. New York: Simon and Schuster, 1985.

——. *From Paralysis to Fatigue: A History of Psychosomatic Disease in the Modern Era*. New York: Free Press, 1993.

Shryock, Richard H. *American Medical Research, Past and Present*. New York: Commonwealth Fund, 1947.

——. *Medical Licensing in America, 1650–1965*. Baltimore: Johns Hopkins University Press, 1967.

Shuch, David J. *Doctor, Be Well: Integrating the Spirit of Healing with Scientific Medicine*. Bloomington, IN: 1st Books, 2003.

Siegel, Bernie. *Love, Medicine, and Miracles: Lessons Learned About Self-Healing from a Surgeon's Experience with Exceptional Patients*. New York: HarperCollins, 1986.

Simpson, James Y. *Homeopathy: Its Tenets and Tendencies, Theoretical, Theological, and Therapeutical*. Philadelphia: Lindsay and Blakiston, 1854.

Simpson, Liz. *The Book of Chakra Healing*. London: Gaia, 2005.

Smith, Christopher U. M. *The Problem of Life: An Essay in the Origins of Biological Thought*. New York: Wiley, 1976.

Smith, Mary Lee, Gene V. Glass, and Thomas I. Miller, *The Benefit of Psychotherapy*. Baltimore: Johns Hopkins University Press, 1980.

Smith, Norman Kemp. *New Studies in the Philosophy of Descartes*. London: Macmillan, 1952.

Song, Cai, and B. E. Leonard. *Fundamentals of Psychoneuroimmunology*. New York: Wiley, 2000.

Sorer, Charles G. *Healing: Biblical, Medical, and Pastoral*. London: Christian Medical Fellowship, 1979.

Spiro, Howard M. *Doctors, Patients, and Placebos*. New Haven, CT: Yale University Press, 1986.

——. *The Power of Hope: A Doctor's Perspective*. New Haven, CT: Yale University Press, 1998.

Spiro, Howard M., Enid Peschel, Mary G. Curnen, and Deborah St. James, eds. *Empathy and the Practice of Medicine: Beyond Pills and the Scalpel*. New Haven, CT: Yale University Press, 1996.

Spitzer, Mkanfred. *The Mind Within the Net*. Cambridge, MA: MIT Press, 1999.

Starr, Paul. *The Social Transformation of American Medicine*. New York: Basic Books, 1982.

Stein, Howard F. *American Medicine as Culture*. Boulder, CO: Westview Press, 1990.

Steiner, Rudolf. *Anthroposophy: An Introduction*. London: Anthroposophical Publishing, 1961.

——. *Rudolf Steiner: An Autobiography*. Blauvelt, NY: Steiner, 1977.

Steiner, Rudolf, and Christopher Bamford. *What Is Anthroposophy? Three Perspectives on Self Knowledge*. Great Barrington, MA: Anthroposophic Press, 2002.

Sternberg, Ester M. *The Balance Within*. New York: Freeman, 2001.

Stevens, Andrew, Keith R. Abrams, and John Brazier. *The Advanced Handbook of Methods in Evidence Based Healthcare*. London: Sage, 2001.

Stevens, Rosemary. *American Medicine and the Public Interest: A History of Specialization*. New Haven, CT: Yale University Press, 1971.

Stigler, Stephen M. *The History of Statistics: The Measurement of Uncertainty Before 1900*. Cambridge, MA: Harvard University Press, 1986.

Still, Andrew Taylor. *Osteopathy: Research and Practice*. Kirksville, MO: self-published, 1910.

——. *The Philosophy and Mechanical Principles of Osteopathy*. Kirksville, MO: Osteopathic Enterprises, 1986.

——. *Philosophy of Osteopathy*. Kirksville, MO: Still, 1899.

Stone, Eric. *Medicine Among the American Indians*. New York: Hafner, 1962.

Stone, Julie. *An Ethical Framework for Complementary and Alternative Therapists*. New York: Routledge, 2002.

Study of Administered Prices in the Drug Industry, Report of the Subcommittee on Antitrust and Monopoly of the Senate Judiciary Committee, Pursuant to Senate Resolution 52, Eighty-Seventh Congress, First Session. Washington, DC: US Government Printing Office, 1961.

Sutherland, Adah S. *With Thinking Fingers: The Story of William Garner Sutherland, D.O.* Portland, OR: Ruda Press, 1998.

Tessier, Jean-Paul. *Clinical Researches Concerning the Homeopathic Treatment of Asiatic Cholera. Preceded by a Review on the Abuse of the Numerical Method in Medicine*. New York: Radde, 1855.

——. *Lectures on Clinical Medicine, Delivered in the Hospital Saint-Jacques, of Paris*. London: New Sydenham Society, 1872.

Thomas, Kate. *National Survey of Access to Complementary Health Care Via General Practice*. Sheffield, UK: Medical Care Research Unit, Sheffield University, 1995.

Thomas, Lewis. *The Youngest Science: Notes of a Medicine Watcher*. New York: Viking Press, 1983.

Thompson, W. Grant. *The Placebo Effect and Health: Combining Science with Compassionate Care*. Amherst, MA: Prometheus Books, 2005.

Thorn, Wendy Anne Fairfax. "The Relationship of Situational and Personality Variables to Placebo Reaction." PhD diss., University of London, King's College, 1968.

Timmermans, Stefan, and Marc Berg. *The Gold Standard: The Challenge of Evidence-Based Medicine and Standardization in Health Care*. Philadelphia: Temple University Press, 2003.

Totman, Richard. *The Social Causes of Illness*. London: Souvenir Press, 1987.

Tröhler, Ulrich. "Quantification in British Medicine and Surgery, 1750–1830, with Special Reference to Its Introduction Into Therapeutics." PhD diss., University of London, 1978.

Trowbridge, Carol. *Andrew Taylor Still: 1828–1917*. Kirksville, MO: Thomas Jefferson University Press, 1991.

Turner, Bryan S. *Theories of Modernity and Postmodernity*. London: Sage, 1990.

Turner, Roger N. *Naturopathic Medicine: Treating the Whole Person*. Wellingborough, UK: Thorsons, 1984.

Tyler, Richard. *Alternative Chiropractic: A Clinician's Manual on Diversified Diagnostic and Therapeutic Applications in Conservative Health Care*. 2nd ed. Santa Cruz, CA: On Target, 2005.

Ullman, Dana. *Discovering Homeopathy: Your Introduction to the Science and Art of Homeopathic Medicine*. Berkeley, CA: North Atlantic Books, 1991.

US Department of Commerce. *Historical Statistics of the United States: Colonial Times to 1970*. Vol. 2: *Work and Welfare*. Washington, DC: US Department of Commerce, 1975.

Usui, Mikao, and Frank Arjava Petter. *The Original Reiki Handbook of Dr. Mikao Usui*. Twin Lakes, WI: Lotus Press, 2002.

Vanderpool, Harold Y., ed. *The Ethics of Research Involving Human Subjects: Facing the 21st Century.* Frederick, MD: University Publishing Group, 1996.

Veatch, Robert M. *A Theory of Medical Ethics.* New York: Basic Books, 1981.

Vithoulkas, George. *The Science of Homeopathy.* New York: Grove Press, 1980.

Wall, Patrick D. *Pain: The Science of Suffering.* New York: Columbia University Press, 2000.

Wall, Patrick D., and R. Melzak, eds. *Text Book of Pain.* Edinburgh: Churchill Livingston, 1999.

Wallis, Roy, ed. *On the Margins of Science: The Social Construction of Rejected Knowledge. Monograph 27.* Staffordshire, UK: University of Keele, 1979.

Walsh, James J. *Cures: The Story of the Cures That Fail.* New York: Appleton, 1924.

Wardwell, Walter. *Chiropractic: History and Evolution of a New Profession.* St. Louis: Mosby, 1992.

Warner, John Harley. *The Therapeutic Perspective: Medical Practice, Knowledge, and Identity in America, 1820–1885.* Cambridge, MA: Harvard University Press, 1986.

Watkins, Alan D., ed. *Mind–Body Medicine: A Clinician's Guide to Psychoneuroimmunology.* New York: Churchill Livingstone, 1997.

Wayne, Michael. *Quantum-Integral Medicine: Towards a New Science of Healing and Human Potential.* Saratoga Springs, NY: iThink Books, 2005.

Weil, Andrew. *Eight Weeks to Optimum Health: A Proven Program for Taking Full Advantage of Your Body's Natural Healing Power.* New York: Knopf, 1997.

——. *Health and Healing: The Philosophy of Integrative Medicine.* Boston: Houghton Mifflin, 2004.

——. *Health and Healing: Understanding Conventional and Alternative Medicine.* Boston: Houghton Mifflin, 1983.

——. *Natural Health, Natural Medicine: A Comprehensive Manual for Wellness and Self-Care.* Boston: Houghton Mifflin, 1990.

——. *The Natural Mind: A Revolutionary Approach to the Drug Problem.* New York: Houghton Mifflin, 1972.

Weintraub, Michael I., and Mark S. Micozzi. *Alternative and Complementary Treatment in Neurologic Illness.* New York: Churchill Livingstone, 2001.

Weiss, R. F. *Herbal Medicine.* Beaconsfield, UK: Beaconsfield, 1991.

Wendel, Paul. *Standardized Naturopathy: The Science and Art of Natural Healing.* Brooklyn: Paul Wendel, 1951.

West, Ruth. *Alternative Medicine: A Bibliography of Books in English.* London: Victoria Park, 1984.

White, Leonard, Bernard Tursky, and Gary E. Schwartz, eds. *Placebo: Theory, Research, and Mechanisms.* New York: Guilford Press, 1985.

Whitehead, Anne. *Meta-analysis of Controlled Clinical Trials.* Chichester, UK: Wiley, 2002.

White House Commission on Complementary and Alternative Medicine Policy. *Final Report, March 2002.* Washington, DC: White House Commission on Complementary and Alternative Medicine Policy, 2002.

Whorton, James C. *Nature Cures: The History of Alternative Medicine in America.* Oxford: Oxford University Press, 2002.

Wilkinson, James Garth. *Epidemic Man and His Visitations*. London: Speirs, 1893.

———. *Swedenborg Among the Doctors: A Letter to Robert T. Cooper, M.D.* London: Speirs, 1895.

Wilson, John R. *The Double Blind*. New York: Doubleday, 1960.

Wood, Garth. *The Myth of Neurosis: Overcoming the Illness Excuse*. New York: Harper and Row, 1986.

Wood, Matthew. *The Magical Staff: The Vitalist Tradition in Western Medicine*. Berkeley, CA: North Atlantic Books, 1992.

———. *Vitalism: The History of Herbalism, Homeopathy, and Flower Essences*. Berkeley, CA: North Atlantic Books, 2000.

Workshop on Alternative Medicine. *Alternative Medicine: Expanding Medical Horizons—a Report to the National Institutes of Health on Alternative Medical Systems and Practices in the United States*. Bethesda, MD: National Institutes of Health, 1995.

World Medical Association. *Declaration of Helsinki*. Ferney-Voltaire, France: World Medical Association, 1989.

———. *Declaration of Helsinki*. Ferney-Voltaire, France: World Medical Association, 1996.

———. *Declaration of Helsinki*. Ferney-Voltaire, France: World Medical Association, 2000.

———. *Declaration of Helsinki*. Ferney-Voltaire, France: World Medical Association, 2013.

———. *Ethical Principles for Medical Research Involving Human Subjects*. Helsinki: World Medical Association, 2000.

Wrobel, Arthur. *Pseudo-science and Society in Nineteenth-Century America*. Lexington: University Press of Kentucky, 1987.

Wunderlich, Carl Auguste. *On the Temperature in Diseases: A Manual of Medical Thermometry*. London: New Sydenham Society, 1871.

Wundt, Wilhelm. *Grundzüge der physiologischen Psychologie* (Principles of physiological psychology). Leipzig: Engelmann, 1874.

Zellner, William W. *Countercultures: A Sociological Analysis*. New York: St. Martin's Press, 1995.

Zilboorg, Gregory. *A History of Medical Psychology*. New York: Norton, 1941.

Zweig, Stefan. *Mental Healers: Franz Anton Mesmer, Mary Baker Eddy, Sigmund Freud*. New York: Viking Press, 1932.

INDEX